In Vitro Toxicology

In Vitro Toxicology

Editor

Shayne Cox Gad, Ph.D.
Director of Toxicology
SYNERGEN
Boulder, Colorado

Raven Press　　New York

Raven Press, Ltd., 1185 Avenue of the Americas, New York, New York 10036

Made in the United States of America

Library of Congress Cataloging-in-Publication Data
In vitro toxicology / editor, Shayne Cox Gad.
    p. cm.
    Includes bibliographical references and index.
    ISBN 0–88167–974–7 ✓
    1. Toxicity testing—In vitro. I. Gad, Shayne C., 1948–
    [DNLM: 1. Toxicology—methods. 2. Cells, Cultured—drug effects.
QV 602 I354 1994]
RA1199.4.I5I53   1994
615.9'07—dc20
DNLM/DLC
for Library of Congress   93–31938
                                            CIP

Contents

Contributors

Daniel Acosta   *Division of Pharmacology and Toxicology, College of Pharmacy, The University of Texas at Austin, Austin, Texas 78712*

Katherine L. Allen   *Human Liver Research Facility, SRI International, Menlo Park, California 94025*

Meg Bason   *Department of Dermatology, University of California at San Francisco, San Francisco, California 94143*

Douglas E. Brenneman   *Laboratory of Developmental Neurobiology, National Institute of Child Health and Human Development, National Institutes of Health, Bethesda, Maryland 20892*

Elaine M. Faustman   *Department of Environmental Health, University of Washington, Seattle, Washington 98195*

Shayne Cox Gad   *Toxicology, SYNERGEN, Boulder, Colorado 80301*

P. D. Gautheron   *Merck Sharp & Dohme Research Laboratories, 63203 Riom, France*

Robin S. Goldstein   *Department of Investigative Toxicology, SmithKline Beecham Pharmaceuticals, King of Prussia, Pennsylvania 19406*

V. C. Gordon   *In Vitro International, Irvine, California 92714*

Peggy J. Guzzie   *Pfizer, Inc., Groton, Connecticut 06340*

Jeff Harvell   *Department of Dermatology, University of California at San Francisco, San Francisco, California 94143*

A. P. Li   *Surgical Research Institute, St. Louis University Medical School, St. Louis, Missouri 63110*

Howard Maibach   *Department of Dermatology, University of California at San Francisco, San Francisco, California 94143*

Phillip G. Nelson   *Laboratory of Developmental Neurobiology, National Institute of Child Health and Human Development, National Institutes of Health, Bethesda, Maryland 20892*

Kenneth Ramos   *Department of Physiology and Pharmacology, College of Veterinary Medicine, Texas A & M University, College Station, Texas 77843*

J. F. Sina   *Merck Sharp & Dohme Research Laboratories, West Point, Pennsylvania 19486*

Joan B. Tarloff   *Department of Pharmacology and Toxicology, Philadelphia College of Pharmacy and Science, Philadelphia, Pennsylvania 19104*

Stephen G. Whittaker   *Department of Environmental Health, University of Washington, Seattle, Washington 98195*

Patricia D. Williams   *Investigative Toxicology, Medical Research Division, American Cyanamid Company, Pearl River, New York 10965*

Preface

Toxicology has made tremendous strides in the sophistication of the models used to identify and understand the mechanisms of agents that can harm or kill humans and other higher organisms. Early on, other people were used as surrogates for monarchs or others. Other animals then came to be used, and, until recently, this use, while becoming increasingly refined, also came to serve as the "gold standard" against which truth (at least in regulatory, legal, and economic senses) was judged.

Nonanimals or *in vitro* models timely started to gain significant use in the 1960s. For reasons of concern about animal welfare, economics, and the need for greater sensitivity and understanding of mechanisms, interest in *in vitro* models has increased.

As the contents of this volume demonstrate, there now exists a broad range of *in vitro* models for use in either identifying or understanding most forms of toxicity. The availability of *in vitro* models spans both the full range of endpoints (irritation, sensitization, lethality, mutagenicity, and developmental toxicity) and the full spectrum of target organ systems (skin, eye, heart, liver, kidney, nervous system, etc.). This volume devotes chapters to each of these specialty areas from a perspective of presenting the principal models and their uses and limitations.

Chapters that overview the principles involved in the general selection and use of models, and that address the issues of safety concerns and regulatory acceptance of these methods are also included.

By the time this book sees print, as in any such volume, portions will be dated but not obsolete. The authors and I hope this will provide a sound basis for broad understanding and utilization of these models.

Shayne Cox Gad

In Vitro Toxicology,
edited by Shayne Cox Gad.
Raven Press, Ltd., New York, © 1994.

1

Introduction

Shayne Cox Gad

Toxicology, SYNERGEN, Boulder, Colorado 80301

Toxicology, in the sense used in this volume, is the science concerned with identifying and understanding the mechanisms of agents which adversely affect the health of man, other animals, and living portions of the environment. Most of it, however, is concerned with those man-made chemical agents which adversely affect the health of man.

The current test methods designed and used to evaluate the potential of man-made materials to cause harm to the people who make, transport, use, or otherwise come in contact with them hold a unique and ambivalent place in our society. On one hand, our society is not only critically dependent on technological advances to improve and/or maintain standards of living, but is also intolerant of risks real or potential to life and health which are seemingly avoidable. On the other hand, the traditional tests (with both their misuse and misunderstanding of their use) have served as the rallying point for those concerned about the humane and proper use of animals. This has caused all testing using animals to come under question on both ethical and scientific grounds, and has provided a great stimulus for the development of alternatives and innovations.

In recent years, tremendous progress has been made in our understanding of biology down to the molecular level. This has translated to multiple modifications and improvements in *in vivo* testing procedures which now give us tests that (a) are more reliable, reproducible, and predictive of potential hazards in humans, (b) use fewer animals, and (c) are considerably more humane than earlier test forms. At the same time, a multitude of *in vitro* test systems have been proposed, developed, and "validated" to at least some extent. Yet the perception persists that little has changed in how toxicology testing is performed.

It is hoped that this volume will serve to make more people aware of both the range of new techniques which are available and the means and extent of their application. But more importantly it is hoped that the whole process involved in testing will continually be modified so that only what needs to be done will be and that those tests which are done will answer the desired questions in a manner which maximizes efficiency, effectiveness, scientific quality, and dependability while limiting any discomfort or suffering in animals.

The entire product safety assessment process, in the broadest sense, is a multistage process in which none of the individual steps is overwhelmingly complex, but the integration of the whole process involves fitting together a large complex pattern of pieces. This volume as a whole seeks to address the questions of the current state of the art of *in vitro* methods and how they can be used. How the data generated by the various test systems and models described elsewhere in this volume can be used by government and private enterprise to provide for a safe product life cycle is the subject of the next chapter. As will be seen, it calls for a modification of the approach to the general product safety assessment problem, and it will be addressed by starting with the general case and progressing to specific plans and a means for changing the process in an iterative fashion. Along the way, limitations of current models and approach and places where testing and research data could be made more practically useful will be pointed out. Particularly with an understanding of mechanisms becoming increasingly important in both product design and evaluating the relevance of findings, the integration of *in vitro* methodologies into the product safety assessment process has become essential (4).

DEFINITIONS

Various terms are used to describe the different kinds of testing and research performed in terms of the model systems used. By and large, *in vivo* (though technically implying the use of living organisms) is used to denote the use of intact higher organisms (vertebrates).

In vitro, meanwhile, is used to describe those tests which use other than intact vertebrates as model systems. These include everything from lower organisms (planaria and bacteria) to cultured cells and computer models. The next section looks in more detail at the different "levels" of *in vitro* models and at their advantages and disadvantages.

In between clearly *in vivo* and *in vitro* models (and overlapping both of them) are the "alternatives." This term has different meanings to different people. In its broadest sense, it incorporates everything which reduces higher animal usage and suffering in the existing traditional test designs. This definition includes the following range of situations:

1. Use of a reduced volume of test material in a rabbit eye irritation test
2. Use of an "up-and-down" method or a limited test design to characterize lethality in the rat
3. Use of earthworms instead of rats or mice for lethality testing
4. Use of fish instead of rats or mice for carcinogenicity bioassays
5. Use of computerized structure activity models for predicting toxicity
6. True *in vitro* models

This volume, however, will concentrate on *in vitro* models.

TABLE 1. *Levels of models for toxicity testing and research*

Level/model	Advantages	Disadvantages
In vitro (intact higher organism)	Full range of organismic responses similar to that of target species.	Costs. Ethical/animal welfare concerns. Species-to-species variability.
Lower organisms (earthworms, fish)	Range of integrated organismic responses.	Frequently lack responses of higher organism. Animal welfare concerns.
Isolated organs	Intact yet isolated tissue and vascular system. Controlled environmental and exposure conditions.	Donor organism still required. Time-consuming and expensive. No intact organismic responses. Limited length of viability.
Cultured cells	No intact animals directly involved. Ability to carefully manipulate system. Low costs. Wide range of variables can be studied.	Instability of system. Limited enzymatic capabilities and viability of system. No or limited integrated multicell and/or organismic responses.
Chemical/ biochemical systems	No donor organism problems. Low cost. Long-term stability of preparation. Wide range of variables can be studied. Specificity of response.	No *de facto* correlation to *in vivo* system. Limited to investigation of single defined mechanism.
Computer simulations	No animal welfare concerns. Speed and low per evaluation cost.	Problematic predictive value beyond narrow range of structures. Expensive to establish.

LEVELS

As the definitions above illustrate, there are many approaches to having a predictive model for use in toxicology. One way to classify these approaches is presented in Table 1, which looks at the different levels of models in terms of their complexity. Each level of approach has advantages and disadvantages, some of which are very specific to the concerns and viewpoints of the user. Each of these levels represents a different approach to a problem set.

There are several approaches to *in vitro* toxicity or target organ models. The first and oldest is that of the isolated organ preparation. Perfused and superfused tissues and organs have been used in physiology and pharmacology since the late 19th century. There is a vast range of these available, and a number of them have been widely used in toxicology (ref. 10 presents an excellent overview). Almost any end point can be evaluated in most target organs (the central nervous system being a notable exception), and these are closest to the *in vivo* situation and therefore generally the easiest to extrapolate or conceptualize from. Those things which can be measured or evaluated in the intact organism can largely also be evaluated in an isolated tissue or organ preparation. The drawbacks or limitations of this approach are also compelling, however.

An intact animal generally produces one tissue preparation. Such a preparation is viable generally for a day or less before it degrades to the point of losing utility. As a result, such preparations are useful as screens only for agents which have rapidly reversible (generally pharmacologic or biochemical) or acute mechanisms of action. They are superb for evaluating mechanisms of action at the organ level for agents which act rapidly, but are generally not useful for evaluating cellular effects or for evaluating agents which act over a course of more than a day.

The second approach is to use tissue or organ culture. Such cultures are attractive due to maintaining the ability for multiple cell types to interact in at least a near-physiological manner. They are generally not as complex as the perfused organs, but are stable and useful over a longer period of time, increasing their utility as screens somewhat. They are truly a middle ground between the perfused organs and the cultured cells. Only for relatively simple organs (such as the skin and bone marrow) are good models which perform in a manner representative of the *in vitro* organ available.

The third and most common approach is that of cultured cell models. These can be either primary or transformed (immortalized) cells, but the former have significant advantages in use as predictive target organ models. Such cell culture systems can be utilized to identify and evaluate interactions at the cellular, subcellular, and molecular level on an organ- and species-specific basis (1). The advantages of cell culture are as follows: (a) Single organisms can generate multiple cultures for use, (b) these cultures are stable and useful for protracted periods of time, and (c) effects can be studied very precisely at the cellular and molecular level. The disadvantages are that isolated cells cannot mimic the interactive architecture of the intact organ, and will respond over time in a manner which becomes decreasingly representative of what happens *in vivo*. An additional concern is that, with the exception of hepatocyte cultures, the influence of systemic metabolism is not factored in unless extra steps are taken. Stammati et al. (15) and Tyson and Stacey (16) present some excellent reviews of the use of cell culture in toxicology. Any such cellular systems would be more likely to be accurate and sensitive predictors of adverse effects if their function and integrity were evaluated while they were operational. For example, cultured nerve cells should be excited while being exposed and evaluated.

HISTORY

The key assumptions underlying modern toxicology are as follows: (a) Other organisms can serve as accurate predictive models of toxicity in man, (b) selection of an appropriate model to use is key to accurate prediction in man, and (c) understanding the strengths and weaknesses of any particular model is essential to understanding the relevance of specific findings to man. The nature of models and their selection in toxicologic research and testing have only recently become the subject of critical scientific review. Usually in toxicology when we refer to "models" we really have meant test organism, though in fact the ways in which parameters are measured (and which parameters are measured to characterize an end point of interest) are also critical parts of the model (or, indeed, may actually constitute the "model").

Though there have been accepted principles for test organism selection, these have not generally been the final basis for such selection. It is a fundamental hypothesis of both historical and modern toxicology that adverse effects caused by chemical entities in higher animals are generally the same as those induced by those entities in man. There are many who point to individual exceptions to this and conclude that the general principle is false. Yet, as our understanding of molecular biology advances and we learn more about the similarities of structure and function of higher organisms at the molecular level, the more it becomes clear that the mechanisms of chemical toxicity are largely identical in humans and animals. This increased understanding has caused some of the same people who question the general principle of predictive value to in turn suggest that our state of knowledge is such that mathematical models or simple cell culture systems could be used just as well as intact animals to predict toxicities in man. This last suggestion also missed the point that the final expressions of toxicity in man or animals are frequently the summation of extensive and complex interactions at cellular and biochemical levels. Zbinden (18) has published extensively in this area, including a very advanced defense of the value of animal models. Lijinsky (9) has reviewed the specific issues about the predictive value and importance of animals in carcinogenicity testing and research. Though it was once widely believed (and still is believed by many animal rights activists) that *in vitro* mutagenicity tests would entirely replace animal bioassays for carcinogenicity, this is clearly not the case on either scientific or regulatory grounds. Though there are differences in the responses of various species (including man) to carcinogens, the overall predictive value of such results (when tempered by judgment) is clear. At the same time, well-reasoned use of *in vitro* or other alternative test model systems is essential to the development of a product safety assessment program which is both effective and efficient (5).

The subject of intact animal models (and of their proper selection and use) has been addressed elsewhere by this author (6) and will not be further addressed here. However, alternative models which use other than intact higher organisms are seeing increasing use in toxicology for a number of reasons.

The Four R's

The first and most significant factors behind the interest in so-called *in vitro* systems has clearly been political—an unremitting campaign by a wide spectrum of individuals concerned with the welfare and humane treatment of laboratory animals (14). The historical beginnings of this were in 1959, when Russell and Burch (13) first proposed what have come to be called the three R's of humane animal use in research: replacement, reduction, and refinement. These have served as the conceptual basis for reconsideration of animal use in research.

Replacement means utilizing methods which do not use intact animals in place of those that do. For example, veterinary students may use a canine cardiopulmonary-resuscitation simulator, Resusci-Dog, instead of living dogs. Cell cultures may replace mice and rats that are fed new products to discover substances poisonous to humans. In addition, using the preceding definition of animal, an invertebrate (e.g., a horseshoe crab) could replace a vertebrate (e.g., a rabbit) in a testing protocol.

Reduction refers to the use of fewer animals. For instance, changing practices allow toxicologists to estimate the lethal dose of a chemical with as few as one-tenth the number of animals used in traditional tests. In biomedical research, long-lived animals, such as primates, may be used in multiple sequential protocols assuming that they are not deemed inhumane or scientifically conflicting. Designing experimental protocols with appropriate attention to statistical inference can lead to either decreases or increases in the numbers of animals used. Through coordination of efforts among investigators, several tissues may be simultaneously taken from a single animal. Reduction can also refer to the minimization of any unintentionally duplicative experiments, perhaps through improvements in information resources.

Refinement entails the modification of existing procedures so that animals are subjected to less pain and distress. Refinements may include: administration of anesthetics to animals undergoing otherwise painful procedures; administration of tranquilizers for distress; humane destruction prior to recovery from surgical anesthesia; and careful scrutiny of behavioral indices of pain or distress, followed by cessation of the procedure or the use of appropriate analgesics. Refinements also include the enhanced use of noninvasive imaging technologies that allow earlier detection of tumors, organ deterioration, or metabolic changes and the subsequent early euthanasia of test animals.

Progress towards these first three R's has been previously reviewed (5). However, there is a fourth R, *responsibility*, that was not in Russell and Burch's initial proposal. To toxicologists this is the cardinal R. They may be personally committed to minimizing animal use and suffering, and to doing the best possible science of which they are capable, but at the end of it all, toxicologists must stand by their responsibility to be conservative in ensuring the safety of the people using or exposed to the drugs and chemicals produced and used in our society.

During the past decade, issues of animal use and care in toxicologic research and testing have become one of the fundamental concerns of both science and the public. Are our results predictive of what may or may not be seen in man? Are we using too many animals, and are we using them in a manner which gets the answer we need with as little discomfort on the part of the animals as possible? How do we balance the needs of man against the welfare of animals?

In 1984, the Society of Toxicology (SOT) held its first symposium and addressed scientific approaches to these issues. The last such symposium for SOT was in 1988. Each year that passes has brought new regulations, attempts at federal and state legislation, and demonstrations which directly affect the practice of toxicology. Increasing amounts of both money and scientific talent have been dedicated to progress in this area. At the same time, the public clearly supports animal use in research when they see a need and benefit. This is shown in Table 2.

During the same time frame, interest and progress in the development of *in vitro* test systems for toxicity evaluations have also progressed. Early reviews by Hooisma (8), Neubert (11), and Williams et al. (17) record the proceedings of

TABLE 2. *Public opinion on animal use in research*

A 1989 survey conducted for the American Medical Association (2) sampled almost 1500 households and found that:
- Sixty-four percent opposed organizations attempting to stop the use of animals in research testing.
- Seventy-seven percent thought animal research was necessary for progress in medicine.
- Other polls have given the same results in terms of medical research or general issues of animal research and testing. But a majority has been found to oppose animal testing of cosmetics, regarding it as unwarranted (3).

conferences on the subject, but Rofe's 1971 review (12) was the first found by this author. Though it is hoped that in the long term some of these (or other) *in vitro* methods will serve as definitive tests in place of those which use intact animals, at present it appears more likely that their use in most cases will be as screens. Goldberg and Frazier (7) give a current overview of the general concepts and status of *in vitro* alternatives.

DRIVING FORCES

There are a number of reasons that are driving toxicology towards a broader use of *in vitro* test systems. These can generally be summarized as political, financial, and technological.

The political reasons are the need to deal with the pressures of the animal welfare movement and its influence on the public and regulators. The economic reasons are based on the rapidly increasing costs of laboratory animals and their upkeep, which translates to spiraling costs for traditional *in vivo* models. The technological reasons encompass all the requirements for having better (i.e., in this case more predictive of effects in man) and faster answers.

With increasing scientific need for alternatives to animal experimentation and increasing perception of the potential scientific, ethical, and commercial value of *in vitro* techniques in toxicology, scientific effort in this area has increased dramatically over the past few years. It is essential, however, that the potential for the reduction in (or avoidance of) whole-animal experiments should not force irrational acceptance of unvalidated tests. It is also important that the value of some *in vitro* approaches should be recognized as complementary to whole-animal experiments at the current state of our knowledge.

The single most important advantage of *in vitro* tests, with a potential which has not yet been realized, is that they allow comparisons of the effects of cellular and organ exposure to drugs and chemicals to be extrapolated across species to include man himself through the use of human cell cultures from necropsy or biopsy material. In other words, such techniques have the potential to allow the toxicological evaluation of compounds in animals and man on an equal basis, which cannot be achieved in classical *in vivo* toxicological testing. However, the difficulties experienced by many laboratories in obtaining human tissue cannot be ignored and are a serious impedance to progress in this area. The comparison across species may be extended further to the establishment of cultured cell lines which can allow scientists in different laboratories to compare results and permit the necessary standardization which is fundamental to good scientific practice.

In the opinion of the author it is essential to establish standards of methodology which will allow parallel assessment by independent laboratories of *in vitro* parameters of closest relevance to the *in vivo* situation. Certainly much is at stake, both in terms of safety and in terms of expensive commercial risk, in interpretations of *in vitro* data which may "kill" a perfectly valid development compound or alternatively allow an unacceptably toxic compound to proceed, with ultimate adverse effects in man.

This leads inevitably to questions on the predictive value of positive or negative results *in vitro*, but the weighing given to such tests can only be established with the experience of time and hard data, by relating *in vitro* observations to proven *in vivo* effects with well-studied compounds. It is clearly important that the aim of all laboratories should be to establish *in vitro* end points which will bear the closest possible relationship to responses obtained *in vivo*. If this is not achieved, *in vitro* parameters will not gain the required scientific and regulatory acceptance in relation to their relevance to ultimate safety *in vivo* in man.

Although there has been a predominance of work in the field of genotoxicity testing, *in vitro* approaches are moving into the field of immunotoxicology and will inevitably expand to the study of all potential target organs. However, the continuing debate concerning the validity of many genotoxicity tests, particularly in terms of their ability to predict potential carcinogens, emphasizes the rigorous evaluation which must be applied to *in vitro* approaches if they are to gain acceptance by the scientific community.

Following the thalidomide tragedy and the establishment of regulatory authorities to consider new drugs and other chemicals, the pharmaceutical and other industries set up more formal toxicological evaluation procedures. "In house" toxicology departments were soon supplemented by contract research organizations, and a series of standard "regulatory" tests became an international requirement for all new compounds which might be taken by man (and other animals) either deliberately or accidentally. The objective of these rather stereotyped studies was to identify the nature of the toxicity of a compound and to assess the potential risks by extrapolation from toxic responses at various dose levels to the therapeutic dose in man, with the highest "no-effect" dose in animals being used as the basis of the so-called "therapeutic ratio."

Although the therapeutic ratio is a valid concept, one of the fundamental guiding principles of the toxicologist is that he is *not* trying to demonstrate that a potential drug or other chemical is nontoxic. The fact that *all* chemicals are toxic has been well recognized for centuries.

If we accept that all chemicals have some potential hazard, it follows that toxicologists are not looking at a compound to see whether it is toxic but to find out the degree of toxicity and the nature of the toxicity. What is important in the development of drugs is the ratio between the therapeutic and the toxic doses or blood levels and between the desired and unwanted effects. The "regulatory" tests achieve this with a degree of certainty.

Another important guiding principle for the toxicologist is that toxicology is essentially a predictive science. We study the nature of the toxic effect in order to assess the risk to man. Unfortunately, there have been sufficient instances of toxic effects arising only after wide exposure to man of compounds which have fully satisfied international regulatory requirements with regard to animal testing to raise questions in the minds of many as to the predictability of "standard" tests for many substances.

The toxicologist is going to administer increasingly higher doses of compound to experimental animals in order to identify target organs or other limiting toxicity. After this in collaboration with colleagues in other disciplines, he has to make risk assessments and contribute to the development and selection of other candidate compounds. Once target organ or limiting toxicity is identified, mechanistic studies are required and it is here that *in vitro* techniques are now becoming widely and increasingly used.

Subject to the validation which has been discussed above, these tests must surely take their place alongside, for example, biochemical or pharmacological tests *in vitro* at the subcellular, cellular, or organ level which are currently used together with *in vivo* tests in forming an overall, and more complete, scientific picture of a new test compound.

Very often whole-animal studies may not be appropriate for mechanistic studies because in many cases the adverse effect becomes apparent only after very long periods of chronic dosing.

It has often been possible to demonstrate that risk to humans is not likely once the mechanism of action of the adverse effect in the experimental animals has been understood. Sometimes the species specificity of toxic effects have been confirmed by utilizing cell cultures from several species, including humans. When the mechanism of an adverse effect seen in whole-animal studies has been studied and is considered possibly to be predictive of risk in humans, the compound may have its development curtailed. However, other candidate compounds may need evaluation in short-term models designed to detect potential adverse effects when only small amounts of compound are available. *In vitro* techniques are frequently the most appropriate means of doing this. In both economic terms and use of animals, such early comparative tests with different compounds in *in vitro* systems must be attractive. The extension of this to multicompound screening is a matter of individual research and development strategy. Such short-term models may also be used in drug design, since when playing "molecular roulette," potency data in biological or pharmacological assays provide only part of the information required by the medicinal chemist. A modern cost-effective approach to drug design must take into account toxicological potential as well as inherent biological activity.

We anticipate that the progress of the science of toxicology in the pharmaceutical, agrochemical, and other similar industries will lead increasingly to mechanistic approaches to toxicology and increasing use of *in vitro* techniques and models.

Contributors to this book have covered almost every area of toxicology and have utilized a full range of *in vitro* techniques ranging from mammalian cell lines (including human) at one end of the spectrum to abbatoir material (eyes) and classical pharmacological isolated organ techniques (hearts) at the other. Whether chicken eggs used for studies on chorioallantoic membranes or whole-rat embryos are *in vitro* or *in vivo* are moot points, but they certainly represent humane alternatives to the use of whole animals and provide elegant investigational tools and models for toxicological study.

It is clear that this volume should provide a valuable reference for scientists involved in the toxicological investigation and evaluation of potential new drugs, agrochemicals, food additives, and so on. It should interest graduate and postgraduate students and research workers in toxicology as this subject becomes an integral part of the training of toxicologists, particularly since individual chapters not only cover the philosophy and strategy of the use of *in vitro* models but also give attention to detailed methodology.

REFERENCES

1. Acosta D, Sorensen EMB, Anuforo DC, et al. An *in vitro* approach to the study of target organ toxicity of drugs and chemicals. *In Vitro Cellular Dev Bio* 1985;21:495–504.
2. American Medical Association. Public support for animals in research. *Ann Med News* 1989; June 9.
3. Cowley G, Hager M, Drew L, et al. The battle over animal rights. *Newsweek* 1988; Dec 26.
4. Gad SC. A tier testing strategy incorporating *in vitro* testing methods for pharmaceutical safety assessment. *Humane Innovations and Alternatives in Animal Experimentation* 1989;3:75–79.
5. Gad SC. Recent developments in replacing, reducing and refining animal use in toxicologic research and testing. *Fundam Appl Toxicol* 1990;15(1):8–16.
6. Gad SC, Chengelis CP. *Animal Models in Toxicology*. New York: Marcel Dekker, 1992.
7. Goldberg AM, Frazier JM. Alternatives to animals in toxicity testing. *Sci Am* 1989;261:24–30.
8. Hooisma J. Tissue culture and neurotoxicology. *Neurobehav Toxicol Teratol* 1982;4:617–622.
9. Lijinsky W. Importance of animal experiments in carcinogenesis research. *Envir Mol Mutagen* 1988;11:307–314.
10. Mehendale HM. Application of isolated organ techniques in toxicology. In: *Principles and methods of toxicology*. Hayes AW, ed. New York: Raven Press, 1989;699–740.
11. Neubert D. The use of culture techniques in studies on prenatal toxicity. *Pharmacol Ther* 1982; 18:397–434.
12. Rofe PC. Tissue culture and toxicology. *Food Cosmet Toxicol* 1971;9:685–696.
13. Russell WMS, Burch RL. *The principles of humane experimental technique*. London: Methuen & Co., 1959.
14. Singer P. *Animal liberation: a new ethic for our treatment of animals*. New York: Random House, 1975.
15. Stammati AP, Silano V, Zucco F. Toxicology investigations with cell culture systems. *Toxicology* 1981;20:91–153.
16. Tyson CA, Stacey NH. *In vitro* screens from CNS, liver and kidney for systemic toxicity. In: Mehlman, M, ed. *Benchmarks: alternative methods in toxicology*. Princeton, NJ: Princeton Scientific, 1989;111–136.
17. Williams GM, Dunkel VC, Ray VA, eds. Cellular systems for toxicity testing. *Ann NY Acad Sci* 1983;407.
18. Zbinden G. *Predictive value of animal studies in toxicology*. Carshalton, UK: Centre for Medicines Research, 1987.

In Vitro Toxicology,
edited by Shayne Cox Gad.
Raven Press, Ltd., New York, © 1994.

2

General Principles for *In Vitro* Toxicology

Shayne Cox Gad

Toxicology, SYNERGEN, Boulder, Colorado 80301

As was introduced in the last chapter, *in vitro* methods actually encompass a broad range of techniques and models for use in toxicity testing. These techniques have varying degrees of reliability and acceptance. Some may be directly substituted in place of existing *in vivo* models, while others are currently suitable only as screens or adjunct tests (1). The challenge to the practicing toxicologist over the upcoming decades will be appropriate and timely selection and utilization of new models and methodologies. The essential starting place for such decisions is a knowledge of the objective behind any testing program, along with an understanding of the entire safety assessment process.

The entire product safety assessment process, in the broadest sense, is a multi-stage process in which none of the individual steps is overwhelmingly complex, but the integration of the whole process involves fitting together a large complex pattern of pieces. The single most important part of this product safety evaluation program is, in fact, the initial overall process of defining and developing an adequate data package on the potential hazards associated with the product life cycle (the manufacture, sale, use, and disposal of a product and associated process materials). To do this, one must ask a series of questions in a highly interactive process, with many of the questions designed to identify and/or modify their successors. First, what is the objective of the testing (i.e., what question is being asked) being conducted?

Required here are (a) an understanding of the way in which a product is to be made and used and (b) an awareness of the potential health and safety risks associated with exposure of humans who will be associated with these processes or the product's use. Such an understanding and awareness is the basis of a hazard and toxicity profile. Once such a profile is established, then the available literature should be searched to determine what is already known.

Taking into consideration this literature information and the previously defined exposure profile, a tier approach (Fig. 1) has traditionally been used to generate a list of tests or studies to be performed. What goes into a tier system is determined by (a) regulatory requirements imposed by government agencies, (b) the philosophy of the parent organization, (c) economics, and (d) available technology. How such

TIER TESTING			
Testing tier	Mammalian Toxicology	Genetic Toxicology	Remarks
0	Literature review	Literature review	Upon initial identification of a problem database of existing information and particulars of use of materials are established
1	Cytotoxicity screens Dermal sensitization Acute systemic toxicity Lethality screens	Ames test *In vitro* SCE *In vitro* cytogenetics Forward mutation/CHO	R&D material and low volume chemicals with severely limited exposure
2	Subacute studies Metabolism Primary dermal irritation Eye irritation	*In vivo* SCE *In vivo* cytogenetics	Medium volume materials and/or those with a significant change of human exposure
3	Subchronic studies Reproduction Developmental toxicology Chronic studies Mechanistic studies		Any materials with high volume or a potential for widespread or long term human exposure or one which gives indications or specific long-term effects

FIG. 1. The usual way of characterizing the toxicity of a compound or product is to develop information in a tiered manner. More information is required (i.e., a higher tier level is attained) as the volume of production and potential for exposure increase. A common scheme is shown.

tests are actually performed is determined on one of two bases. The first (and most common) is the menu approach: selecting a series of standard design tests as "modules" of data, then modifying the design of each module to meet the specifics of the particular case. The second is an interactive/iterative approach, where strategies are developed and studies are designed based both on needs and on what has been learned to date about the product. This process has been previously examined in some detail (4,7). Our interest here, however, is in the specific portion of the process involved in generating data (namely, the test systems), and we are also interested in how *in vitro* systems may be incorporated.

TEST SYSTEMS: CHARACTERISTICS, DEVELOPMENT AND SELECTION

Any useful test system must be sufficiently sensitive that the incidence of false-negatives is low. Clearly a high incidence of false-negatives is intolerable. In such a situation, large numbers of dangerous chemical agents would be carried through extensive additional testing only to find that they possess undesirable toxicological properties after the expenditure of significant time and money. On the other hand, a test system which is overly sensitive will give rise to a high incidence of false-positives which will have the deleterious consequence of rejecting potentially beneficial chemicals. The "ideal" test will fall somewhere between these two extremes and thus provide adequate protection without unnecessarily stifling development.

The "ideal" test should have an end-point measurement which provides data such that dose–response relationships can be obtained. Furthermore, any criterion of effect must be sufficiently accurate in the sense that it can be used to reliably resolve the relative toxicity of two test chemicals which produce distinct (in terms of hazard to humans) yet similar responses. In general, it may not be sufficient to classify test chemicals into generic toxicity categories. For instance, a test chemical which falls into an "intermediate" toxicity category, yet is borderline to the next more severe toxicity category, should be treated with more concern than a second test chemical which falls at the less toxic extreme of the same category. Therefore, it is essential for any credible test system to be able to both place test chemicals in an established toxicity category and rank materials relative to others in the category.

The end-point measurement of the "ideal" test system must be objective. This is important so that a given test chemical will give similar results when tested using the standard test protocol in different laboratories. If it is not possible to obtain reproducible results in a given laboratory over time or between various laboratories, then the historical database against which new test chemicals are evaluated will be time/laboratory-dependent. If this condition is the case, then there will be significant limitations on the application of the test system because it could potentially produce conflicting results. From a regulatory point of view, this possibility would be highly undesirable. Along these lines, it is important for the test protocol to incorporate internal standards to serve as quality controls. Thus, test data could be represented utilizing a reference scale based on the test system response to the internal controls. Such normalization, if properly documented, could reduce inter-test variability.

From a practical point of view, there are several additional features of the "ideal" test which should be satisfied. *In vitro* alternatives to current *in vivo* test systems basically should be designed to evaluate the observed toxic response in a manner as closely predictive of the outcome of interest in man as possible. In addition, the test should be fast enough that the turnaround time for a given test chemical is reasonable for the intended purpose (very rapid for a screen, timely for a definitive test). Obviously the speed of the test and the ability to conduct tests on several chemicals simultaneously will determine the overall productivity. The test should be inexpensive so that it is economically competitive with current testing practices. And finally, the technology should be easily transferred from one laboratory to another without excessive capital investment (relative to the value of the test performed) for test implementation.

It should be kept in mind that though some of these practical considerations may appear to present formidable limitations for any given test system at the present time, the possibility of future developments in testing technology could overcome these obstacles. In the real-world environment, these practical considerations are grounds for consideration of multiple new candidate tests on the basis of competitive performance. The most predictive test system in the universe of possibilities will never gain wide acceptance if it takes years to produce an answer or costs substantially more than other test systems which are only marginally less predictive.

The point is that these characteristics of the "ideal" test system provide a general framework for evaluation of alternative test systems in general. No test system is likely to be "ideal." Therefore, it will be necessary to weigh the strengths and weaknesses of each proposed test system in order to reach a conclusion on how "good" a particular test is.

In both theory and practice, *in vivo* and *in vitro* tests have potential advantages. Tables 1 and 2 summarize their advantages. How then might the proper tests be selected, especially in the case of the choice of staying with an existing test system or adopting a new one? The next section will present the basis for selection of specific tests.

Considerations in Adopting New Test Systems

Conducting toxicological investigations in two or more species of laboratory animals is generally accepted as being a prudent and responsible practice in developing a new chemical entity, especially one that is expected to receive widespread use and to have exposure potential over human lifetimes. Adding a second or a third species to the testing regimen offers an extra measure of confidence to the toxicologist and

TABLE 1. *Rationale for using* in vivo *test systems*

1. They provide evaluation of actions/effects on intact animal and organ/tissue interactions.
2. Either neat chemicals or complete formulated products (complex mixtures) can be evaluated.
3. Either concentrated or diluted products can be tested.
4. They yield data on the recovery and healing processes.
5. They are the required statutory tests for agencies under such laws as the Federal Hazardous Substances Act (unless data are already available), Toxic Substances Control Act, Federal Insecticides, Fungicides, and Rodenticides Act (FIFRA), Organization for Economic Cooperation (OECD), and Food and Drug Administration (FDA) laws.
6. Quantitative and qualitative tests with scoring system are generally capable of ranking materials as to relative hazards.
7. They are amenable to modifications to meet the requirements of special situations (such as multiple dosing or exposure schedules).
8. They have an extensive available database and cross-reference capability for evaluation of relevance to human situation.
9. They involve the ease of performance and relative low capital costs in many cases.
10. Tests are generally both conservative and broad in scope, providing for maximum protection by erring on the side of overprediction of hazard to man.
11. Tests can be either single end point (such as lethality, corrosion, etc.) or shot-gun (also called multiple end point, and include such test systems as a 13-week oral toxicity study).

TABLE 2. *Limitations of in vivo testing systems which serve as a basis for seeking in vitro alternatives for toxicity tests*

1. Complications and potential confounding or masking findings of *in vivo* systems.
2. *In vivo* systems may only assess short-term site of application or immediate structural alterations produced by agents. Specific *in vivo* tests may only be intended to evaluate acute local effects (however, this may be a purposeful test system limitation).
3. Technician training and monitoring are critical (particularly due to the subjective nature of evaluation).
4. *In vivo* tests in animals do not perfectly predict results in humans if the objective is to exclude or identify severe-acting agents.
5. Structural and biochemical differences between test animals and humans make extrapolation from one to the other difficult.
6. Lack of standardization of *in vivo* systems.
7. Variable correlation with human results.
8. Large biological variability between experimental units (i.e., individual animals).
9. Large, diverse, and fragmented databases which are not readily comparable.

the other professionals who will be responsible for evaluating the associated risks, benefits, and exposure limitations or protective measures. Although undoubtedly broadening and deepening a compound's profile of toxicity, the practice of enlarging on the number of test species is an indiscriminate scientific generalization as has been demonstrated in multiple points in the literature (as reviewed in ref. 8). Moreover, such a tactic is certain to generate the problem of species-specific toxicoses. These are defined as toxic responses or inordinately low biological thresholds for toxicity that are evident in one species or strain, while all other species examined are either unresponsive or strikingly less sensitive. Species-specific toxicoses usually imply that different metabolic pathways for converting or excreting xenobiotics are involved or that anatomical differences are involved. The investigator confronting such findings must be prepared to address the all-important question, Are humans likely to react positively or negatively to the test agent under similar circumstances? Assuming that numerical odds prevail and that humans automatically fit into the predominant category would be scientifically irresponsible, whether on the side of being safe or at risk. Such a confounded situation can be an opportunity to advance more quickly into the heart of the search for predictive information. Species-specific toxicoses can frequently contribute toward a better understanding of the general case if the underlying biological mechanism either causing or enhancing toxicity is defined and especially if it is discovered to uniquely reside in the sensitive species.

The designs of our current tests appear to serve society reasonably well (i.e., significantly more times than not) in identifying hazards that would be unacceptable. However, the process can just as clearly be improved from the standpoint of both improving our protection of society and doing necessary testing in a manner that uses fewer animals in a more humane manner.

There are substantial potential advantages in using an *in vitro* system in toxicological testing; these include (a) isolation of test cells or organ fragments from homeostratic and hormonal control, (b) accurate dosing, and (c) quantitation of results. It should be noted that, in addition to the potential advantages, *in vitro* systems per se also have a number of limitations which can contribute to their not being acceptable models. Findings from an *in vitro* system which either limit their use in predicting *in vivo* events or make them totally unsuitable for the task include wide differences in the doses needed to produce effects or differences in the effects elicited. Some reasons for such findings are detailed in Table 3.

Tissue culture has the immediate potential to be used in two very different ways in industry. Firstly, it has been used to examine a particular aspect of the toxicity of a compound in relation to its toxicity *in vivo* (i.e., mechanistic or explanatory studies). Secondly, it has been used as a form of rapid screening to compare the toxicity of a group of compounds for a particular form of response. Indeed, the pharmaceutical industry has used *in vitro* test systems in these two ways for years in the search for new potential drug entities.

The theory and use of screens in toxicology has previously been reviewed by this author (4–6). Mechanistic and explanatory studies are generally called for when a traditional test system gives a result that is unclear or for which the relevance to the real-life human exposure is doubted. *In vitro* systems are particularly attractive for such cases because they can focus on well-defined single aspects of a problem or pathogenic response, free of the confounding influence of the multiple responses of

TABLE 3. *Possible interpretations when* in vitro *data do not predict results of* in vivo *studies*

1. Chemical is not absorbed at all, or is poorly absorbed, in *in vivo* studies.
2. Chemical is well absorbed but is subject to "first-pass effect" in the liver.
3. Chemical is distributed so that less (or more) reaches the receptors than would be predicted on the basis of its absorption.
4. Chemical is rapidly metabolized to an active or inactive metabolite that has a different profile of activity and/or different duration of action than the parent drug.
5. Chemical is rapidly eliminated (e.g., through secretory mechanism).
6. Species of the two test systems used are different.
7. Experimental conditions of the *in vitro* and *in vivo* experiments differed and may have led to different effects than expected. These conditions include factors such as temperature or age, sex, and strain of animal.
8. Effects elicited *in vitro* and *in vivo* by the particular test substance in question differ in their characteristics.
9. Tests used to measure responses may differ greatly for *in vitro* and *in vivo* studies, and the types of data obtained may not be comparable.
10. The *in vitro* study did not use adequate controls (e.g., pH, vehicle used, volume of test agent given, samples taken from sham-operated animals), resulting in "artifacts" of method rather than results.
11. *In vitro* data cannot predict the volume of distributional central or peripheral compartments.
12. *In vitro* data cannot predict the rate constants for chemical movement between compartment.
13. *In vitro* data cannot predict the rate constants of chemical elimination.
14. *In vitro* data cannot predict whether linear or nonlinear kinetics will occur with specific dose of a chemical *in vivo*.
15. Pharmacokinetic parameters (e.g., bioavailability, peak plasma concentration, half-life) cannot be predicted based solely on *in vitro* studies.
16. *In vivo* effects of chemical are due to an alteration in the higher-order integration of an intact animal system, which cannot be reflected in a less complex system.

an intact higher-level organism. Note, however, that first one must know the nature (indeed the existence) of the questions to be addressed. It is then important to devise a suitable model system which is related to the mode of toxicity of the compound.

There is currently much controversy over the use of *in vitro* test systems: Will they find acceptance as "definitive test systems," or only be used as preliminary screens for such final tests? Or in the end, not be used at all? Almost certainly, all three of these cases will be true to some extent. Depending on how the data generated are to be used, the division between the first two is ill-defined at best.

Before trying to definitively answer these questions in a global sense, each of the end points for which *in vitro* systems are being considered should be overviewed and considered against the factors outlined up to this point.

TARGET ORGAN TOXICITY MODELS

This final model review section addresses perhaps the most exciting potential area for the use of *in vitro* models—as specific tools to evaluate and understand discrete target organ toxicities. Here the presumption is that there is reason to believe (or at least suspect) that some specific target organ (nervous system, lungs, kidney, liver, heart, etc.) is or may be the most sensitive site of adverse action of a systemically absorbed agent. From this starting point, a system that is representative of the target organ's *in vivo* response would be useful in at least two contexts.

First, as with all the other end points addressed in this chapter, a target organ predictive system could serve as a predictive system (in general, a screen) for effects in intact organisms, particularly man. As such, the ability to identify those agents with a high potential to cause damage in a specific target organ at physiologic concentrations would be extremely valuable.

The second use is largely specific to this set of *in vitro* models. This is to serve as tools to investigate, identify, and/or verify the mechanisms of action for selective target organ toxicities. Such mechanistic understandings then allow for one to know if such toxicities are relevant to man (or to conditions of exposure to man), to develop means to either predict such responses while they are still reversible or to develop the means to intervene in such toxosis (i.e., first aid or therapy), and, finally, to potentially modify molecules of interest to avoid unwanted effects while maintaining desired properties (particularly important in drug design).

In the context of these two uses, the concept of a library of *in vitro* models (5,6) becomes particularly attractive. If one could accumulate a collection of "validated," operative methodologies that could be brought into use as needed (and put away, as it were, while not being used), this would represent an extremely valuable competitive tool. The question becomes one of selecting which systems/tools to put into the library, and how to develop them to the point of common utility.

Additionally, one must consider what forms of markers are to be used to evaluate the effect of interest. Initially, such markers have been exclusively either morphological (in that there is a change in microscopic structure), observational (Is the cell/preparation dead or alive, or has some gross characteristic changed?), or functional (Does the model still operate as it did before?). Recently, it has become clear that more sensitive models do not generate just a single end-point type of data, but rather a multiple set of measures which in aggregate provide a much more powerful set of answers.

A wide range of target-organ-specific models have already been developed and utilized. Their incorporation into a library-type approach requires that they be evaluated for reproducibility of response, ease of use, and predictive characteristics under the intended conditions of use. These evaluations are probably at least somewhat specific to any individual situation. The remaining chapters in this volume address each of these applications in some detail.

SENSITIVITY AND PREDICTIVE VALUE

Two of the key issues that must be confronted when considering any new test system are predictive value and sensitivity. These (along with the general scientific requirement of reproducibility) are points which must be evaluated for an *in vitro* system. Both these characteristics are essential for a test system to be able to identify situations (in statistical terms, "population elements") which are different in some specified manner or another.

Sensitivity determines how much "power" a test has: How much different does an end point need to be before it is identified as different (or an effect is detected)? Predictive value determines how selective a test is in determining that an effect is present. A highly specific test will detect only "real" effect with a high level of confidence. These two characteristics are not independent. That is, changes in one result in changes in the other, all other factors being held constant. This relationship is made clear by first considering possible test outcome.

Test Outcome	True Result	
	Positive	Negative
Positive	a	b
Negative	c	d

Sensitivity is then defined as $a/(a + c)$, where a is all true-positives detected by a test and $a + c$ represents all true-positives.

Specificity is then equal to $d/(b + d)$. Predictive value can now be defined as $a/(a + b)$—that is, the percent of cases identified as positive which are actually positive (2). Increases in sensitivity must bring with them some degree of cost in terms of type II error—that is, an increase in the number of false-positives. The statistical characteristics of test performance have been discussed elsewhere (5).

If the operating technology or basis of interpretation of a test system is changed, of course this redefines the basic operating characteristics. Thus, for example, cultured cell systems which directly incorporate some form of metabolic activation into their operations (say by being based on coculture with hepatocytes) have potentially more favorable values for a, b, c, and d as a starting place.

PROBLEMS IN INTERPRETATION AND EXTRAPOLATION

Perhaps the principal barrier against more widespread use of existing *in vitro* tests (and against gaining support for development of new ones) is the difficulty in interpreting the outcome of tests (especially when one considers issues of sensitivity and predictive value presented earlier) and in extrapolating these results to potential effects in people. What changes are looked at in a model (say cell culture) system to provide prediction of a specific intact animal end point? Simple lethality to a cell-based system does not imply target organ toxicity simply because the cells in question are those that constitute the organ in question. It may simply be cytotoxicity which is meaningful only if the cells in question are selectively more sensitive than other cell types. Alterations in functionality that is specific to the cell type (or organ/tissue in question) is more likely to be predictive of a selective toxicity. It is also important that the concentrations of toxicant which yield a positive outcome in the media of an *in vitro* system be relevant to (and hopefully in a known manner, likely related to) those tissue or plasma concentrations which cause effects in intact animals. If it takes higher levels *in vitro* to produce a toxicity than it does *in vivo*, the relevance of the model should be questioned. This also means, by the way, that pharmacokinetic data are of significant value in designing and interpreting *in vitro* test systems.

At the same time, *in vitro* systems will tend to respond differently than the intact animal in some ways which will concern traditional toxicologists. For example, concentration responses of cultured cell systems tend to be fairly sharp (somewhat "all or none") even though in animal or man one for the same target organ end point will see a graded dose response. This is because the cells in a culture system are much more homogeneous than those in a group of animals (or even the cells which compare the target organ of a single animal) because they are near-clonal—they have been derived from a small number of parent cells.

Extrapolation to outcome in man requires a knowledge of the (at least projected) pharmacokinetics of the compound in question and an appreciation of the limitation (time course or limits on cell-to-cell or organ-to-organ interactions) of the *in vitro* system in question. The most likely reasons for failure in such extrapolation were presented earlier in Table 3.

Both interpretation and extrapolation can be made less error-prone if proper controls are incorporated into a test system. During development it is optimal if agents for which there are data in intact animals (the donor species for the *in vitro* system) and humans are available and if a human cell or tissue-based system can also be evaluated. Using this approach, standard (i.e., known positive and negative response compounds) should be established. Subsequent use of the new test system must incorporate regular reference back to the response of these compounds. Likewise, simple osmolarity and cell preparation viability controls should also be included.

VALIDATION

Validation is a somewhat ill-defined concept which currently is the principal stumbling block impeding use of *in vitro* tests for many. It is ill-defined because there is no fixed process and many people mean "regulatory (or peer) acceptance" when they say validation. The issues and considerations involved in conducting a validation have been most recently (and extensively) covered by Frazier (3), and the interested reader is referred to that source for a detailed discussion. In general, the major points to consider are as follows:

1. Is the method reproducible (will it give the same results to all who use it)? This reproducibility must be established both intralab and interlab.
2. Is the method predictive of the outcome in the species of concern? It is not essential that it give results the same as those of established animal tests, but they should be close.
3. Are the ways the method fails known?

Historically, new test systems in the biomedical sciences were proposed in the literature. If they withstood the tests of peer review and being reproduced by others, they were used by more and more people until they became the "accepted method" and were eventually picked up in guidelines and regulations. This was the traditional scientific process, but is now viewed as not being defined, rigorous, and timely enough.

REFERENCES

1. Bennenuto AJ, Cohen R. A realistic role for non-animal tests. *Pharm Exec* 1990;June.
2. Cooper JA, Saracci R, Cole P. Describing the validity of carcinogen screening test. *Br J Cancer* 1979;39:87–89.
3. Frazier JM. *Scientific criteria for validation of in vitro toxicity tests*. Brussels: Organization for Economic Co-Operation and Development, 1990.
4. Gad SC, ed. *Handbook of Product Safety Evaluation*. New York: Marcel Dekker, 1988.
5. Gad SC. Statistical analysis of screening studies in toxicology: with special emphasis on neurotoxicity. *J Am Coll Toxicol* 8(1):171–183.
6. Gad SC. A tier testing strategy incorporating *in vitro* testing methods for pharmaceutical safety assessment. *Humane Innovations and Alternatives in Animal Experimentation* 1989;3:75–79.
7. Gad SC. Industrial application for *in vitro* toxicity testing methods: a tier testing strategy for product safety assessment. In: Frazier J, ed. *In vitro toxicity testing*. New York: Marcel Dekker, 1991.
8. Gad SC, Chengelis CP. *Acute Toxicology: Principles and Methods*. Caldwell, NJ: Telford Press, 1988.

In Vitro Toxicology,
edited by Shayne Cox Gad.
Raven Press, Ltd., New York, © 1994.

3

Ocular Toxicity Assessment *In Vitro*

J. F. Sina* and P. D. Gautheron†

*Merck Sharp & Dohme Research Laboratories, West Point, Pennsylvania 19486; and
†Merck Sharp & Dohme Research Laboratories, 63203 Riom, France*

Given the number of chemicals to which people are exposed each day, a real need exists to identify potential hazards associated with this exposure. For predicting ocular irritation potential, the Draize method (1) has been, and continues to be, a standard procedure, despite a number of criticisms. These drawbacks include a substantial intra- and interlaboratory variability (2), subjectivity of the scoring, questions of extrapolation to humans, and animal welfare concerns. In view of these problems, much work has been done in recent years to find modifications or alternatives for the Draize test. These have centered around both modifications to the *in vivo* test and the search for *in vitro* or *ex vivo* techniques. In this chapter we will deal primarily with alternative (i.e., non-whole animal) tests, though a discussion of the *in vivo* assay is necessary to develop some of the issues faced when developing alternative methods.

IN VIVO IRRITATION TESTING

Since only key points will be discussed here, the reader is referred to the review of Chan and Hayes (3) for a more detailed examination of the standard Draize methodology, as well as modifications. Basically, the Draize assay is a subjective test in which 0.1 ml of a liquid or 0.1 g of a solid test material is placed into the conjunctival sac of one eye of a rabbit, with the other eye serving as the control. At various times after dosing, observations are made and a numerical score assigned based on the extent and severity of corneal opacity, redness of the iris, chemosis of the conjunctiva, and discharge. The bulk of the score (80 of a possible 110) comes from observations of corneal opacity. The maximal score for conjunctival changes is 20, and 10 for effects on the iris. Based on the total score, chemicals are classified as nonirritating, mild, moderate, severe, or extreme.

Many different scoring systems have been developed to try to more precisely or reproducibly describe the irritation potential of chemicals (see, for instance, ref. 4; see also cosmetic, AFNOR, and OECD as cited in ref. 5). And the number of distinct irritation categories varies from a 1 to 10 scale (6), to a four-category (non-irritating, mild, moderate, severe) classification by Green et al. (7), to the FHSA scale (8) in which a material is either irritating or nonirritating. This diversity in scoring methods and categorization of chemicals has contributed to sometimes significant discrepancies in comparing irritation potential among chemicals and has highlighted the subjective character of the test.

In an attempt to eliminate some of this subjectivity, many investigators have attempted to measure some parameter which would more precisely relate to irritation potential. One end point which has been the focus of much attention is measurement of corneal thickness or swelling. According to a number of investigators (9–11) this parameter correlates quite well with the irritation category derived from the traditional Draize scoring method. Although this end point is more objective, one drawback is that special equipment and expertise is required to reproducibly and effectively make such measurements, and the technique does not appear to be widespread. In addition, the method still requires the use of living animals and thus does not address animal welfare concerns.

To address some of these animal welfare issues and other scientific issues, various modifications to the *in vivo* test have been proposed. A good discussion of the pros and cons of some of these variations is presented in an ECETOC monograph (12) on irritation testing. One such modification is the use of anesthetics during the test period, although there is concern that this could interfere with the response of the animal and thus compromise the validity of the data obtained. Other measures proposed as ways to decrease animal suffering include (a) irrigation of the eye at various times after dosing and (b) screening out compounds of extreme pH, making the assumption that these are severe irritants without testing. Another approach has been the development of the low-volume Draize test (13) in which the animal is exposed to one-tenth the dose of the standard Draize test. This method is said not only to cause less discomfort to the test animals, but also to correlate better with data on human exposure.

But perhaps the best way to address concerns with the *in vivo* test would be to develop an *in vitro* model system which would objectively quantitate specific parameters of the irritation index. To develop such a model, one needs to ask what the Draize test is really measuring—that is, what is the mechanism(s) of irritation. The answer is complex because in all likelihood multiple mechanisms of action lead to the clinical signs identified with varying degrees of ocular irritation. For instance, Igarashi (14) has suggested that opacity may be due to precipitation of proteins in the cornea. This hypothesis is based on observations with surfactants which coagulated egg white solutions, where the extent of coagulation paralleled the ability of the compounds to cause corneal opacity. The author noted, however, that some anionic surfactants produced entirely opposite results suggesting that opacity cannot be fully explained on the basis of protein precipitation.

Since clarity of the cornea is in large part due to the tightly layered organization of the epithelium and/or the integrity of the endothelium, one could easily hypothesize that disruption of these structures by any mechanism (cell death, disruption of junctional complexes, osmotic imbalance, altered ion fluxes, etc.) can result in opacification. For instance, Duke-Elder and Leigh (15), in discussing corneal lesions, cite examples of endothelial trauma resulting in either transient or permanent corneal opacity.

With respect to epithelial damage, Basu (16) has presented data suggesting that damage to the peripheral cells of the cornea results in altered fluid permeability, which leads to distortion of the corneal layers and altered transparency. Additionally, Burstein and Klyce (17) studied the effects of some components of ophthalmic preparations (benzalkonium chloride, thimerosal, amphotericin B, etc.) on morphology and electrophysiologic parameters of isolated corneas. These authors found that many of these test materials (which can be irritants in high enough concentrations) can cause destruction of the epithelial cell layers followed by alteration in transport properties of the cornea. These data support the idea that parameters such as altered cell morphology or viability and ion or water transport may be early indicators of irritation potential.

And, although corneal damage is important, there are other responses to irritants which need to be considered in modeling *in vivo* irritation. For instance, to provide a basis for developing alternative methods, Parish (18) attempted to define the histological features associated with irritants. He found that mild to moderate chemicals caused a thinning (through exfoliation) of the corneal epithelium, but no irreversible damage. Furthermore, the conjunctiva showed edema, leukocyte infiltration, and congestion of the blood vessels, suggesting that damage to this tissue may also need to be examined.

In addition, inflammation is a major clinical sign recorded in scoring the Draize assay and may be either a cause of or a response to irritation. If necrosis of the corneal epithelium or conjunctiva occurs, autolysis of the cells may release factors which initiate an acute inflammatory response to "clean up" the area of damage, resulting in a secondary response. Alternatively, it has been demonstrated (19) that neutrophil or macrophage infiltration of either the endothelial or epithelial corneal surface can cause substantial damage resulting in cell loss as well as separation of the cell layers and consequent opacification.

From the discussion above, it should be clear that ocular irritation is most likely due to multiple mechanisms causing distinct clinical signs (opacity, inflammation, congestion, necrosis, etc.). Opacification could be due to altered ion fluxes, protein precipitation, or cross-linking, etc., whereas inflammation may involve chemotactic factors or other components of the arachidonic acid cascade. And the cells involved could be the epithelial or endothelial cells of the cornea, stromal cells, or conjunctiva. The question that arises, then, is which end point and/or target tissue should be the focus of attempts to define alternative test methods.

DEVELOPMENT OF ALTERNATIVES

If one could develop a method for testing ocular irritation potential in a non-whole animal system using an objective measurement(s), it would be a major improvement over the current rabbit eye test. A rather extensive list of models proposed as alternatives to the Draize test has been compiled by Frazier et al. (20). But while this might serve as a starting point, none of these is well enough developed or validated for general use. There are also a number of "nonexperimental" methods for predicting irritation potential—computer databases, structure–activity models, etc. Given this wide range of choices, how does one proceed?

One strategy for approaching this problem is to determine what information is already available upon which a prediction of ocular irritation may be made (i.e., assessment based on no further biological testing). If the data are insufficient, and further testing is required, one must determine which biological parameters will best define the *in vivo* response to irritants, then develop a model which adequately measures these end points. For the purposes of this chapter, we will discuss some of the types of information that might be used to predict ocular irritation without further testing, then we will discuss *in vitro* models which are being developed to measure the various parameters assessed *in vivo* in a Draize test.

PREDICTION FROM PREEXISTING DATA

Because of the diversity of chemicals to be tested and the number of different ways in which the results will be used (worker safety, transportation regulation, consumer product safety, possible litigation), it is important to find out as much as possible about the test substance. And because of the large number of chemicals which need to be tested, one needs to proceed as quickly as practical without sacrificing accuracy. As a starting point, then, it would be practical to ask whether there is any information already available that can be used for making predictions?

Databases

Using ocular irritation data previously collected by other scientists and published in the literature or contained in computer databases seems like a reasonable place to start investigating a new chemical entity. The problem, however, is that such data are limited. Since the Draize test is a routine assay, not contributing new expertise, irritation data are not often published. Some effort is being made to provide a forum for this type of data, for instance in the Acute Toxicity Data section of the *Journal of the American College of Toxicology*, but to date there is a limited amount of information available. Where data exist, for instance in the publications of Carpenter and Smyth (6), they are reduced to an arbitrary scale (in this case 1 to 10), and since the data in this example were collected over a number of years, discrepancies in scoring tend to increase (due to variations in individuals performing the test, animals, test protocols, etc.). Contributing to the discrepancies are the variability and lack of strict reproducibility in the first place [as shown by the study of Weil and Scala (2)]. Furthermore, in view of the number of different scoring methods (cited above), making comparisons from lab to lab is very difficult. And when the data are reduced to irritating or nonirritating, or to a broad category, there is no way that a more specific appraisal can be made or that a reader can make an independent evaluation and reconcile any apparent discrepancies.

Computer databases suffer from these same sorts of problems, but magnified. In order to be useful, such databases need to incorporate as much information as possible. This means that there are even more laboratories involved, with the attendant variability in performance of the assay and in scoring. And the personnel establishing the database generally have no means of making an assessment as to the quality of the data going in.

In-house databases may provide the most appropriate information available. Usually the raw data are available, and generally the methodology is more consistent so that test results and scoring change less with time or personnel performing the test. Another potential advantage is that within an industry group, the compounds comprising the databases are more likely to have similarities with the unknowns that need to be examined. However, this can also be a drawback in that the materials tested by, for instance, a cosmetics company may have no practical relevance to those tested by a pharmaceutical company, and therefore some in-house data may be too specific for general application. Thus, though it is a good idea to examine databases, it is likely that the data will be useful for flagging a potential problem, but not adequate for making a decision as to irritation potential.

Computer Modeling

Computer modeling is an alternative that has been proposed by many people. Such models are based generally on computer databases, and while modeling may be of some use, it suffers from the same drawbacks as do databases; that is, a computer simulation is only as reliable as the data used to generate the mathematical equations. Health Designs Inc. has developed such a model (TOPKAT), which is available commercially. The model was developed by quantitating various parameters, then comparing these measurements with the irritation potential of known materials to determine which end points correlate best. This allows one to weight each measurement as to its importance for irritation, and to develop a mathematical model. Thus the equations and model are only as accurate as the underlying data.

According to their own literature (21; TOPKAT manual), it has been difficult to construct this model due to the inherent variability in compound classification. The model that was generated has two sets of equations. In a first step, nonirritating compounds are separated from all other materials. Then a second set of equations is used to distinguish severe materials from the rest of the materials. The result is a three-category estimate: nonirritating, severe, or other. A further problem is that the developers predict that approximately 30% of materials cannot be handled by this model.

Some investigators are, however, using models based on their own in-house data with more success than was found with commercially available packages. This is logical since it is likely that within a particular company many of the materials making up the database might be generally related to the unknowns being tested. Thus, while these individual models might not be useful for as broad a range of materials as one might like (i.e., for screening across different industries), they may be practical for use within an individual company or within an industry group (pharmaceuticals, soaps and detergents, toiletries, specialty chemicals, etc.).

Physical/Chemical Data

As alluded to above, in constructing a model one looks at various measurements that might correlate with irritation potential and then attempts to determine which are truly important (causal) and which are secondary. Various parameters have been examined. For instance, many investigators look first at pH, assuming that compounds at the pH extremes (e.g., <3 or >12) are severe irritants which do not need animal testing. Support for this can be found in Walz (22) and Guillot et al. (5), where materials at pH extremes were generally very irritant (although there were exceptions). Extending this idea, a study sponsored by the Soap and Detergent Association has found that the alkalinity of a test material (i.e., the strength of the acid or base) may be the key point rather than a simple measure of pH (23).

Other physical/chemical parameters have been proposed as possibly predictive of irritation potential. For instance, a compound possessing surfactant properties generally is given close scrutiny because many surfactants are severe irritants, though again exceptions exist (Tween 20, for instance, is mild). Octanol:water partition coefficients have been proposed as an indicator of hazard because a material which tends to partition out of the aqueous phase may penetrate the eye more deeply. But although data are available to suggest that the octanol:water partition coefficient may correlate with cytotoxicity in some cases (24,25), there are no solid data to suggest that this parameter correlates with the ocular irritation potential of a chemical. And this is a general problem with using physical/chemical parameters for prediction of irritation. While some correlations and hypotheses exist, the data to adequately support the use of the various parameters are lacking. Thus, although certain characteristics of a chemical may be used to raise a warning flag, or to set testing priorities, at this time prediction of irritation potential cannot be based solely on physical or chemical data.

Data from Other Tests

Since multiple toxicity tests (acute and chronic) are generally performed on most chemicals, the question arises as to whether the results from these tests could predict ocular irritation and eliminate the need for a Draize test. Comparisons have been made between dermal and ocular irritation data under the hypothesis that if a material is irritating to the skin, it will also be irritating to the eye.

For instance, Gad et al. (26) found some correlation between ocular and dermal irritation, but the degree of correlation was dependent upon the *in vivo* classification scale used. When chemicals were classified as either irritating or nonirritating, the correlation between ocular and dermal data was better than when a categorical ranking (nonirritating, mild, moderate, severe) was used. Gilman et al. (27), on the other hand, found that a reliable correlation between ocular and dermal irritation could not be established for a series of petrochemicals and consumer products. Guillot et al. (5,28) examined both ocular and dermal irritation scored by different protocols. Correlating the data in the two articles, one finds that all dermal irritants (11 chemicals) were ocular irritants, but the degree of ocular irritation was not predictable from the dermal data. Only 18 of 45 nonirritating to slightly irritating materials dermally were nonirritating to slightly irritating in the eye. The remaining 27 compounds showed ocular irritation ranging from mild/moderate to extreme. And Williams (29,30) reported similar results. He found that 65% (39 of 60) of severe dermal irritants tested were severe ocular irritants, while 10% were moderate and 25% were mild or nonirritating.

These data suggest that if a compound is a severe dermal irritant, it is likely that it will be an ocular irritant as well. However, a significant number of exceptions (false-positives in the ocular test) exist. And, the fact that a compound is nonirritating or mild on the skin does not appear to correlate with lack of ocular irritation. Thus, while dermal irritation data may be of some utility, they cannot be relied upon to adequately predict ocular irritation potential.

IN VITRO MODELS

If a decision cannot be made based upon preexisting data, the next step is to use *in vitro* models for testing. Since the biological system which one is trying to model (the eye and its myriad responses to irritants) is quite complex, a multifaceted approach probably has the most chance of success with a broad range of test materials. The major parameters scored *in vivo* are corneal opacity, inflammation, and necrosis, so it is logical to begin the development of *in vitro* methods by establishing assays for one or more of these parameters. In this section we review some of the approaches being taken, as well as their advantages and disadvantages.

Opacity

Since corneal opacity is the most heavily weighted component of the Draize score, it is important to account for this response in an *in vitro* system. And yet relatively few proposed alternatives have attempted to directly address this end point. One method reported by Price and Andrews (31) uses whole isolated rabbit eyes with measurement of corneal thickness as the end point. The authors found this a reliable test, showing a good correlation with *in vivo* irritation potential for the 60 compounds tested.

Muir (32,33) reported the development of an opacity assay, using isolated bovine cornea, in which decreases in light transmission through the cornea were monitored as the end point. His work with surfactants and some industrial chemicals indicated a good correlation between the *in vivo* and *in vitro* data. Igarashi et al. (34) have developed a variation on this method in which isolated porcine corneas (with endothelial cells removed) are exposed to test compounds. Changes in voltage across the corneal epithelium are used as a measure of opacification.

In our own laboratory, we have extended the technique of Muir and have developed a bovine corneal opacity assay coupled with a fluorescein permeability test (35). This assay is described in more detail below.

The BCO-P assay uses corneas obtained from an abattoir as the target tissue, and measures both opacification and the penetration of fluorescein dye through the cornea as end points. Briefly, corneas are dissected free of the eye and mounted in plastic holders which allow access to both sides of the cornea. The isolated corneas are allowed to equilibrate in culture medium containing 1% serum for 1 hr, then the posterior compartment is filled with fresh culture medium containing 1% serum, while the anterior chamber is filled with test compound in either medium or polyethylene glycol 400. After an appropriate exposure period, the exposure medium is replaced with fresh medium, and the opacity of the treated cornea is measured relative to control without removal of the corneas from the holders. This measurement is done in an opacitometer (which is similar to a dual beam spectrophotometer), with a control cornea in one compartment and the treated one in another. The difference in light transmission is a measure of the chemically induced increase in opacity of the treated cornea.

We have tested approximately 45 commercially available chemicals as well as 43 in-house materials representative of a broad range of chemical classes, and have found that the correlation between the opacity measurement and *in vivo* Draize score is very good. This model also allows the assessment of recovery from injury, by simply continuing incubation of the cornea in fresh medium after taking the initial opacity reading. Readings taken at various times thereafter would give an indication of reversibility of the lesion.

We have found that some compounds cause sloughing of epithelial cells from the cornea, resulting in false-negative readings. (Since the damaged corneas had fewer cell layers, a greater transmittance of light was detected than might be expected.) To measure this type of damage, we adapted the fluorescein dye penetration concept of Tchao (36). After opacity readings were taken, the posterior compartment (endothelial cell side) was filled with fresh medium while the anterior compartment received sodium fluorescein in buffer. Following a 90-min incubation, the amount of dye in the posterior compartment was determined by spectrophotometric measurement at 490 nm. Since the epithelial layers of the cornea form a barrier resistant to chemical penetration, the amount of dye penetrating through to the posterior chamber should be directly proportional to the degree of damage to the epithelium.

We have found this two end-point assay (BCO-P) to be quite reliable for assessing irritation potential of manufacturing intermediates and raw materials. And we have found relatively few limitations with this method. For instance, working with insoluble materials is difficult in most *in vitro* assays. With the BCO-P assay, however, we are able to test most materials because the corneas can be exposed in the holders in a horizontal position. This allows material in suspension to settle out onto the cornea and to interact with the cells. The only problem we have encountered has been with a compound which was hydrophobic as well as insoluble. The material floated on the medium, never coming into contact with the cornea, and thus was not available to interact with the corneal cells.

One other potential problem would occur if a compound caused minimal irritation *in vivo* for some period of time (24–36 hr), but then induced increasing irritation over time. This type of delayed reaction would be difficult to detect with most *in vitro* assays, and the BCO-P would be no exception. However, if the basic protocol was modified so that readings for opacity were made over the course of 24–48 hr, one might be able to account for this delayed reaction.

Another assay which has been put forth as an alternative measure of corneal opacification is the Eytex assay. This method stems from the observations that transparency of the cornea depends on the hydration and organization of proteins, and that the presence of high-molecular-weight aggregates of protein caused opacity (37). Basically, the test measures the reduction in light transmission resulting from precipitate caused by interaction of the test material with a proprietary protein matrix (38). In certain applications, this method has proven quite useful (39,40), giving good correlations with *in vivo* results. On the other hand, Sanders et al. (41) and Bruner et al. (42) found that the correlation of Eytex data with *in vivo* data was unsatisfactory, and that other *in vitro* tests gave better correlations.

Part of the reason for this discrepancy may be in the type of materials tested. For instance, Thomson et al. (43) tested materials from a number of consumer product lines. Good correlation between Eytex data and *in vivo* results was seen for surfactant blends and eye area use products. However, the correlation was not as good when alcohol-containing formulations were tested. Further modifications of the basic Eytex method have been developed for testing specific product types, and the correlations are reportedly better if an appropriate modification is used (Dickens et al., reported in ref. 44). While the use of specific modifications is an advantage for testing within chemical categories, it can be a drawback for general screening. If the test compounds come from a variety of chemical classes, one may not be able to determine *a priori* which modification will give acceptable results and which will produce artifacts.

Another potential drawback of this assay is that if a chemical exerts its irritant effects by a mechanism other than protein precipitation or coagulation, the test would give false results. And Igarashi (14) did point out that for some materials (anionic surfactants) the ability to coagulate protein did not correlate well with irritation potential.

Cytotoxicity

The majority of assays proposed as alternatives to the Draize test are cytotoxicity tests. Usually these methods are simple, straightforward, and relatively rapid, with a defined end point which can be reproducibly and accurately measured. Many of the assays make use of immortalized cell lines as the target tissue, so no use of animals is required. Disadvantages include the fact that the assays are not usually mechanistically based and therefore may not provide information as to why and how a chemical causes irritation. Additionally, if the measured end point is not causally related to irritation, any correlation with *in vivo* data for one group of compounds may be due to chance and may not hold for another type of chemical. In this section we will consider some methods that are widely cited in the literature, in order to point out specific uses and limitations of this type of assay.

Table 1 lists a number of end points which have been used to assess the correlation of *in vitro* cytotoxicity with *in vivo* ocular irritation. Most are reported to give relatively good rank correlations within the group of chemicals tested. Two points are clear from the table. First, essentially any cell line can be used as the target for cytotoxicity testing. This point was directly tested and confirmed by Borenfreund and Borrero (45) and by Shopsis et al. (46). In these two cited studies, all five lines tested gave approximately equivalent rank correlations.

The second point is more disconcerting. Most of the testing was performed with products within a single chemical or product class (mostly with surfactants). This leaves unanswered the question of what correlation would be obtained in attempting to rank diverse compounds against each other. Indeed, Shopsis (reported in ref. 44) has shown that if chemicals are grouped together regardless of class, the correlation between *in vivo* and *in vitro* data breaks down. This may result from different mechanisms of toxicity among different chemical classes, or from any other expla-

TABLE 1. *End points used to assess the correlation of in vitro cytotoxicity with in vivo ocular irritation*

End point	Compounds	Cell type	References
Altered morphology; colony-forming efficiency	34, mostly alcohols	5 cell lines	45
Altered morphology; uridine uptake	22, weighted toward alcohols (13)	3 cells lines	46
Uridine uptake	Alcohols (14)	Balb/c 3T3	47
Colony-forming efficiency	13 surfactants	SIRC	48
Fluorescein diacetate/ ethidium bromide	11 detergent products	LS mouse fibroblasts	49
Trypan blue uptake	16 surfactants	V79	50
Fluorescein diacetate/ ethidium bromide; alkaline phosphatase release	11 detergents	HEp2, HeLa	51
MTT dye reduction	22 cosmetic products	Living dermal equivalent	52
MTT dye reduction; PGE_2 release	3 product formulations	Living dermal equivalent	53
Cellular metabolism (silicon microphysiometer)	17, mainly surfactants	Human keratinocytes	54

nation that the reader can imagine. But it raises the larger issue of how universally applicable cytotoxicity assays will be as alternatives for ocular irritation testing in animals.

This point can be illustrated by examining a specific cytotoxicity assay, the neutral red assay developed by Borenfreund and Puerner (55,56). This test has been widely used and has been adapted to a commercial test kit (57). The basis of the test is the sequestration of the vital dye neutral red into the lysosomes of viable cells. Nonviable cells are unable to retain the dye during harvesting, and thus the amount of dye per test culture (determined spectrophotometrically) is proportional to the number of viable cells per culture.

This assay has been used by a number of laboratories, and reportedly gives good correlations with *in vivo* ocular irritation data (42,58,59). However, most of the compounds tested in these studies were cosmetic ingredients, alcohols, or surfactant-based products. The correlations between neutral red data and *in vivo* irritation tend to break down when comparisons are made across chemical classes. For instance, Thomson et al. (60) reported that correlations within certain chemical groupings were substantially better than for other chemical types, and that the overall correlation of the assay with 94 compounds was relatively poor. They concluded that for their purposes this assay had limited usefulness. And we have had a similar experience in our own laboratory. Testing a number of diverse materials in V79 and rabbit corneal epithelial cells, we found that the overall correlation between the neutral red end point and ocular irritation *in vivo* was relatively poor ($r = -0.33$) (61). However, if the rank correlation was limited to alcohols, the correlation improved greatly, giving a correlation coefficient (r) of -0.67.

Another type of cytotoxicity end point is measured in dye penetration assays. This end point monitors the integrity of a cell sheet as a measure of penetration of a test material into the tissue of the cornea. The hypothesis is that a compound which destroys cell-to-cell connections will penetrate the cornea and potentially cause extensive damage. For example, Brooks and Maurice (62) have developed a proptosed mouse eye permeability test in which eyes of freshly sacrificed mice are exposed to test agent and sulforhodamine B penetration is measured. Unfortunately, few compounds have been tested, and it is thus difficult to assess the overall utility of the assay.

Another example of a dye penetration assay is the method developed by Tchao (36). In this model, Madin–Darby canine kidney (MDCK) cells, a cell line which forms tight junctions at confluence, are grown on a filter which separates two compartments, so that polarity of the monolayer is established and the sides can be separated. Fluorescein is placed in the inner chamber (analogous to the external surface of the cornea), and the passage of the dye through the cell sheet to the other chamber is monitored. When an intact monolayer covers the filter, the passage of fluorescein through the cell is restricted. If a chemical damages the cells, extensive leakage of fluorescein occurs. Tchao's work with five surfactants showed a good correlation between fluorescein penetration and irritation *in vivo*. Work with this method in our laboratory, however, indicated that the assay correctly identified only severe irritants. Mild and moderate compounds, as well as some severe irritants (which presumably act by a mechanism other than junctional disruption), showed no increased penetration. Used in combination with our opacity end point, this method was valuable (as described above), but by itself the penetration end point was of limited utility.

This brings us back to the question of when and how cytotoxicity assays could be used to estimate ocular irritation potential. It is clear that cytotoxicity assays are applicable in some situations (46,48,50), but it is equally clear that in many instances the ability of *in vitro* cytotoxicity assays to predict *in vivo* irritation is inadequate (58,63,64). The data suggest that if testing is being performed within a limited range of chemical classes or product lines, a cytotoxicity assay by itself might be practical. But, if a number of diverse chemicals need to be tested, cytotoxicity assays are not likely to be predictive.

However, data in the literature appear to support the use of cytotoxicity end points as a complementary component of a multiple-end-point model (e.g., the BCO-P assay) or in a battery of tests. If one were to test the same set of chemicals (from diverse classes) in a number of different cytotoxicity assays, multivariate analysis of the data might suggest a series of tests in which those compounds incorrectly classified by one end point might be detected in another assay.

Inflammation

The inflammation component is another important aspect of the Draize score which needs to be addressed in any attempt to develop *in vitro* alternatives. And the mechanistic rationale for the involvement of inflammation in ocular irritation and damage has been amply demonstrated. For instance, Elgebaly et al. (19,65) have shown that leukocytes, attracted to an inflammation site by the release of chemotactic factors, can cause significant damage to the corneal epithelium or endothelium. Bazan et al. (66) have demonstrated that after cryogenic injury to rabbit cornea, both prostaglandins and hyroxyeicosatetraenoic acids (HETEs) are released from epithelium, stroma, and endothelium. Srinivasan and Kulkarni (67) have demonstrated that prostaglandins and prostacyclin are involved in mediating the polymorphonuclear leukocyte response to different types of corneal injury. And Bhattacherjee et al. (68) have reported that both prostaglandins and leukotrienes are important in the development of ocular inflammation, inducing both vascular and cellular changes in ocular tissue.

But one of the problems in trying to develop an inflammation model *in vitro* is our limited understanding of the interactions among cells and molecules (prostaglandins, leukotrienes, histamine, serotonin, thromboxane, etc.) involved in inflammation. That is to say, it is clear that certain cells and molecules are present at the site of inflammation, and thus are likely to be involved early in the response, while others are involved in modulation of the response. The difficulty is to define which molecules are most likely to be reproducible and quantitative indicators of a chemical effect. The studies cited above suggest two possible end points to evaluate —chemotaxis and the release of eicosanoids.

The approach to assessing chemotaxis, taken by Elgebaly et al. (69), obviates the need to identify the individual factors involved. Based on Elgebaly's work showing that chemotactic factors are released from a variety of tissues in response to injury, she has developed a bovine corneal cup model. In this assay, corneas (bovine, rabbit, or human) are put into holders such that the epithelial surface forms the inside of a cup. Exposures are made by adding compounds into this cup, allowing an incubation time for release of factors involved in inflammation into the medium, and then measuring the chemotactic activity of the exposure medium to neutrophils. Metwally et al. (70) have performed preliminary characterization of the chemotactic factor(s) released in response to injury; however, the advantage of the system is that it does not matter what the specific attractant factor(s) is. One can measure the chemotactic response without specifically identifying the causative agent. To date the method has not been extensively validated, but the approach holds promise.

Another approach is that taken by Benassi et al. (71) in which they evaluated the release of inflammatory mediators by use of high-performance liquid chromatography (HPLC) and fluorescence. Using a bovine eye cup model, they measured the release of specific mast cell mediators (histamine, serotonin, and leukotrienes) after exposure of ocular tissue to test compounds. Quantification of the released mediators was performed by HPLC analysis of mediators derivatized with fluorescamine. While this is a promising approach, the model has only been tested with two compounds.

Along these same lines, others have sought to correlate the release of specific eicosanoids with *in vivo* irritation potential. Dubin and co-workers (72,73) used radioimmunoassay (RIA) methods to examine the release of four prostanoids from rat vaginal tissue in response to alcohols. Their data indicate that the mild irritant ethanol induces the release of PGE_2, $PGF_{2\alpha}$, 6-keto-$PGF_{1\alpha}$, and thromboxane B_2, and that longer chain alcohols, which are generally more irritating, caused a greater amount of prostanoid to be released. The next step would be to determine whether the correlation holds for a more extensive series of materials.

This approach of measuring specific eicosanoids has also been taken by others for the study of dermal as well as ocular irritation (53,74,75). In our own laboratory we are examining inflammation *in vitro* with a combination of RIA and HPLC techniques. Since it is not yet clear which components of the arachidonic acid cascade can be quantitatively or qualitatively correlated with ocular irritation, we have chosen to let the data indicate the appropriate molecule(s). We have therefore developed HPLC methods [based on the work of Powell (76) and Peters et al. (77)] to identify and quantitate as many eicosanoids as possible in a single run. Once a pattern develops such that one or more changes in the profile appear to correlate with the severity of irritation caused by a chemical, we can examine the specific molecules effected by RIAs. Preliminary evidence (based on a limited number of compounds) suggests that the appearance of HETEs may correlate with irritation potential better than does the release of specific prostaglandins or leukotrienes.

Another type of assay which has been proposed as an indicator of inflammation (although a degree of toxicity or necrosis is also included) is the chorioallantoic membrane (CAM) assay (78,79) and various modifications of this test, including CAMVA (80–82), BECAM (83), and HET/CAM (84,85). Basically the assay scores alterations (vascularity, necrosis, etc.) in the CAM of chicken eggs upon exposure to test compounds. As proposed by Leighton et al. (79), the scoring system is quite subjective and covers a wide range of observations made after a 3-day exposure to compound. In contrast, the HET/CAM assay concentrates the scoring on effects on blood vessels of the CAM and the egg albumen, and scoring is performed after only 0.5 to 5 min of exposure to test material. The BECAM assay scores alterations primarily to the blood vessels of the CAM, with scoring and timing of exposure similar to the HET/CAM technique. But in addition, this assay combines the CAM observations with observations of opacity and fluorescein permeability made in isolated bovine eye.

The CAMVA assay is a modification of the original CAM assay developed at Colgate–Palmolive. Early evaluation efforts (80) indicated that the correlation of the standard CAM with Draize data was not always satisfactory. A modification was made such that exposures were limited to 30 min, and scoring was focused on changes in vascularity (hemorrhaging, capillary injection, ghost vessels). Using this modification (termed CAMVA), Bagley et al. (82) have found good correlation between the results from this assay and irritation data from a traditional Draize score for surfactant-based materials.

As with most of the other assays discussed here, the CAM assay has proven useful in some applications but inadequate in others. The reason(s) for this discrepancy may be due to the compound classes tested, or to various methodological differences between laboratories. For instance, Lawrence and co-workers (86,87) found the CAM assay inadequate for their purposes. When they tested nine materials (surfactants, alcohols, miscellaneous), they found that in only four cases were they able to predict the *in vivo* irritation potential from the CAM data. They hypothesize that this may be due to observations that indicate that inflammation in the rabbit conjunctiva differs mechanistically from inflammation in the CAM, with the former being associated with infiltration of neutrophils and macrophages while the latter is basically chemically induced necrosis. Price et al. (88) also reported that the CAM assay was of limited value for their applications. Using a protocol with short exposure times (similar to HET/CAM), they found that while the assay was capable of accurately predicting 23 of 30 materials as to whether they were irritating or nonirritating, the degree of irritation could not be assessed based on the CAM response. Perhaps in other applications, this positive or negative categorization would be more appropriate.

A final point that needs to be mentioned with regard to testing on the CAM is that, as indicated by Lawrence (86), the technique is considered to be an *in vivo* procedure in the United Kingdom and therefore would not be an acceptable "animal alternative."

USING ALTERNATIVES

Given the array of methods available, how does one approach reducing or replacing *in vivo* ocular irritation testing in a practical situation? It should be clear from the discussion above that different assays measure different components or mechanisms of the *in vivo* response. Therefore it seems highly unlikely that a single test, measuring a single end point, will prove to be an adequate alternative. Rather, as has been suggested in the literature (12,89,90), it seems reasonable to perform a battery of tests. For instance, one approach would be to gather as much data as possible from structure–activity relationships, databases, physical/chemical characteristics, or other toxicity studies, then supplement this with *in vitro* or *ex vivo* testing. Only if these steps were still inadequate would an animal assay be performed. This is similar to the approach being taken by Procter and Gamble Co. as reported by Yam and Winters (91). But, this still leaves a number of practical questions: Which assays and how many assays should be performed? What are the criteria for defining a clear negative, clear positive, or equivocal response? Are some types of assays or data mechanistically irrelevant (or misleading) for assessment of ocular irritation? How does one reconcile the data if different responses are obtained in different assays? Unfortunately, the answers to questions such as these are elusive and may not be universally applicable. In the following section, we will try to provide some points for consideration.

In deciding how to structure an overall approach, one needs to specifically frame the question(s) to be addressed. One such question would be: How precisely does irritation potential need to be determined? For instance, three scenarios come to mind: (i) a simple irritating versus nonirritating determination, (ii) a ranking of greater or lesser irritation potential relative to a known irritant(s), or (iii) a continuous scale ranking from nonirritating through severe. The number of tests necessary and the precision required of each will likely depend upon the question asked. For determining whether a compound is irritating or not, one needs an end-point measurement which provides clear-cut, objective data where a distinct "threshold" of effect versus no effect can be defined. For continuous scale ranking, this might be totally inadequate, while an assay providing a more subjective end point might be acceptable. In both of these cases, two or more different assays may need to be performed to provide confirmation of the results. On the other hand, for a measurement of irritation potential relative to a known irritant, a single assay may suffice, since any variation within the test would likely affect both known and unknown similarly.

Another question that needs to be answered is: What types of materials will be tested in the alternative assay(s)? For example, if testing is to be done on a new entity about which little is known, one would likely need to perform not only more assays, but more diverse types of assays, than when testing a material which is essentially a reformulation of previously tested components.

A third consideration, and perhaps the major question, is: How will the test results be applied in a decision-making scheme? For instance, an alternative test may be used (a) to set priorities for subsequent *in vivo* testing, (b) to screen out any irritating materials, which would be labeled without further testing, while mild or equivocal materials would be confirmed *in vivo*, or (c) to actually identify the irritation potential of a material with no testing at all to be done in animals. If the purpose is to completely replace animal testing (as opposed to reduction or refinement), one would probably need to do a more extensive battery of tests in order to reach a level of confidence in the test results, compared to the case in which the *in vitro* testing would be for pre-screening (i.e., establishing an approximation of irritation potential) with an *in vivo* test to confirm the results at a later time.

Related to this is the question of the purpose for obtaining the irritancy data. For instance, if the testing is to be done for worker safety on unknown compounds (where exposure would usually be limited but might be acute), the *in vitro* assay would have to be quite conservative. That is to say, false-positives, while undesirable, would be more acceptable than false-negatives which could have drastic consequences in the workplace. Since exposure to potentially hazardous materials could be limited in an occupational setting, perhaps a single, sensitive test would be appropriate for establishing a level of precaution. If, on the other hand, the testing was to be done on a ocular product where exposure to the eye would be deliberate, or on a consumer product where a larger population would be potentially exposed, a more definitive irritancy ranking might be necessary. The extent of exposure could no longer be controlled, and therefore equivocal irritation results could not be handled by providing more individual protection (as in the workplace). Therefore a greater number of more sophisticated and definitive assay methods would be necessary.

In view of these types of considerations, it seems likely that no single approach to alternative testing can be universally applied, but that the varying concerns of each laboratory need to be addressed in deciding on an appropriate test battery. So while these concepts provide a general framework, we are still left to determine which assay(s) would work best in a given situation. One therefore needs to obtain information on the strengths and weaknesses of the various tests which have been proposed as assays of ocular irritation potential.

For this purpose, one can look in the literature at the various evaluation studies which have been conducted, or perhaps perform such a study on one's own chemical entities. For instance, Bruner et al. (42) have evaluated seven proposed ocular testing alternatives (silicon microphysiometer, luminescent bacteria, neutral red, total protein, *Tetrahymena* motility, BE/CAM, or Eytex) with test materials relevant to their own situation (emphasis on surfactants). The assays selected covered a range of end points and potential mechanisms of action, and suggested those methods which would be applicable for their consumer products. They concluded that all of the tests, except BE/CAM and Eytex, had some utility as screens prior to limited confirmation studies *in vivo*. Sanders et al. (41) took a similar approach with a series of cosmetic formulations. In their studies, they wanted to select assays which would give a reliable distinction between irritating and nonirritating materials. They found that for the test chemicals chosen, the CAMVA, Microtox, *Tetra-*

reported that by using complementary aticals or plasticizers can be ranked for of animal testing needed. And Lawrenc expect that the test would produce an lated whole eye preparations for assessus scale if it was only validated for does not address questions of recovery c in both instances.

case, for worker safety testing, we have can truly "validate" a test for general P assay (35). If the material is moderated to individual situations. The litera-lished in our validation studies, we willrs clear that some end points work well tions in the workplace. To be conservatnadequate for others, and that a single nonirritating *in vitro* results in a limitecom acute versus chronic exposure, re-and comfort with the *in vitro* test, we wmed with a clear question in mind. For confirmation step for the greater majoright ask whether assay x or y correlates

What we are seeing, then, is that la) of chemicals. This is much easier to methods where practical, recognizing tlgeneral use, since as more people use a teries of methods are being used to overll try to use it in a way that the devel-generally accepted tests are not availabl include in their validation.

he test materials used in the validation

ssible to the characteristics of the un-

VALIrature, for instance, that many cytotox-

n vivo irritancy data for surfactants, but

Evaluation studies help to define theounds from other chemical classes are used, but they don't address fully the qudifferent utility for different persons or *tion* evokes different meanings for diffate potential methods under conditions one can simplify the process to a singlation. Although some have proposed a tained so that one is comfortable using sed in the validation of all assays, our say, one has to explicitly define criterin in performance characteristics of the acceptable for routine usage, and measertainly to perform an interlaboratory meet these criteria. pounds to be tested is appropriate. But

Good overall reviews of points to bene's own situation, it is more logical to presented in OECD monograph no. 36 ¢t likely need to be tested in the future in workshop (98). Some of these points wi ing section. ds tested, number of different laborato-

In the simplest sense, validation is an be done before an assay is considered evaluation study with different assays arewhat subjective, but we would suggest correlate well with *in vivo* data, the next that a specific hazard assessment judg-large number of compounds in the most ce based on the assay results. The extent compounds are still acceptable, one mig one wants from the test. If one needs a say that enough compounds with differelevel may be reached after 50 chemicals had been tested to give the user confidendetermine nonirritating, mild, moderate, mean? Critically speaking, it only meansategory may need to be tested, resulting similar to those used for validation, theyled overall.

vitro test which predicts with some accurgainst which the *in vitro* test should be *in vivo* study. What it does not mean is tbe acceptable. For instance, it is well or that the test can be used in ways unrebbit is subjective and varies significantly tion. For example, if the test was validaton as to how often the rabbit data do not predict the human experience. Yet for the majority of chemicals, the rabbit studies are the only data available; thus essentially all of the proposed *in vitro* alternatives are being compared to ocular irritation data generated in rabbits. Given this variability in the *in vivo* data, one would not expect a 100% correlation between *in vivo* and *in vitro* data (nor would such a correlation mean that the *in vitro* assay would be 100% predictive of the potential human hazard). We would argue that at this point the Draize rabbit database is the only adequate database available for comparison, but that appropriate leeway needs to be included in *in vivo–in vitro* comparisons to account for the subjectivity of the animal data.

No matter what the scoring system or *in vitro* test, there will always be the question of dividing lines between irritation categories: When is a compound mild and when is it moderate? How precisely can the cutoff be defined? Is it necessary to define it? What are we willing to accept? Thus, what is a reasonable level of correlation to expect in order for an assay to be judged an acceptable alternative? Obviously there are no hard and fast answers, and the answer comes back to the question of individual confidence levels. These are, however, issues that need to be addressed by developers as well as users of *in vitro* alternative assays.

A number of validation or evaluation projects are currently underway within various organizations, as well as within the laboratories of individuals working with specific assays. These studies illustrate the different approaches taken to validation. For instance, the BGA in Germany has chosen to investigate only two alternatives, the neutral red/kenacid blue assay and the HET/CAM assay, but to conduct the study among 12 different laboratories with 32 compounds from diverse chemical classes (99–101). The intent of this study is to determine "whether and to what extent" these assays can be used to predict eye irritation potential.

Similarly, Blein et al. (102) chose to examine three very different tests (the low-volume Draize test, HET/CAM, and neutral red uptake) to determine which correlated best with the standard eye irritation assay. Six laboratories were involved in testing 40 compounds from diverse chemical classes, and interlaboratory, as well as intralaboratory, variability was assessed.

On the other hand, MEIC (103) has not attempted to predetermine the appropriate assays. They have constructed a battery of 50 reference materials for which a variety of animal and human toxicity data are available. Anyone with an *in vitro* alternative assay can test this battery and report the results to MEIC. They then analyze the data for correlation with some category of *in vivo* toxicity, with the view toward determining batteries of tests with the best predictive value for the various measures of human toxicity (acute, chronic, target organ, local irritancy, etc.).

A similar approach has been taken by the SDA, but it is focused specifically on ocular irritation alternatives. They conducted a preliminary study with a limited number of test materials to choose the most promising assay among 14 different alternative tests (94). In a second phase, the number of different assays was reduced whereas the number of compounds tested in each was increased, thus testing the predictive value and versatility of the individual tests (23).

The CTFA has focused on determining the strengths and weaknesses of a number of alternatives for different classes of chemicals (95,96). Participants test 10 different agents from a single class (Phase I—ethanol-based materials; Phase II—oil/water emulsions; etc.), in assays with which they have experience. The result is that data have been generated in approximately 25 potential alternative tests for the compound battery. This approach recognizes that some assays will provide better prediction for one type of material than for others, and it aims to determine the most appropriate method(s) for different testing needs.

The key expectation of any validation study is that the strengths and weaknesses of proposed alternative assays will be identified, so that a user of the assay(s) can have confidence in the interpretation and reliability of the data generated. This comfort level can only be achieved by performing some parallel testing in one's own laboratory with compounds similar to those likely to be evaluated as unknowns, even if some other group has "validated" a test previously. It seems apparent that one test or group of tests will not suffice for all purposes, and thus a specific battery should not be prescribed by regulatory agencies (as noted in ref. 104). Because of the amount of work needed to test various assays (and combinations) with a diversity of chemical classes, the validation process will be a long, somewhat tedious project, but will be necessary before *in vitro* alternatives can be used responsibly.

CONCLUSIONS

We have tried to briefly outline the range of approaches being used to reduce or eliminate animal testing for ocular irritation. A number of alternative assays have been reported in the literature, each with its own uses and limitations. But given the complexity of the *in vivo* response being modeled, it is not reasonable to depend upon a single test, measuring a single end point, to be predictive of *in vivo* ocular irritation potential in all cases. The broad approach of using a tiered testing system, gathering as much data as practical before making predictions, is likely to be the most fruitful in the long term.

One such tiered approach might consist of first evaluating any data available on the test material or on structurally related compounds (dermal or ocular irritation, acute or chronic toxicity, etc.). Next, physical/chemical data could be evaluated. These preliminary steps should provide a general idea of the properties of the chemical, and may be sufficient to allow a prediction of irritation potential. Should the data be insufficient, one could then select one or more *in vitro* assays to perform.

The battery of *in vitro* tests that could be used should be as flexible as possible to allow evaluation of a broad range of materials (e.g., different chemical classes, different physical forms, etc.). And the individual components of the battery need to be fully evaluated such that both their weaknesses and strengths are known. In this way one would know when to use a particular method and when it might not be applicable. Also, knowing both strengths and weaknesses allows one to better determine complementarity among assays and thus determine what would comprise the best battery of methods. This type of information will arise from "evaluation" studies carried out with multiple chemical classes, in multiple laboratories.

Only if these previous steps were inadequate to make a decision with confidence would an *in vivo* test be performed. And even if an *in vivo* test becomes necessary, given the information that would already have been obtained in the first steps of the tier, it might be possible to use a modified Draize test (e.g., single animal, low volume, use of anesthetics, etc.) and thereby further limit the use of animals.

Finally, if *in vitro* models are to be as fully effective as possible, the underlying mechanisms of ocular irritation need to be better defined. Many of the *in vitro* assays proposed as alternatives to *in vivo* testing are based on correlations rather than mechanisms of irritation (i.e., the *in vitro* end point correlates with an *in vivo* response), but the reason for the agreement is unclear and may be fortuitous for the compounds evaluated. The ideal assay would monitor biochemical or biological events specifically evoked in the whole animal by irritants. If events which are actually causal to irritation are measured, the probability of false results would decrease. Until we fully understand the mechanisms of the irritant response seen in whole eye, a battery of tests aimed at evaluating as many biological events as possible is likely to be the best approach.

REFERENCES

1. Draize JH, Woodard G, Calvery HO. Methods for the study of irritation and toxicity of substances applied topically to the skin and mucous membranes. *J Pharmacol Exp Ther* 1944;82:377–390.
2. Weil CS, Scala RA. Study of intra- and interlaboratory variability in the results of rabbit eye and skin irritation tests. *Toxicol Appl Pharmacol* 1971;19:276–360.
3. Chan P-K, Hayes AW. Assessment of chemically induced ocular toxicity: a survey of methods. In: Hayes AW, ed. *Toxicology of the eye, ear, and other special senses*. New York: Raven Press, 1985;103–143.
4. Kay J, Calandra J. Interpretation of eye irritation tests. *J Soc Cosmetic Chem* 1962;13:281–289.
5. Guillot JP, Gonnet JF, Clement C, Caillard L, Truhaut R. Evaluation of the ocular-irritation potential of 56 compounds. *Food Chem Toxicol* 1982;20:573–582.
6. Carpenter CP, Smyth HF. Series of papers in *J Indust Hyg (Arch Indust Hyg)* 1944–1974.
7. Green WR, et al. *A systematic comparison of chemically induced eye injury in the albino rabbit and rhesus monkey*. New York: The Soap and Detergent Association, 1978.
8. FHSA. Code of federal regulations, Title 16: subchapter C—Federal Hazardous Substances Act, Part 1500.42, revised January 1, 1981 (test for eye irritants).
9. Conquet P, Durand G, Lallier J, Plazonnet B. Evaluation of ocular irritation in the rabbit: objective versus subjective assessment. *Toxicol Appl Pharmacol* 1977;39:129–139.
10. Morgan RL, Sorenson SS, Castles TR. Prediction of ocular irritation by corneal pachymetry. *Food Chem Toxicol* 1987;25:609–613.
11. Kennah HE, Hignet S, Laux PE, Dorko JD, Barrow CS. An objective procedure for quantitating eye irritation based upon changes of corneal thickness. *Fundam Appl Toxicol* 1989;12:258–268.
12. ECETOC. *Eye irritation testing*. Monograph no. 11, Brussels, 1988;1–65.
13. Griffith JF, Nixon GA, Bruce RD, Reer PJ, Bannan EA. Dose–response studies with chemical irritants in the albino rabbit eye as a basis for selecting optimum testing conditions for predicting hazard to the human eye. *Toxicol Appl Pharmacol* 1980;55:501–513.
14. Igarashi H. The opacification of the bovine isolated cornea by surfactants and other chemicals—a process of protein denaturation? *ATLA* 1987;15:8–19.
15. Duke-Elder S, Leigh AG. *Diseases of the outer eye*, vol VIII, part 2. London: Henry Kimpton, 1965.

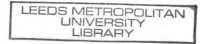

16. Basu PK. Toxic effects of drugs on the corneal epithelium: a review. *J Toxicol—Cutan Ocular Toxicol* 1983;2:205–227.
17. Burstein NL, Klyce SD. Electrophysiologic and morphologic effects of ophthalmic preparations on rabbit cornea epithelium. *Invest Ophthalmol Vis Sci* 1977;16(10):899–911.
18. Parish WE. Ability of *in vitro* (corneal injury, eye organ, and chorioallantoic membrane) tests to represent histopathological features of acute eye inflammation. *Food Chem Toxicol* 1985;23:215–227.
19. Elgebaly SA, Gillies C, Forouhar F, Hahem M, Baddour M, O'Rourke J, Kreutzer DL. An *in vitro* model of leukocyte mediated injury to the corneal epithelium. *Curr Eye Res* 1985;4:31–41.
20. Frazier JM, Gad SC, Goldberg AM, McCulley JP. A critical evaluation of alternatives to acute ocular irritation testing. In: Goldberg AM, ed. *Alternative methods in toxicology*, vol 4. New York: Mary Ann Liebert, 1987.
21. *HDI Toxicology Newsletter*, no. 6. Rochester, NY: Health Designs Inc., 1987.
22. Walz D. Irritant action due to physico-chemical parameters of test solutions. *Food Chem Toxicol* 1985;23:299–302.
23. Booman KA, De Prospo J, Demetrulias J, Driedger A, Griffith JF, Grochoski G, Kong B, McCormick WC, North-Root H, Rozen MG, Sedlak RI. The SDA alternatives program: comparison of *in vitro* data with Draize test data. *J Toxicol—Cutan Ocular Toxicol* 1989;8:35–49.
24. Halle W, Baeger I, Ekwall B, Spielmann H. Correlation between *in vitro* cytotoxicity and octanol/water partition coefficient of 29 substances from the MEIC programme. *ATLA* 1991;19:338–343.
25. Babich H, Borenfreund E. Structure–activity relationship (SAR) models established *in vitro* with the neutral red cytotoxicity assay. *Toxicol In Vitro* 1987;1:3–9.
26. Gad SC, Walsh RD, Dunn BJ. Correlation of ocular and dermal irritancy of industrial chemicals. *J Toxicol—Cutan Ocular Toxicol* 1986;5:195–213.
27. Gilman MR, Jackson EM, Cerven DR, Moreno MT. Relationship between primary dermal irritation index and ocular irritation. *J Toxicol—Cutan Ocular Toxicol* 1983;2:107–117.
28. Guillot JP, Gonnet JF, Clement C, Caillard L, Truhaut R. Evaluation of the cutaneous-irritation potential of 56 compounds. *Food Chem Toxicol* 1982;20:563–572.
29. Williams SJ. Prediction of ocular irritancy potential from dermal irritation test results. *Food Chem Toxicol* 1984;22:157–161.
30. Williams SJ. Changing concepts of ocular irritation evaluation: pitfalls and progress. *Food Chem Toxicol* 1985;23:189–193.
31. Price JB, Andrews IJ. The *in vitro* assessment eye irritancy using isolated eyes. *Food Chem Toxicol* 1985;23:313–315.
32. Muir CK. A simple method to assess surfactant-induced bovine corneal opacity *in vitro*: preliminary findings. *Toxicol Lett* 1984;22:199–203.
33. Muir CK. Opacity of bovine cornea *in vitro* induced by surfactants and industrial chemicals compared with ocular irritancy *in vivo*. *Toxicol Lett* 1985;24:157–162.
34. Igarashi H, Katsuta Y, Nakazato Y, Kawasaki T. The use of an opacitometer to compare the *in vitro* cornea opacifying effects of timolol with and without benzalkonium chloride. *ATLA* 1991;19:263–270.
35. Gautheron P, Dukic M, Aliz D, Sina JF. The bovine corneal opacity and permeability test: an *in vitro* assay of ocular irritancy. *Fundam Appl Toxicol* 1992;18:442–449.
36. Tchao R. Trans-epithelial permeability of fluorescein *in vitro* as an assay to determine eye irritants. In: Goldberg AM, ed. *Alternative methods in toxicology*, vol 6. New York: Mary Ann Leibert, 1988;271–283.
37. Kelly C. EYTEX: an *in-vitro* method of predicting ocular safety. *Pharmacopeial Forum* 1989; Jan–Feb:4815–4824.
38. Gordon VC, Kelly CP. An *in vitro* method for determining ocular irritation. *Cosmet Toiletries* 1989;104:69–73.
39. Lawrence-Beckett EM, James JT. Initial experience with the Eyetex *in vitro* irritation test system. *Toxicologist* 1991;10:259.
40. Soto RJ, Servi MJ, Gordon VC. Evaluation of an alternative method for ocular irritation. In: Goldberg AM, ed. *Alternative methods in toxicology*, vol 7. New York: Mary Ann Liebert, 1989; 289–296.
41. Sanders C, Swedlund TD, Stephens TJ, Silber PM. Evaluation of six *in vitro* toxicity assays: comparison with *in vivo* ocular and dermal irritation potential of prototype cosmetic formulations. *Toxicologist* 1991;11:282.

42. Bruner LH, Kain DJ, Roberts DA, Parker RD. Evaluation of seven *in vitro* alternatives for ocular safety testing. *Fundam Appl Toxicol* 1991;17:136–149.
43. Thomson MA, Dickens MS, Gordon VC. Evaluation of the Eytex biochemical assay for use in determining cosmetic product ocular irritancy. CAAT Symposium Poster, April 4–5, 1989.
44. Flint OP. *In vitro* alternatives to ocular toxicity testing: report of a meeting organized by the Industrial *In Vitro* Toxicology Group. *In Vitro Toxicol* 1990;3:281–291.
45. Borenfreund E, Borrero O. *In vitro* cytotoxicity assays: potential alternatives to the Draize ocular irritancy test. *Cell Biol Toxicol* 1984;1:33–39.
46. Shopsis C, Borenfreund E, Walberg J, Stark DM. *In vitro* cytotoxicity assays as potential alternatives to the Draize ocular irritancy test. In: Goldberg AM, ed. *Alternative methods in toxicology*, vol 2. New York: Mary Ann Liebert, 1984;103–114.
47. Shopsis C, Sathe S. Uridine uptake inhibition as a cytotoxicity test: correlations with the Draize test. *Toxicology* 1984;29:195–206.
48. North-Root H, Yackovich F, Demetrulias J, Gacula M, Heinze JE. Evaluation of an *in vitro* cell toxicity test using rabbit corneal cells to predict the eye irritation potential of surfactants. *Toxicol Lett* 1982;14:207–212.
49. Kemp RB, Meredith RWJ, Gamble S, Frost M. A rapid cell culture technique for assessing the toxicity of detergent-based products *in vitro* as a possible screen for eye irritancy *in vivo*. *Cytobios* 1983;36:153–159.
50. Tachon P, Cotovio J, Dossou KG, Prunieras M. Assessment of surfactant cytotoxicity: comparison with the Draize eye test. *Int J Cosmet Sci* 1989;11:233–243.
51. Scaife MC. An *in vitro* cytotoxicity test to predict the ocular irritation potential of detergents and detergent products. *Food Chem Toxicol* 1985;23:253–258.
52. Gay R, Jadlos S, Marenus K. The living dermal equivalent (LDE) as an assay for ocular irritation potential. Presented at the 7th Annual CAAT Symposium, 1989.
53. Harnett C, Class T, Swiderek M, Gay R. Induction of prostaglandin E_2 in TESTSKIN as an indicator of irritation potential. Presented at the 7th Annual CAAT Symposium, 1989.
54. Bruner LH, Miller KR, Owick JC, Parce JW, Muir VC. Testing ocular irritancy *in vitro* with the silicon microphysiometer. *Toxicol In Vitro* 1991;5:277–284.
55. Borenfreund E, Puerner JA. A simple quantitative procedure using monolayer cultures for cytotoxicity assays. *J Tissue Culture Methods* 1984;9:7–9.
56. Borenfreund E, Puerner JA. Short-term quantitative *in vitro* cytotoxicity assay involving an S-9 activating system. *Cancer Lett* 1987;34:243–248.
57. Triglia D, Wegener PT, Harbell J, Wallace K, Matheson D, Shopsis C. Interlaboratory validation study of the keratinocyte neutral red bioassay from Clonetics Corporation. In: Goldberg AM, ed. *Alternative methods in toxicology*, vol 7. New York: Mary Ann Liebert, 1989;357–365.
58. Bracher M, Faller C, Spengler J, Reinhardt CA. Comparison of *in vitro* cell toxicity with *in vivo* eye irritation. *Mol Toxicol* 1987;1:561–570.
59. Shopsis C. Validation study: ocular irritancy prediction with the total cell protein, uridine uptake, and neutral red assays applied to human epidermal keratinocytes and mouse 3T3 cells. In: Goldberg AM, ed. *Alternative methods in toxicology*, vol 7. New York: Mary Ann Liebert, 1989;273–287.
60. Thomson MA, Hearn LA, Smith KT, Teal JJ, Dickens MS. Evaluation of the neutral red cytotoxicity assay as a predictive test for the ocular irritancy potential of cosmetic products. In: Goldberg AM, ed. *Alternative methods in toxicology*, vol 7. New York: Mary Ann Liebert, 1989;297–305.
61. Sina JF, Ward GJ, Laszek MA, Gautheron PD. Assessment of cytotoxicity assays as predictors of ocular irritation of pharmaceuticals. *Fundam Appl Toxicol* 1992;18:515–521.
62. Brooks D, Maurice D. A simple fluorometer for use with a permeability screen. In: Goldberg AM, ed. *Alternative methods in toxicology*, vol 5. New York: Mary Ann Liebert, 1987;173–177.
63. Flower C. Some problems in validating cytotoxicity as a correlate of ocular irritancy. In: Goldberg AM, ed. *Alternative methods in toxicology*, vol 5. New York: Mary Ann Liebert, 1987;269–274.
64. Kennah HE, Albulescu D, Hignet S, Barrow CS. A critical evaluation of predicting ocular irritancy potential from an *in vitro* cytotoxicity assay. *Fundam Appl Toxicol* 1989;12:281–290.
65. Elgebaly SA, Forouhar F, Gillies C, Williams S, O'Rourke J, Kreutzer DL. Leukocyte-mediated injury to corneal endothelial cells: a model of tissue injury. *Am J Pathol* 1984;116:407–416.
66. Bazan HEP, Birkle DL, Beuerman RW, Bazan NG. Inflammation-induced stimulation of the synthesis of prostaglandins and lipoxygenase-reaction products in rabbit cornea. *Curr Eye Res* 1985;4:175–179.

67. Srinivasan BD, Kulkarni PS. The role of arachidonic acid metabolites in the mediation of the polymorphonuclear leukocyte response following corneal injury. *Invest Ophthalmol Vis Sci* 1980; 19:1087–1093.
68. Bhattacherjee P, Hammond B, Salmon JA, Stepney R, Eakins KE. Chemotactic response to some arachidonic acid lipoxygenase products in the rabbit eye. *Eur J Pharmacol* 1981;73:21–28.
69. Elgebaly SA, Forouhar F, Kreutzer DL. *In vitro* detection of cornea-derived leukocytic chemotactic factors as indicators of corneal inflammation. In: Goldberg AM, ed. *Alternative methods in toxicology*, vol 5. New York: Mary Ann Liebert, 1987;257–268.
70. Metwally F, Cohen A, Rossomando EF, Elgebaly SA. High performance liquid chromatography analysis of the novel neutrophil chemoattractants "Nourin" released from alkali-burned corneas. In: Goldberg AM, ed. *Alternative methods in toxicology*, vol 6. New York: Mary Ann Liebert, 1988; 207–213.
71. Benassi CA, Angi MR, Salvalaio L, Bettero A. Ocular irritancy evaluated *in vivo* by conjunctival lavage technique and *in vitro* by bovine eye cup model. In: Goldberg AM, ed. *Alternative methods in toxicology*, vol 5. New York: Mary Ann Liebert, 1987;235–242.
72. Dubin NH. Prostaglandin production as an index of *in vitro* cytotoxicity. In: Goldberg AM, ed. *Alternative methods in toxicology*, vol 3. New York: Mary Ann Liebert, 1985;45–51.
73. Dubin NH, Ghodgaonkar RB, Parmley TH. Differential response of *in vitro* vaginal tissue to various test agents. In: Goldberg AM, ed. *Alternative methods in toxicology*, vol 6. New York: Mary Ann Liebert, 1988;153–158.
74. Cohen C, Dossou G, Rougier A, Roguet R. Measurement of inflammatory mediators produced by human keratinocytes *in vitro*: a predictive assessment of cutaneous irritation. *Toxicol In Vitro* 1991;5:407–410.
75. Osborne R, Perkins MA. *In vitro* skin irritation testing with human skin cell cultures. *Toxicol In Vitro* 1991;5:563–567.
76. Powell WS. Reversed-phase high-pressure liquid chromatography of arachidonic acid metabolites formed by cyclooxygenase and lipoxygenases. *Anal Biochem* 1985;148:59–69.
77. Peters SP, Schulman ES, Liu MC, Hayes EC, Lichtenstein LM. Separation of major prostaglandins, leukotrienes, and monoHETEs by high performance liquid chromatography. *J Immunol Methods* 1983;64:335–343.
78. Leighton J, Nassauer J, Tchao R, Verdone J. Development of a procedure using the chick egg as an alternative to the Draize rabbit test. In: Goldberg AM, ed. *Alternative methods in toxicology*, vol 1. New York: Mary Ann Liebert, 1983;165–177.
79. Leighton J, Nassauer J, Tchao R. The chick embryo in toxicology: an alternative to the rabbit eye. *Food Chem Toxicol* 1985;23:293–298.
80. Kong BM, Viau CJ, Rizvi PY, De Salva SJ. The development and evaluation of the chorioallantoic membrane (CAM) assay. In: Goldberg AM, ed. *Alternative methods in toxicology*, vol 5. New York: Mary Ann Liebert, 1987;59–73.
81. Bagley DM, Rizvi PY, Kong BM, De Salva SJ. An improved CAM assay for predicting ocular irritation potential. In: Goldberg AM, ed. *Alternative methods in toxicology*, vol 6. New York: Mary Ann Liebert, 1988;131–138.
82. Bagley DM, Kong BM, De Salva SJ. Assessing the eye irritation potential of surfactant-based materials using the chorioallantoic membrane vascular assay (CAMVA). In: Goldberg AM, ed. *Alternative methods in toxicology*, vol 7. New York: Mary Ann Liebert, 1989;265–272.
83. Weterings PJJM, Van Erp YHM. Validation of the Becam assay—an eye irritancy screening test. In: Goldberg AM, ed. *Alternative methods in toxicology*, vol 5. New York: Mary Ann Liebert, 1987;515–521.
84. Luepke NP. Hen's egg chorioallantoic membrane test for irritation potential. *Food Chem Toxicol* 1985;23:287–291.
85. Luepke NP. HET-chorionallantois test: an alternative to the Draize rabbit eye test. In: Goldberg AM, ed. *Alternative methods in toxicology*, vol 3. New York: Mary Ann Liebert, 1985;592–605.
86. Lawrence RS. The chorioallantoic membrane in irritancy testing. In: Atterwill CK, Steele CE, eds. *In vitro methods in toxicology*. New York: Cambridge University Press, 1987;263–278.
87. Lawrence RS, Groom MH, Ackroyd DM, Parish WE. The chorioallantoic membrane in irritation testing. *Food Chem Toxicol* 1986;24:497–502.
88. Price JB, Barry MP, Andrews IJ. The use of the chick chorioallantoic membrane to predict eye irritants. *Food Chem Toxicol* 1986;24:503–505.

89. Fielder RJ, Gaunt IF, Rhodes C, Sullivan FM, Swanston DW. A hierarchial approach to the assessment of dermal and ocular irritancy: a report by the British Toxicology Society working party on irritancy. *Hum Toxicol* 1987;6:269–278.
90. Williams PD, Sina JF, Smolarek TA. The application of *in vitro* techniques in drug safety assessment. In: Gad SC, ed. *Safety assessment for pharmaceuticals*. New York: Van Nostrand Reinhold, 1992.
91. Yam J, Winters R. Development of alternatives in a consumer product company. In: Goldberg AM, ed. *Alternative methods in toxicology*, vol 7. New York: Mary Ann Liebert, 1989;23–31.
92. Bulich AA, Tung KK, Scheibner G. The luminescent bacteria toxicity test: its potential as an *in vitro* alternative. *J Biolumin Chemilumin* 1990;5:71–77.
93. Bell E, Parenteau N, Gay R, Nolte C, Kemp P, Bilbo P, Ekstein B, Johnson E. The living skin equivalent: its manufacture, its organotypic properties and its responses to irritants. *Toxicol In Vitro* 1991;5:591–596.
94. Booman KA, Cascieri TM, Demetrulias J, Driedger A, Griffith JF, Grochoski GT, Kong B, McCormick WC, North-Root H, Rozen MG, Sedlak RI. *In vitro* methods for estimating eye irritancy of cleaning products phase I: preliminary assessment. *J Toxicol—Cutan Ocular Toxicol* 1988;7:173–185.
95. Gettings SD, McEwen GN. Development of potential alternatives to the Draize eye test: the CTFA evaluation of alternatives program. *ATLA* 1990;17:317–324.
96. Gettings SD, Di Pasquale LC, Bagley DM, Chudkowski M, Demetrulias JL, Feder PI, Hintze KL, Marenus KD, Pape W, Roddy M, Schnetzinger R, Silber P, Teal JJ, Weise SL. The CTFA evaluation of alternatives program: an evaluation of *in vitro* alternatives to the Draize primary eye irritation test (Phase I) hydro-alcoholic formulations; a preliminary communication. *In Vitro Toxicol* 1990;3:293–302.
97. Frazier JM. *Scientific criteria for validation of in vitro toxicity tests*. OECD monograph, no. 36, 1990.
98. Balls M, Blaauboer B, Brusick D, Frazier J, Lamb D, Pemberton M, Reinhardt C, Roberfroid M, Rosenkranz H, Schmid B, Spielmann H, Stammati A, Walum E. Report and recommendations of the CAAT/ERGATT workshop on the validation of toxicity test procedures. *ATLA* 1990;18:313–337.
99. Kalweit S, Gerner I, Spielmann H. Validation project of alternatives for the Draize eye test. *Mol Toxicol* 1987;1:597–603.
100. Kalweit S, Besoke R, Gerner I, Spielmann H. A national validation project of alternative methods to the Draize rabbit eye test. *Toxicol In Vitro* 1990;4:702–706.
101. Spielmann H, Gerner I, Kalweit S, Moog R, Wirnsberger T, Krauser K, Kreiling R, Kreuzer H, Lupke N-P, Miltenburger HG, Muller N, Murmann P, Pape W, Siegemund B, Spengler J, Steiling W, Wiebel FJ. Interlaboratory assessment of alternatives to the Draize eye irritation test in Germany. *Toxicol In Vitro* 1991;5:539–542.
102. Blein O, Adolphe M, Lakhdar B, Cambar J, Gubanski G, Castelli D, Contie C, Huber F, Latrille F, Masson P, Clouzeau J, Le Bigot JF, De Silva O, Dossou KG. Correlation and validation of alternative methods to the Draize eye irritation test (OPAL project). *Toxicol In Vitro* 1991;5:555–557.
103. Bondesson I, Ekwall B, Hellberg S, Romert L, Stenberg K, Walum E. MEIC—a new international multicenter project to evaluate the relevance to human toxicity of *in vitro* cytotoxicity tests. *Cell Biol Toxicol* 1989;5:31–34.
104. Balls M, Atkinson KA, Gordon VC. Complementation in the development, validation, and use of non-animal test batteries, with particular reference to ocular irritancy. *ATLA* 1991;19:429–431.

In Vitro Toxicology,
edited by Shayne Cox Gad.
Raven Press, Ltd., New York, © 1994.

4

In Vitro Methods to Predict Dermal Toxicity

V. C. Gordon,* Jeff Harvell,† Meg Bason,† and Howard Maibach†

*In Vitro International, Irvine, California 92714; and †Department of Dermatology,
University of California at San Francisco, San Francisco, California 94143*

Skin absorption occurs through a process of binding, partitioning, and diffusion of test materials on and into the skin. Penetration has been assessed *in vivo* by measuring at different times the amount of test substances at different layers of the skin. Blood levels of the test sample have been measured in this test.

A complicated series of chemical and physiological responses result in primary skin irritation. When skin is exposed to toxic substances, the Draize rabbit skin test, first outlined by John Draize in 1944, remains an important source of safety information for government and industry (1). In this test, the dermal irritation caused by a substance is investigated by observing changes ranging from erythema and edema to ulceration produced in rabbit skin when irritants are applied. These skin reactions are produced by diverse physiologic mechanisms, although they are easily observed visually and by palpitation.

In vivo laboratory methods for sensitization have been performed on 20–40 albino guinea pigs. The methods for performing the test have varied widely, preventing comparative evaluation of the test. Observations do not provide adequate differentiation between weak sensitization and irritation. As a result of high concentrations used in guinea pigs, many materials have been overestimated. Human volunteers are also used for repeat patch testing.

The applicability of irritation or sensitization evaluation based on the visual assessment of reactions in animals has been a source of controversy for many years (2,3). Levels of skin damage are judged by observation, a procedure that has long been noted as highly subjective and unreliable, leading to problems of interlaboratory variability and calling the accuracy of the data into question (3). Also, the differing skin reactions exhibited by varying species has cast doubt on the applicability of the results derived from animal studies as they pertain to human irritation (2). Furthermore, the fact that the guinea pig and rabbit *in vivo* system yields little information about the physiologic mechanisms underlying skin irritation has contributed to the search for objective *in vitro* investigational methods. Recent concerns about the humane treatment of animals have galvanized these efforts to develop improved methods of *in vitro* toxicology evaluation.

Thus, in response to scientific and sociological issues, research on *in vitro* dermal toxicology methods has recently been very active. Many investigators are developing *in vitro* irritation systems that elicit more specific information about actual mechanisms involved in the complicated cascade of events causing irritation or sensitization.

In vitro methods are based on years of laboratory and clinical research determining the basic features of skin penetration, irritation, and sensitization. The targets are so complex that the effect of toxic substances on the structure of the skin is poorly understood.

Studies have elucidated considerable information about the mechanisms of damage and repair that occur in skin. Typical events identified in the dermal irritation process include protein denaturation, epidermal cells lysis, cytotoxicity, enzyme leakage, and production of epidermal antigens and cytokines (4–7). The means of evaluating the evidence of damage include examining morphology, signs of the inflammatory reaction initiation, cellular toxicity, and electrical properties (8). Also, synthetic models of epithelium have been designed to mimic irritant damage characteristics (9). Some investigators have combined two or more of these modalities and compared them to assess the differences.

Helman et al. (10) compared the morphologic responses of *in vitro* and *in vivo* skin exposed to chemicals with light microscopy. They found that the absence of an intact vascular system in *in vitro* skin specimens did not interfere significantly with the ability to detect graded microscopic epidermal lesions and concluded that the morphologic response of skin maintained in organ culture is an accurate indicator of skin toxicity. In addition to the altered histology seen with light microscopy, electron-microscopic analysis of irritant-damaged skin reveals characteristic changes, including spongiosis of epidermis, disappearance of tonofilament–desmosome complexes, and dissolution of the horny cells (11,12).

Enzyme leakage may provide a means for detecting sublethal cell injury which might not be observed histologically. Skin in organ culture has been analyzed to determine quantifiable parameters to assess injury such as cellular enzyme leakage, glucose metabolism, DNA synthesis, water loss, and changes in electrolyte concentration (10). Rat skin *in vivo* exposed to toxicants causes release of acid phosphatase, lactate dehydrogenase, and N-acetylglucosaminidase, which is associated histologically with epidermal edema and an increase in dermal leukocytes (8).

Irritation has been evaluated by analyzing epidermal edema with other techniques. Sodium lauryl sulfate produced swelling in *in vitro* skin discs prepared from excised human skin and dermal calf collagen (13,14). In an *in vitro* system without skin, tritiated water uptake (i.e., swelling) of a collagen film was proportional to the degree of *in vivo* irritation in a series of surfactants (14).

CURRENT *IN VITRO* METHODS

Proposed *in vitro* methods are based on cell cytotoxicity, inflammatory or immune system response, alterations of cellular, bacterial or fungal physiology, cell

TABLE 1. *Current* in vitro *methods*

1. Physicochemical analysis
2. Target macromolecular and biochemical responses
3. Cell culture techniques
4. Microorganism studies
5. Human tissue equivalents
6. Isolated tissue techniques
7. Computer modeling (structure–activity relationships)
8. Human volunteer studies

morphology, biochemical end points, macromolecular targets, and structure activity analysis (15–20). With a decrease in animal testing, additional *in vitro* testing has been more often utilized in a comprehensive toxicology program. These methods can be broadly placed in eight categories (see Table 1). Human volunteer studies are *in vivo* studies but are often used to replace *in vivo* animal test methods.

DESCRIPTION OF CURRENT *IN VITRO* METHODS

Physicochemical Test Methods

Analysis of the physicochemical properties of test substances, including the pH, absorption spectra, partition coefficients, and other parameters, often indicates potential dermal toxicity. According to OECD guidelines, substances with a pH of less than 2 or greater than 11 do not need to be tested for irritancy *in vivo* (21). The potential effects of acids and bases to produce irritancy has been well established.

Physicochemical analysis has evaluated the particular chemical properties of test substances which have been identified as key structural components contributing to penetration, irritation, or sensitization. Absence of absorption in the ultraviolet (UV) range also has been used to suggest lack of photoirritant potential (22). Physicochemical tests are rapid, cost-effective, easily standardized, and transferable to outside laboratories. For penetration, a partition coefficient of the test sample provides a useful guide. The size of a chemical is also indicative of potential penetration. Many of the physicochemical properties of surfactants have been found to be potential indicators of their action on skin (23).

Target Macromolecular and Biochemical Systems

Test methods which utilize the analysis of biochemical reactions or changes in organized macromolecules evaluate toxicity at a subcellular level. Because of their simplicity, they can be readily standardized and transferred to outside laboratories to provide yardstick measurements for varying degrees of dermal toxicity.

One *in vitro* irritation prediction method that utilizes nonbiological, nonliving substances can be described as a biomembrane-barrier–macromolecular-matrix system. This method is known as the SKINTEX system. The SKINTEX system makes use of a two-compartment physicochemical model incorporating a keratin/collagen membrane barrier and an ordered macromolecular matrix (24). The effect of irritants on this membrane is detected by changes in the intact barrier membrane through the use of an indicator dye attached to the membrane. The dye is released following membrane alteration or disruption, which can occur when the synthetic membrane barrier is exposed to an irritant. A specific amount of dye corresponding to the degree of irritation can be liberated and quantified spectrophotometrically. The second compartment within the system is a reagent macromolecular matrix that responds to toxic substances by producing turbidity. This second response provides an internal detection for materials which disrupt organized protein conformation after passing through the membrane barrier (24).

Test samples can be applied directly to the barrier membrane as liquids, solids, or emulsions and inserted into the liquid reagent. The results are directly compared to the Draize dermal irritation results.

More than 5300 test samples have been studied in the SKINTEX system, including petrochemicals, agrochemicals, household products, and cosmetics. The reproducibility with standard deviations of 5–8% is excellent. New protocols applicable to very low irritation test samples and alkaline products have increased the applicability of this method. SKINTEX validation studies resulting in an 80–89% correlation to the Draize scoring have been reported by Yves Rocher, S. C. Johnson & Son, and the Food and Drug Safety Center (25–27).

Thus far, most *in vitro* irritation methods, including SKINTEX, have relied heavily on the vast Draize rabbit skin database for validation. As previously discussed, the discrepancies in the information generated by the Draize system raise questions about the applicability of this information to irritation reactions in man.

A new SKINTEX protocol called the "human response assay" optimizes the model to predict human irritation. A collaborative study with Dr. Howard Maibach and co-workers at the University of California at San Francisco demonstrated good correlations to human response for pure chemicals with diverse mechanisms of dermal toxicity. Ongoing studies have evaluated pure chemicals, surfactants, vehicles, and fatty acids (28–30).

The SKINTEX test is a rapid, standardized approach with well-refined protocols and an extensive database. The results produced are contiguous with the historical *in vivo* database. However, the method cannot predict immune response, penetration, or recovery after the toxic response.

Cell Culture Techniques

In vitro cytoxicity tests that indicate basic cell toxicity by measuring parameters such as cell viability, proliferation, membrane damage, DNA synthesis, or metabolic effects have been used as indicators of dermal toxicity (31–34).

The most commonly used approaches are the Neutral Red assay (cell viability, membrane damage), the Lowry (labeled proline) Coomassie Blue and Kenacid Blue assays (cell proliferation, total cell protein), the MTT or tetrazolium assay (mitochondrial function), and the intracellular lactate dehydrogenase activity test (cell lysis).

In the Neutral Red (cell viability) and total protein (cell proliferation) assays, cells are treated with various concentrations of a test substance in Petri or multiwell dishes; after a period of exposure, the substance is washed out of the medium. (An analytical reagent is added in the case of protein measurements.) Neutral Red is a supra-vital dye which accumulates in the lysosomes of viable, uninjured cells, and it can be washed out of cells which have been damaged. In the protein test, Kenacid Blue is added and reacts with cellular protein. Controlled cells are dark blue; killed cells are lighter colored. The IC_{50} (the concentration which inhibits by 50%) is determined; the test can be rapidly performed with automation. However, materials must be solubilized into the aqueous cell media for analysis. For many test materials this will require large dilutions which eliminate properties of the materials which cause irritation (31).

The MTT test assays mitochondrial function by measuring reduction of the yellow MTT tetrazolium salt to a blue insoluble product. It has been compared with the Neutral Red technique for testing the cytotoxicity of 28 test substances, including drugs, pesticides, caffeine, and ascorbic acid. With the mouse BALB/c 3T3 fibroblast cell line, for any given cell density the two assays ranked the test substances with a correlation coefficient of 0.939, on the basis of IC_{50} concentrations. The two assays did differ in sensitivity for a few test agents, suggesting that a combination of the two might be most effective (32).

Some cytotoxicity tests are likely to underestimate the toxicity of chemicals which are metabolically activated in the body, but this problem can be overcome by the addition of liver enzymes, preferably from a human source to eliminate species differences.

Inhibition of mitogen-stimulated thymidine incorporation in human peripheral blood mononuclear cells has been reported as a method for screening for photosensitisers (33). Cells from at least three volunteers were used for testing each chemical.

Microorganism Studies

An important method using a fungi is Daniels' test for phototoxicity, which utilizes the yeast *Candida albicans* as the test organism. A 1988 study compared favorably the results of this test with the results of photo-patch testing in volunteers for samples from six furocoumarin-containing plants (34). Many test materials which produce an erythemic response in the photoirritant test are not analyzed as positive in this test. A new test method, SOLATEX-PI, has demonstrated capability to predict the potential for photoirritation of materials in this class as well as that of other well-known *in vivo* photoirritants (35). SOLATEX-PI utilizes the two-compartment physicochemical model of SKINTEX to predict the interactive effects of specific chemicals and UV radiation. SOLATEX-PI is being validated by FRAME and the BGA (Zebet) as an *in vitro* test to predict photoirritants.

Human Tissue Equivalents

Human skin equivalents have been developed by several laboratories. One equivalent, TESTSKIN, consists of human keratinocytes seeded onto a collagen base or collagen–glycosaminoglycan matrix containing human fibroblasts. In many respects, the epidermis which develops resembles epidermis *in vivo*. The tissue culture system survives for several weeks and may be useful in studying skin penetration. TESTSKIN is a commercially produced skin equivalent system marketed by Organogenesis, Inc. (Cambridge, Massachusetts); it is currently being assessed for use in skin penetration studies. Several companies launched studies of TESTSKIN during 1990 and 1991 (36).

Marrow-Tech, Inc. (Elmsford, New York), has also developed a human skin model. Marrow-Tech's skin equivalent consists of (a) a dermal layer of fibroblasts and naturally secreted collagen and (b) an epidermal layer of keratinocytes separated by a dermal–epidermal junction. Whereas TESTSKIN uses bovine collagen, Marrow-Tech's skin model consists solely of human tissue.

Both of these skin equivalent methods permit higher concentrations of test samples to be studied. However, dilutions are still necessary which alter the physical chemistry of the test sample which may be responsible for irritation. Many protocols and end points have been evaluated as predictive of eye or skin irritation (37).

Isolated Tissue Methods

Skin isolated from rats, rabbits, and humans has been monitored *in vitro* to predict penetration and irritation. The rat epidermal slice technique has been validated as a screen for corrosive substances. The electrical impedance changes as the integrity of the stratum corneum is altered. The use of this technique to predict irritancy is being investigated in the United Kingdom (38). Another method studies enzyme changes when a substance is applied to a slice whose lower surface is bathed in culture medium. Enzyme changes separate irritant and nonirritant chemicals (39).

Human cadaver skin has also been studied *in vitro*. Human skin shows a higher threshold of sensitivity than does rat skin. The excised or full-thickness slices are also studied in Fran 2 diffusion chambers to evaluate diffusion or absorption characteristics of test materials. Changes in the amount of a test material at different times and different depths are monitored and are very useful in predicting penetration rates for simple solutions and solvents.

These methods are difficult to implement in routine testing. Epidermal slices can be stored for 4 weeks, but the thicker slices deteriorate quickly. All tissues must be prescreened for damage prior to use.

Human Volunteer Studies

Human volunteer studies are widely used to assess skin irritation, penetration, and sensitization.

Many industries regularly conduct repeat insult patch tests on human volunteers to evaluate topical irritancy. Groups of human volunteers are patched with test substance. One to five concentrations can be tested simultaneously, which is a wide enough range to yield results relevant to the usage. Cumulative skin irritancy is measured by applying patch applications each day for 3 weeks (30). Skin irritation is usually assessed visually, but blood flow and skin temperature can be measured objectively by laser doppler flowmetry, ultrasound doppler, heat flow disc measurement, sensitive thermocouple devices, or noncontact infrared radiative techniques. In these tests, dose–response curves can be obtained. Skin thickness can be measured with calipers, as a measure of edema formation.

Human volunteers are also used in many industries in tests for allergic sensitization by cosmetic substances and formulations. The repeat insult patch test includes an induction phase (repeat applications during 3 weeks) and a 2-week rest period (incubation phase), followed by a challenge to see if sensitization has occurred. A pilot study of 20 human volunteers can be followed by more extensive testing (80–100 subjects). Positive results at more than the 10% level in the human volunteers would suggest a major problem with the formulation. User tests with the sensitized individuals and nonreactive matched control subjects can oftentimes determine the importance of these results to end use. Such a procedure may determine whether the sensitivity is significant under normal conditions of product use. Broader tests can be carried out with 250–500 subjects (30).

CONCLUSIONS

Whole-animal tests represent true physiological and metabolic relationships of macromolecules, cells, tissues, and organs which can evaluate the reversibility of toxic effects. However, these tests are costly, time-consuming, insensitive, and difficult to standardize and are sometimes poorly predictive of human *in vivo* response.

New *in vitro* test methods target the behavior of macromolecules, cells, tissues, and organs in well-defined methods which control experimental conditions and standardize experimentation. These tests provide more reproducible, rapid, and cost-effective results. In addition, more information at a basic mechanistic level can be obtained from these tests.

The challenge of the 1990s will be to understand the capabilities and limitations of these methods. Combining information on new molecules obtained from structure–activity relationships with results on macromolecular alterations in SKINTEX that occur for undiluted molecules may provide more information on dermal toxic effects of particular chemical classes. Combining test methods can provide a greater understanding of the mechanisms of toxic molecules. Test batteries evaluating cell cytotoxic responses at high dilutions and changes in macromolecules at low dilutions will be more informative than visual scoring of complex events *in vivo*.

SUMMARY

A wide range of *in vitro* methods based on diverse end points have been developed to provide information on the complicated series of chemical and physiological responses of the skin to toxic substances. This series of responses concentrates on dermal toxicity, which has been studied *in vivo* using the Draize rabbit skin irritation test, the guinea-pig sensitization test, and the skin penetration test.

The study of dermal toxicity has provided information on the absorption of materials into the skin, the production of erythema or edema on contact, and the recognition of test materials by the immune system.

REFERENCES

1. Draize JH, Woodard G, Calvery HO. Methods for the study of irritation and toxicity of substances applied topically to the skin and mucous membranes. *J Pharmacol Exp Ther* 1944;82:377–389.
2. Patrick E, Maibach HI. Comparison of the time course, dose response and mediators of chemically induced skin irritation in three species. In: Frosch PJ, et al., eds. *Current topics in contact dermatitis.* New York: Springer-Verlag, 1989;399–403.
3. Kastner W. Irritancy potential of cosmetic ingredients. *J Soc Cosmet Chem* 1977;28:741–754.
4. Nago S, Stroud JD, Hamada T, et al. The effect of sodium hydroxide and hydrochloric acid on human epidermis: an EM study. *Acta Derm Venereol (Stockh)* 1972;52:11–23.
5. Kanerva L, Lauharanta J. Variable effects of irritants (methylmethacrylate, terphenyls, dithranol and methylglyoxal-bisguanylhadrazone) on the fine structure of the epidermis. *Arch Toxicol* 1986; 9:455.
6. Gibson WT, Teall MR. Interactions of C12 surfactants with the skin: changes in enzymes and visible and histological features of rat skin treated with sodium laurel sulfate. *Fundam Chem Toxicol* 1983;21(5):587–593.
7. SOT Position paper. Comments on the LD 50 and acute eye and skin irritation tests. *Fundam Appl Toxicol* 1989;13:621–623.
8. Oliver GJA, Pemberton MA, Rhodes C, et al. An *in vitro* model for identifying skin-corrosive chemicals. 1. Initial validation. *Toxicol In Vitro* 1988;2:7–17.
9. Bell E, Gay R, Swiderek M, et al. Use of fabricated living tissue and organ equivalents as defined higher order systems for the study of pharmacologic responses to test substances. Presented at the NATO Advanced Research Workshop. Pharmaceutical Application of Cell and Tissue Culture to Drug Transport, Bandol, France, September 4–9, 1989.
10. Helman RG, Hall JW, Kao JV. Acute dermal toxicity: *in vivo* and *in vitro* comparisons in mice. *Fundam Appl Toxicol* 1986;7:94–100.
11. Geller W, Kobel, W, Seifert G. Overview of animal test methods for skin irritation. *Fundam Chem Toxicol* 1985;23(2):165–168.
12. Bloom E, Maibach HI, Tammi R. *In vitro* models for cutaneous effects of glucocorticoids using human skin organ and cell culture. In: Maibach HI, Lowe NJ, eds. *Models dermatology*, vol 4. New York: Karger, 1989;12–19.
13. Blake-Haskins JC, Scala D, Rhein LD, et al. Predicting surfactant irritation from the swelling response of a collagen film. *J Soc Cosmet Chem* 1986;37:199–210.
14. Choman BR. Determination of the response of skin to chemical agents by an *in vitro* procedure. *J Invest Dermatol* 1963;44:177–182.
15. Borenfreund E, Peurner JA. Toxicity determined *in vitro* by morphological alterations and Neutral Red absorption. *Toxicol Lett* 1985;24:119–124.
16. Borenfreund E, Puerner JA. A simple quantitative procedure using monolayer cultures for cytotoxicity assays. *J Tissue Culture Methods* 1984;9:7–9.
17. Bulich AA, Greene MW, Isenberg DL. Reliability of bacterial compounds and complex effluents. In: Branson DR, Dickson KL, eds. *Aquatic Toxicology and hazard assessment.* Philadelphia: American Society for Testing and Materials (ASTM 737), 1981;338–347.

18. Luepke NP, Kemper FH. The HET–CAM test: an alternative to the Draize eye test. *Fundam Chem Toxicol* 1986;24:495–496.
19. Parce JW, Owicki JC, Kercso KM, et al. Detection of cell-affecting agents with silicon biosensor. *Science* 1989;246:243–247.
20. Silverman J. Preliminary findings on the use of protozoa (*Tetrahymena thermophila*) as models for ocular irritation testing rabbits. *Lab Anim Sci* 1983;33:56–58.
21. OECD. *Guidelines for testing chemicals*, Section 404, "Acute dermal irritation/corrosion." Paris: OECD, 1981.
22. Morrison WL, McAuliffe DJ, Parrish JA, Bloch JJ. *In vitro* assay for phototoxic chemicals. *J Invest Dermatol* 1982;78:460–463.
23. Serban GP, Henry SM, Cotty VF, et al. *In vivo* evaluation of skin lotions by electrical capacitance: I. The effect of several lotions on the progression of damage and healing after repeated insult with sodium laurel sulfate. *J Soc Cosmet Chem* 1981;32:407–419.
24. Gordon VC, Kelly CP, Bergman HC. Evaluation of SKINTEX, an *in vitro* method for determining dermal irritation. *Toxicologist* 1990;10(1):78.
25. Soto RJ, Servi MJ, Gordon VC. Evaluation of an alternative method for ocular irritation. In: Goldberg AM, ed. *in vitro toxicology*. New York: Mary Ann Liebert, 1989.
26. Khaiat A. Evaluation of SKINTEX at Yves Rocher. Presented at 1st European *In Vitro* Symposium, Paris, June 1990.
27. Food and Drug Safety Center Report. Presented at JSAAE, Tokyo, Japan, November 1990.
28. Bason M, Gordon VC, Maibach H. Skin irritation *in vitro* assays. *Int J Dermatol* 30:623–626.
29. Bason M, Harvell J, Gordon V, Maibach H. Evaluation of the SKINTEX system. Presented at the Irritant Contact Dermititis Symposium, Groningen, Netherlands, 1991.
30. Harvell J, Bason M, Gordon V, Maibach H. Evaluation of dermal irritation of pure chemicals. *Presented at the* In Vitro *Workshop*, FDA/AAPS Symposium, Washington, DC, December 2, 1991.
31. Clothier RH, Hulme L, Ahmed AB, Reeves HL, Smith M, Balls M. *In Vitro* cytotoxicity of 150 chemicals to 3T3-L1 cells, assessed by the FRAME Kenacid Blue method. *ATLA* 1988;16:84–95.
32. Borenfreund E, Babich H, Martin-Alguacil N. Comparisons of two *in vitro* cytotoxicity assays—the Neutral Red (NR) and tetrazolium MTT tests. *Toxicol In Vitro* 1988;2:1–6.
33. Chan KY. Chemical injury to an *in vitro* ocular system: differential release of plasminogen activator. *Clin Eye Res* 1986;5:357–365.
34. Jackson EM, Hume RD, Wallin RF. The agarose difusion method for ocular irritancy screening: cosmetic products, Part II. *J Toxicol Cutan Ocular Toxicol* 1988;7:187–194.
35. Gordon VC, Acevedo J. SOLATEX-PI, An *in vitro* method to predict photoirritation. Presented at JSAAE, Japan, November 13, 1991.
36. Anonymous. TESTSKIN: an analysis. In: *The alternatives report*, vol 4. Boston, MA: Center for Animals & Public Policy, Tufts School of Veterinary Medicine, 1991;1–6.
37. Naughton GK, et al. A physiological skin model for *in vitro* toxicity studies. In: Goldberg AM, ed. *Alternative methods in toxicology*, vol 7. New York: Mary Ann Liebert.
38. Duffy PA, Irritancy testing—a cultured approach. *Toxicol In Vitro* 1989;3:157–158.
39. Oliver GJA, Pemberton MA, Rhodes C. An *in vitro* skin corrosivity test—modifications and validation. *Food Chem Toxicol* 1986;24:507–512.
40. Daniels F. A simple microbiological method for demonstrating phototoxic compounds. *J Invest Dermatol* 1965;44:259–263.

In Vitro Toxicology,
edited by Shayne Cox Gad.
Raven Press, Ltd., New York, © 1994.

5

Lethality Testing

Peggy J. Guzzie

Pfizer, Inc., Groton, Connecticut 06340

Several assays have been developed over the last decade to evaluate the acute toxicity and lethality of chemicals in an *in vitro* environment. These assays by their nature are simple, rapid indicators of relative toxicity with the intent of predicting the toxic effects of chemicals in animals and man. *In vitro* assays are attractive alternatives to traditional animal tests not only because they limit the use of animals but also because they provide a cost-effective approach for the rapid screening of large numbers of environmental xenobiotics and new drugs in development. There are also advantages to using *in vitro* systems for mechanistic studies. *In vitro* studies are simplistic in that they can be limited to the single target cell or tissue of interest. In addition, culture conditions can be easily controlled without the influence of exogenous factors including diet, drug usage, and environmental chemical exposures, or endogenous systemic factors such as metabolism, immunological status, and hormonal variation.

There are many factors that must be considered when using *in vitro* methods to extrapolate *in vivo* toxicity. The major differences that exist between growth of many cell types in culture and their growth in an intact organ arise from displacement and changes in spatial rearrangement. Normal cells *in situ* grow in a complex three-dimensional arrangement of different cell types, whereas *in vitro* they are forced to grow on a two-dimensional substrate. Not only is the normal spatial architecture of the tissue lost, but as cells spread out they begin to lose their capability for normal cell-to-cell interactions and communications. *In vitro* cultures also lack the hormonal and neural control mechanisms that are required for the normal homeostatic regulations that are inherent *in vivo*. Although *in vitro* systems have their limitations, it should not be the intention to totally replace the need for animal testing with *in vitro* tests, but rather to augment primary quantitative *in vivo* tests and to provide supportive mechanistic information.

Many of the same principles that govern *in vivo* toxicity assessment are also applicable to the study of *in vitro* cytotoxicity. The cytotoxicity of a xenobiotic in an *in vitro* system is dependent upon the quantity of a compound that reaches the cell and the duration of exposure, as is true for *in vivo* toxicity. However, in an *in vitro*

57

test system, chemicals come into direct contact with cell membranes and diffuse into cells without the protection afforded by barriers such as skin and limitations of absorption. In addition, *in vitro* systems have limited metabolic and detoxification mechanisms. *In vitro* systems are therefore highly sensitive and can often exaggerate the magnitude of the response. The *in vitro* cytotoxic properties of a given xenobiotic are also dependent upon the biological system itself and the end points that are evaluated. Thus, it is imperative that the investigator use caution in the experimental design and interpretation of *in vitro* tests. In addition, both the cell system and the end points should be well characterized and validated as a basis for a meaningful interpretation of the results.

CELL SYSTEMS

A variety of cell culture systems have been developed and used to assess *in vitro* toxicity and lethality. Prior to choosing a particular cell system for *in vitro* testing, it is important to understand the fundamental differences between the various sources and types of cultures that are available. Once a cell system is selected, it is then necessary to define the optimal growth conditions for that system.

Primary Cultures

Primary cultures are prepared from tissues or organs taken directly from an organism immediately after necropsy. A single-cell suspension is obtained by mechanical or chemical dispersion of the cells with the use of enzymes such as collagenase. The cells are suspended into growth medium and incubated for at least 24 hr in culture, during which time they may attach to the surface of the vessel or remain in suspension, depending on the growth characteristics of that particular tissue. With the exception of mature hematopoietic cells, most normal cells attach to a substrate, spread, and grow as a monolayer in culture. Transformed cell lines and lines established from tumor cells can proliferate in suspension since they have lost the need for attachment. Viability of the culture is affected by mechanical and/ or enzymatic damage to the cell membrane during cell isolation and by depletion of essential nutrients and/or hormones needed for cell survival. Primary cultures are difficult to reproduce since the viability and growth kinetics of the cells will vary between cultures as a result of individual genetic, hormonal, and age differences. Even replicate cultures derived from the same tissue contain varying proportions of different cell types.

Primary cell cultures are initially heterogeneous and well differentiated, and thus retain many of the complex biochemical functions of the animal tissue from which they are derived. However, primary cultures have limited life spans in culture. Within days in culture, faster growing and more rigorous subpopulations begin to take over and predominate through the selective pressures of the culture conditions in which they are maintained. With time, the cultures become more homogeneous, less differentiated, and begin losing specific cell functions and metabolic capabilities. Thus, most *in vitro* systems are established with permanent cell lines that will grow consistently for relatively long periods of time in culture.

Permanent Cell Lines

Permanent cell lines are usually derived by subculture from a primary culture to form a diploid, continuous (established), or clonal line that may either grow in suspension or attach as a monolayer on the surface of the culture dish. At least 75% of the population of cells in a diploid cell line contain the same normal complement of genetic material as the organism from which it was derived (20) and will usually undergo approximately 40–50 divisions in culture. The typical life cycle of human fibroblast cultures has been characterized into three phases on the basis of growth characteristics in culture (41). The initial phase 1 primary culture has a long population doubling time. After the first subculture, the primary culture is referred to as a cell line. Selection pressures and phenotypic drift gradually change the cell population and growth characteristic of the cell line with each subsequent subculture. By phase 2, the culture has become more stable and hardy and the growth kinetics have changed, resulting in a period of short, consistent population doubling times. Phase 3 is characterized by the onset of senescence, with progressively longer doubling times followed by degeneration and subsequent death.

Continuous or established cell lines are permanent cell lines that are derived from tumor cells by either a spontaneous or induced transformation of a primary culture or diploid cell line that results in immortalization of the line. Transformation can be induced by viruses, chemical mutagens, or irradiation to result in cells with acquired inheritable morphological growth characteristics that are stably transmitted from generation to generation in all of the progeny cells. The genome of continuous cell lines deviates genetically from that of the normal cells from which they originated. Most continuous cell lines are aneuploid and heteroploid compared to the normal, consistently diploid karyotype. Transformed cells are similar to tumor cells in that they have altered morphology and lack contact inhibition, anchorage dependence, and density-dependent inhibition of cell multiplication, which results in unlimited cell division in culture.

Clonal Cell Lines

Clonal cell lines are derived from the mitosis of a single cell of a primary, diploid, or continuous line to form a genetically homogeneous subline termed a *cell strain*. Frequent reisolation and cloning is required to minimize heterogeneity over time produced by genetic drift and thus to maintain a genetically homogeneous population of cells. Cells with specific phenotypic traits or markers can be selected by growing the cells in selection medium containing a drug or chemical that will allow only the clones exhibiting the trait to survive. Alternatively, cells can be cloned by subculturing at a relatively low density, which allows single cells to attach and form colonies that can be selected for their desired phenotypes.

Growth Conditions

To maximize viability and reproducibility, the culture medium and growth conditions must be optimized and standardized for any given cell system. Tissues and cell lines differ in their nutritional requirements and preference for growth in suspension, as a monolayer, or in more specialized three-dimensional matrices such as collagen gel. The cell concentration in a culture can also be critical for adequate cell viability. Normal (untransformed) cells suspend division in culture by a mechanism known as contact inhibition once the cells begin to touch and the culture becomes confluent. Therefore, most cultures that are actively dividing must be regularly subcultured in order to reduce the cell density to an optimal level for growth and cell division. However, the process of subculture itself can adversely affect the viability of the cells due to mechanical or chemical (trypsin) damage to the cell membranes from the methods and agents required to detach cells growing in monolayer. In addition, cell densities that are too low can also adversely affect the viability of the cultures. Cells that are actively growing secrete essential growth factors and chemical messengers into the culture medium that can be taken up by adjacent cells by a mechanism known as cross-feeding. If adequate cell densities cannot be maintained to facilitate cross-feeding, then it is necessary to supplement the culture medium with the necessary growth factors. Cell density can also affect the uptake of compound: as cell density increases with time in culture there is a tendency toward decreased uptake. Decreased uptake may be a function of reduced growth rate and a decreased cell surface area exposure as the result of increased cell-to-cell contacts (75).

In vitro systems, by their nature, experience nonphysiological conditions and periods of hypoxia regardless of how well the system is defined and controlled. Since *in vitro* systems do not have inherent methods of clearance, they are dependent upon regular changes of growth medium, which results in dramatic fluctuations in levels of nutrients and metabolites over the culture period. Buffering the culture medium and providing CO_2 is necessary to minimize extreme fluctuations in pH that can occur in metabolically active cultures. A humidified atmosphere in the incubator is also necessary to minimize evaporation of culture medium that can result in hypertonicity.

Metabolic Activating Systems

Several chemicals are metabolically activated *in vivo* to a more toxic metabolite. Primary cultures of hepatocytes and several hepatocellular tumor cell lines are metabolically competent. However, most cell cultures contain little, if any, cytochrome P-450 mixed function oxidase (MFO) metabolic capability. Cocultivation of these cells with primary hepatocytes is one means of providing P-450 activity. The addition of exogenous metabolic activation systems to the culture medium, similar to those that have been routinely used in established *in vitro* tests for genotoxicity, can also be used to provide some metabolic functions in *in vitro* toxicity assays. These systems can be prepared with either an S9 (9,000 g postmitochondrial supernatant) fraction of liver homogenate, which provides both microsomal and cytosolic enzymes, or with a more purified microsomal fraction, prepared by first centrifuging at 15,000 g and subsequently centrifuging the supernatant at 105,000 g. Either fraction must be mixed with an NADPH-generating cofactor system in order to be metabolically active. Approximately 5 days prior to collecting hepatocytes, the animals can be pretreated with chemicals, such as Aroclor-1254 (a mixture of polychlorinated biphenyls), phenobarbitol, 3-methylcholanthrene, or β-naphthoflavone, which will induce the synthesis of various P-450 isozymes, thus increasing the metabolic activity of the liver fraction.

The use of induced S9 systems has been shown to increase the cytotoxicity of various chemicals such as cyclophosphamide, an antineoplastic agent that is metabolically activated to a cytotoxic and mutagenic metabolite (44). Both S9 fractions and purified microsomal fractions are cytotoxic in themselves. However, the S9 fraction is much more cytotoxic than the microsomal fraction (4), which limits its usage to no more than 2–4 hr. In tests with cyclophosphamide, the microsomal fraction was shown to be approximately twice as active as the S9 fraction in producing the cytotoxic metabolite, with IC_{50} values of 35 μg/ml and 70 μg/ml, respectively (4).

Although these systems have improved the overall correlations with *in vivo* toxicity, they are highly artificial and do not always reflect the level or types of reactive metabolites produced *in vivo*. Since phase 2 conjugation and detoxification enzymes such as glutathione S-transferase, sulphotransferases, and glucuronosyltransferases are not available at sufficient levels in S9 or microsomal fractions, these exogenous activation systems may overestimate toxicity with some chemicals. An apparent decrease in cytotoxicity with S9 is not necessarily indicative of metabolism to a less toxic species but may be a consequence of nonspecific binding to S9 proteins. Toxicity may be either under- or overestimated with some chemicals, depending on species differences in the types and levels of isozymes and differences between induction systems. Discordance with *in vivo* results may still occur even if the appropriate metabolite is generated *in vitro*. For example, paraoxon, the toxic metabolite of parathion *in vivo*, is produced *in vitro* by exogenous activation systems. However, in contrast to what is observed *in vivo*, paraoxon *in vitro* is significantly less toxic than parathion (53). *In vivo*, paraoxon exerts its toxicity by inhibiting cholinesterase in the nervous system, a mechanism that is not relevant *in vitro*.

END POINTS

The goal of most end points that are selected for evaluation is to objectively measure either a cytotoxic or a cytostatic effect. Cytotoxic effects are those that ultimately reduce cell viability, while cytostatic effects are those that inhibit normal cell division without necessarily affecting the viability of the affected cell. However, either can result in toxicity or lethality in an organism if the function of the affected cell is critical and if a significant number of cells are affected.

Cytotoxicity, as perceived *in vitro*, is dependent on the end points and methods used to define it in a given test system. The end point that is measured must be both specific and well-defined. Qualitative and quantitative end points have been used to assess cytotoxicity. Although quantitative end points are advantageous in that they can be objectively measured, qualitative data can also provide a wealth of information if the investigator strictly adheres to a defined evaluation criteria. Although no single *in vitro* assay can totally replace *in vivo* testing, a battery of well-designed complementary *in vitro* assays can augment *in vivo* results and help prioritize compounds for *in vivo* testing and further development.

End points that are most valuable are those which are indicative of a wide variety of chemical damage (68). Cell death is an end point that is easy to define and may result from a diverse array of cellular insults. Xenobiotics can produce cellular lethality by either direct damage to the structural components of the cell or indirectly by interfering with the normal physiology and metabolism of the cell through impaired protein synthesis, respiration, ion exchange, and DNA synthesis capabilities. Thus, cell death, as an end point, is nonspecific and all-or-nothing, providing no opportunity to establish mechanisms or the reversibility of the damage. Various other end points have been used to measure cellular toxicity *in vitro* include those that are characterized by altered cell morphology, abnormal cell behavior and reductions in growth. More specific end points such as those that affect specific metabolic or enzymatic systems may detect compounds that are toxic without necessarily resulting in acute lethality. However, these systems may be overly sensitive at detecting end points of little *in vivo* consequence. Thus, the ideal end point is one that is sensitive only to serious insults, and relevant by any mode of insult (75).

Basal Cytotoxicity

The term *basal cytotoxicity* has been used to describe the toxic effects that a chemical may have on the basic cellular functions and structures that are common and critical to all eukaryotic cells (21). Target organ toxicity has been correlated with the chemical distribution and basal cytotoxicity to that organ *in vivo* (20,21). *In vitro* models may be developed in conjunction with *in vivo* pharmacokinetic data to simulate the distribution and plasma levels of a xenobiotic that may be achieved *in vivo*. In theory, the lowest concentration of a chemical that is toxic to the basal function of all cells *in vitro* can be compared to the concentrations that are toxic to various target tissues to determine a critical concentration for producing toxicity to a particular target organ *in vivo*. Once plasma concentrations have reached this level in a vital target organ *in vivo*, ensuing toxicity would be expected. Thus, the end points that are relevant to basal cytotoxicity may be assessed *in vitro* as a useful method for studying and predicting the toxic effects that are responsible for animal lethality.

VIABILITY

Cell viability has been evaluated using a variety of techniques. Reduced cell numbers can be quantified microscopically using a hemocytometer or by using electronic cell counters. In either case, only a reduction in the number of intact cells produced by cell degeneration or lysis can be accurately obtained. Dead and damaged cells that are still intact are difficult to differentiate from living cell on the basis of cell counts alone. Other methods for assessing cell viability are based on changes in membrane permeability assessed as dye exclusion of viable cells and membrane leakage of dead or damaged cells.

Dye Exclusion/Uptake

Dyes such as trypan blue and nigrosin can be used as vital stains to detect a large portion of dead and membrane-damaged cells that have lost their ability for dye exclusion. Cells with damaged membranes allow the stain to pass into the cytoplasm, whereas undamaged cells are capable of dye exclusion. Conversely, supravital stains such as neutral red can diffuse through the plasma membrane and concentrate in the lysosomes of living cells. Neutral red uptake, measured by extraction and spectrophotometric absorption, has been used as a reliable, reproducible, and inexpensive *in vitro* assay for viability (8,9). Damage to the cell surface or lysosomal membranes leads to lysosomal fragility and ultimately decreased uptake and binding of neutral red. A dual fluorescence technique that combines fluorescein diacetate with diethidium bromide can be used to simultaneously stain living and dead cells using a fluorescence microscope with an epifluorescence condenser (49,77). With this procedure, fluorescein diacetate is converted to fluorescein by cellular esterases in living cells, resulting in a green fluorescence while ethidium bromide, excluded by living cells, can penetrate damaged cell membranes and stain the nuclear component of dead and damaged cells red. Each of these stains can be used in conjunction with manual microscopic counts with a hemacytometer or electronic counts with more sophisticated methods involving flow cytometry or colorimetric analysis using spectrophotometers. With flow cytometry, several thousands of cells per second pass through a laminar flow system, then one by one through a laser beam which is scattered by the cells and the red incident light is absorbed by the trypan blue stain.

Membrane Leakage

Leakage of soluble cellular cytosolic enzymes such as lactate dehydrogenase (LDH) into the cytoplasm has also been used to quantitate lethality. The advantage of this end point is that it quantitates enzyme leakage from cells that have been lysed in addition to those that are dead and damaged with leaky membranes. The amount of enzymes that the dead and damaged cells release into the culture medium can be assayed using sodium pyruvate as a substrate and NADH as a cofactor. In the presence of pyruvate, LDH is assayed by conversion of NADH to NAD^+. The rate of change in NADH absorbance at 340 nm can be measured with a spectrophotometer or by using a microcentrifugal analyzer. The LDH content of the surviving cells can also be assessed by lysing the remaining cells and measuring the levels of enzymes that are subsequently released. Using this technique, enzyme leakage can be presented as the percentage released relative to the total amount of enzyme in the culture. Alternatively, if the number of cells in each culture is variable, enzyme leakage can be presented on the basis of the amount of enzyme per million cells by determining the cell number, the total amount of DNA, or the protein content of each culture.

Total cellular protein can be assayed after treatment using the classic methodology of Lowry (54) or by more recent methodology. With the Lowry procedure, cells are incubated with a solution containing NaOH to lyse the membranes and an alkaline copper sulfate and potassium tartrate solution to produce a colorimetric reaction. Phenol is then added 30 min prior to assaying absorbance at 660 nm with a spectrophotometer. An alternative procedure involves first lysing the cells at 37°C for 60 min with NaOH, then mixing the suspension with Coomassie brilliant blue G-250 dye (52). Absorbance with this procedure is measured at 630 nm with a spectrophotometer or microplate reader. Protein content can also be determined by binding of Kenacid blue dye, as described by Knox et al. (51). This method was shown to be faster and the results less variable than with the Lowry method.

Similar methods have been based on the release of radiolabeled compound, proteins, or DNA into the medium to provide a sensitive and objective measure at relatively low levels of cell damage. Typically, cells are cultured in the presence of the radioactive labeled marker compound for a period of time to allow uptake of the label. The medium containing the label is then removed and the cultures are rinsed to remove surface label. Cells are then treated with the test article and the supernatant medium is harvested and counted in a gamma counter or liquid scintillation counter. If desired, the cells can then be lysed and counted to estimate the counts present in the intact cells. Chromium-51 (^{51}Cr) is a common radiolabel used for the study of cell damage since it can be used to assess cell damage prior to lysis, whereas the [^3H]thymidine- or [^{125}I]deoxyuridine-labeled DNA are only released after nuclear and cellular lysis. Radiochromium-labeled sodium chromate does not covalently bind to cell proteins and other cell constituents as does ^3H- or ^{14}C-labeled thymidine, which are readily incorporated during the synthesis of DNA, RNA, and protein. As a consequence, at least 70% of the radioactivity taken up as ^{51}Cr is subsequently released by dead cells. Hexavalent sodium chromate is reduced to the trivalent form once incorporated into cells and attaches to proteins and other cellular components. Once the chromate is reduced to the trivalent form, it cannot be reutilized by other cells (11,43).

A disadvantage of several of these techniques is that they will only detect the most severely and irreversibly damaged cells, not cells that are otherwise functionally impaired or unable to divide. For example, line 1 carcinoma cells treated with Vibrio cholerae neuraminidase showed no evidence of cytotoxicity using dye (eosin or trypan blue) exclusion techniques but showed a 73–84% reduction in viability when assessed for cell growth by colony formation or ^{3}H-thymidine incorporation (85).

CELL GROWTH

Cloning Efficiency

Cell growth and reproduction are widely used end points for assessing the viability of cells in culture. Cloning efficiency can be determined for cells that grow in monolayers by dispersing a dilute suspension of a known number of cells (100–200) into culture plates. Upon incubating the cells undisturbed for several days in culture, reproductively competent cells form clones that can be visually counted. Changes in cell number can also be used to assess cell growth kinetics in culture. Cells cultured at low densities in buffered, pH-controlled medium will divide logarithmically as long as there are sufficient nutrients available and there is room for growth. By counting the cells at various intervals in culture, one can assess reductions in growth relative to untreated control cultures through differences in cell number. A reduction in cloning efficiency can result from cell death or the impaired ability to reproduce.

DNA Synthesis

Reductions in DNA synthesis can be assessed directly by measuring the uptake of tritium-labeled thymidine (^{3}HTdR). Cells actively involved in DNA synthesis incorporate thymidine as a normal constituent of DNA. To assess effects on DNA synthesis, cells treated with test article are cultured in medium containing ^{3}HTdR. Cells that have retained the ability to synthesize DNA can incorporate the radiolabeled thymidine in place of thymidine. Since released thymidine can be reutilized by the cells, it is necessary to add an excess of cold thymidine prior to harvest to block the reutilization of the labeled thymidine. The DNA is then extracted from the cells and the extracts are counted in a liquid scintillation spectrometer.

An indirect method (6) for measuring the DNA content of the cells can be performed using DNA-specific fluorescence staining procedures (feulgen hydrolysis followed by Schiff-type acriflavine staining). Photometric readings are then obtained for each cell using a microscope photometer. DNA synthesis curves can then be derived for each culture using the distribution of DNA fluorescence readings as described by Walker (79).

Mitogenicity

Mitotic index is another useful end point for assessing the reproductive competence of cells. Not only must the cells be capable of DNA synthesis, but they must also be able to progress through G_2 and the chromatin must be able to condense to form chromosomes. Various methods exist for assessing mitotic index. Cells can be grown in suspension, as monolayers in culture dishes, or directly attached to cover-slips. Cells are treated with the test article 6–48 hr after treatment, and colchicine (or the synthetic, colcemid) is added during the final hours of treatment to arrest the cells in metaphase. Cells grown directly on coverslips can be fixed and stained with Giemsa. Alternatively, cells grown attached to plates are removed by trypsinization and the cell suspensions are fixed and stained. Prior to fixation, cells can be treated briefly with a hypotonic solution of KCl or sodium citrate if optimal chromosome morphology is also desired. At least 1,000 cells are then scored for the proportion that are in mitosis and the mitotic index is calculated as the number of metaphases per 100 cells.

Cell Cycle Kinetics

Many cells that are capable of mitosis may experience treatment-related delays in cell-cycle kinetics at one or more stages of the cell cycle. Various methods are available to assess cell-cycle kinetics, a few of which are based on incorporation of 5-bromo, 2-deoxyuridine (BUdR) during DNA synthesis. BUdR is an analogue of thymidine that can be taken up by the cell and incorporated into DNA in place of thymidine. Cells are treated and grown in the presence of BUdR for approximately two cell cycles. Through semiconservative replication, one strand of DNA will incorporate BUdR with each cell cycle. Thus, after one division, both chromatids of each chromosome will contain one strand that has incorporated BUdR. After a second round of replication in the presence of BUdR, one chromatid will contain one strand of DNA with BUdR and the other chromatid will have BUdR in both strands, resulting in differential staining between the chromatids upon staining with Hoechst fluorescent stain. Cells arrested in metaphase are then scored on the basis of their differential staining patterns for the relative frequency of cells that are in the first (M_1), second (M_2) or third (M_3) division after treatment. The replicative index (RI) of each culture is first calculated as follows: $RI = 1(M_1) + 2(M_2) + 3(M_3)$. The average generation time (AGT) can then be calculated by dividing the total culture time in BUdR by the RI for each culture (45).

More recently, with the advent of monoclonal antibodies, an antibody to BUdR (anti-BUdR) has become available commercially (38). This antibody can be used as a primary antibody for the sensitive detection of BUdR incorporation. A secondary antibody that is selective for the primary antibody and conjugated with an FITC (fluorescein isothiocyanate) stain is then used to attach a fluorescent label to the anti-BUdR/BUdR complex. The amount of fluorescence can then be quantitated using a photometric plate reader or by flow cytofluorometry. With flow cytometry, it is possible to use an improved double-staining method that combines anti-BUdR staining with conventional DNA stains such as propidium iodine or DAPI (6-di-amidino-2-phenylindol dihydrochloride). This method permits quantitation of the proportions of cells in G_1, S, and $G_2 + M$ and establishes the distribution of cells in each phase of the cell cycle (50).

Another method that is useful for assessing cell cycle kinetics involves treatment of the cells with cytochalasin B. Cytochalasin B interferes with the polymerization of actin, which blocks the cytokinesis of the cell without affecting DNA synthesis or mitosis. Cells that appear mononucleate have not yet undergone replication, where as binucleate, and polynucleate cells have undergone one or more replications, respectively. By assessing the proportions of mono-, bi- and poly-nucleated cells relative to a normal untreated control population of cells, one can estimate the amount of treatment-induced cell cycle delay.

CELL AND CULTURE MORPHOLOGY

Cell Morphology

Morphological and cytological evaluation can be performed on cells treated in culture to evaluate cellular toxicity using light and electron microscopy. Techniques for the study of whole cell preparations *in situ* have steadily evolved and have been refined in recent years to include several improvements for fixation, preparation, and viewing using high-voltage electron microscopes. The use of glutaraldehyde as a fixative by Buckley and Porter in 1975 was a major improvement followed by the combination of rapid freezing and freeze-substitution technology more recently (57). To minimize artifacts during dehydration and drying, aldehyde-fixed cells can be adhered to plastic substrates or electron-transparent melamine foil support mediums. These techniques have been shown useful for maintaining cellular topography and improving the study of fine cellular details (81).

Morphological Indicators of Cytotoxicity

Morphological changes in the cell membrane associated with toxicity include changes in size (pycnotic or giantism), shape (blebbing), and integrity of the cell membrane. Morphological changes in the attachment, spreading, and growth patterns of cells that grow in monolayers can also be evaluated as end points of cytotoxicity. Normal cells grown as monolayers display a regular, polar orientation that may be disrupted under toxic conditions. With fluorescence staining, the nucleolar borders of normal cells fluoresce brightly, and nuclei rich in uncondensed euchromatin fluoresce with a ground-glass-like appearance. Conversely, damaged cells lack nucleolar fluorescence and contain more heterochromatic chromatin in the nuclei that progressively becomes more heteropycnotic (condensed) as the cell dies. Toxic effects on the nucleus of the cell and its membrane may appear as blebbing, distribution of the nuclear membrane, reductions in numbers of mitotic figures, chromosome damage, or stickiness, and multinuclearity. Cytoplasmic changes may also be observed, such as vacuolization, condensation or swelling of mitochondria,

precipitation or changes in the distribution of ribosomes, and blebbing of the cytoplasmic membrane. Blebs appear as protrusions of the membrane containing cytosol
and are thought to be a symptom of membrane damage (21). Ultimately, dead cells
lyse upon release of lysosomes or degrade by necrosis. Necrosis is pathologically
characterized *in vivo* by cell swelling, membrane rupture, and disorganized disruption of chromatin. Necrosis can also be observed *in vitro* as an increase in cell
detachment, nuclear debris, and chromatin clumping. Apoptosis, programmed cell
death, can also be induced by toxins and appears as reduced cell volume, dilation of
the endoplasmic reticulum, compaction of organelles, loss of junctional complexes,
membrane blebbing, and condensation and margination of chromatin.

Quantification of Morphological Changes

Although morphological observations are mostly subjective and descriptive, various methods have been employed to make these data more objective and quantifiable. One of the first attempts to categorize and rank cytotoxicity by degree was
proposed by Toplin (78) as a method for standardizing the evaluation of cytotoxicity
of various chemotherapeutic drugs. The Toplin scale ranges from 0 to 4, with a
score of 0 indicating no cellular damage and 4 indicating complete cell degeneration
or cytolysis. Although semiquantitative, this method is based on subjective, qualitative end points.

Morphometric methods employing image analysis coupled with computer digital-
ization have allowed some morphological end points to become quantifiable. One
such procedure considers the volume densities of cells relative to the total number of
cells as opposed to the area of the section being evaluated to convert two-dimensional morphological information into three-dimensional quantitative data that can
be statistically analyzed (74). This procedure was validated using primary hepatocyte cultures treated with cadmium, erythromycin, benoxaprofen, and indomethacin and was demonstrated to be a sensitive index of cell injury even at levels
that caused detachment of a significant percentage of the cells.

Planimetric methods have also been employed as simple and rapid methods for
quantifying gross cytotoxicity by measuring the area occupied by cells on a substratum. To assess viability, cells are cultured as monolayers and evaluated for
plaque formation using a double agar overlay procedure in which the second agar
overlay medium contains neutral red. Neutral red is taken up by living cells while
dead cells remain unstained. Planigraphs are then prepared by tracing the areas of
cytotoxicity (plaques) onto paper and cytotoxicity is quantitated by area measurements which can be automated by using a compensating polar planimeter (69).
Computer-assisted planimetry can be used to further assess changes in shape, orientation, or polarization of the cells.

Cell spreading has been shown to be necessary for the survival, growth, and
movement of many cells that typically grow as monolayers on a substratum (76).
Cell spreading is characterized by cell attachment, flattening, and a subsequent

increase in surface area. Using image analysis, the degree of cell spreading on a substratum can be quantified by measuring the cell perimeter as a function of time (10). Since cell margins are difficult to contrast, the cells are stained with acridine orange (2,8 *bis*-dimethylaminoacridine), a fluorescent stain, to produce a bright fluorescence which appears dark on a photonegative. The basic methodology utilizes a drum scanner as an input device to scan the photonegatives to construct a computer image defined by gray levels.

A sophisticated automated system for assessing more complex cytotoxic end points has been developed using AVEC-DIC (Allen video-enhanced contrast-differential interference contrast) microscopy. DIC microscopy was developed to study phase objects with bright-field by providing shadowcast details at interfaces between membrane and organelles, resulting in gradients of optical paths based on differences in the refractive indices. The AVEC method incorporates a video camera that is especially designed to reject stray light, which can limit contrast and resolution (1). This system has been used to measure microtubule-related motility, changes in the movement of cellular organelles, and the fine structure of organelles (55). AVEC-DIC methodology is particularly well suited for assessing sublethal effects in living cells by providing a quantitative analysis of organelle dynamics at earlier time points and at lower concentrations than those required to produce gross effects. This system has been used to evaluate cytoplasm consistency, the appearance of vacuoles, spikes, blebs, and changes in the number, length, and shape of mitochondria that were vital-stained with a fluorescent rhodamine-123 dye. Several effects, including cell retraction (which precedes detachment), the appearance of blebs, and changes in the number and fine morphology of mitochondria, were detected with this system at concentrations of a toxin that did not increase LDH release or produce cytotoxic changes using conventional morphometric analysis or viability assessments.

CELL FUNCTIONS

While indicative of lethality, morphological changes are often subjective and time-consuming to quantify. Biochemical assays based on vital cell functions are usually easier to quantify, are more objective, and are readily automated. In addition, these assays can often detect subtle impairments in function that may occur long before cell death.

Thermodynamic and Metabolic Function

Adenosine triphosphate (ATP) can be used as an indicator of cytotoxicity since it is the primary energy source at the cellular level. In order for the cell to function optimally it must maintain an intricate balance between energy production and consumption. Several assays for ATP have been developed. A specific and highly sensitive assay for ATP has been developed on the basis of the firefly luciferase bioluminescent reaction which requires ATP as a source of energy to drive the reaction (15). This assay is technically complex, requiring an acid extraction of ATP with perchloric acid, followed by neutralization with KOH and dilution at various concentrations using a luciferin–luciferase test reagent. The intensity of luminescence, which correlates with ATP content, can be measured with a luminometer. To quantitate levels of ATP, a standard curve with known concentrations of ATP must be constructed.

A simpler technique using ^{14}C-labeled ATP has been shown to correlate well with ATP levels as measured by the luciferin–luciferase method (71). A few hours prior to treatment, ATP pools are labeled by adding [^{14}C]adenine to the culture medium. The amount of uptake can be verified by lysing a sample of cells with Triton X-100 and determining the amount of radioactivity in the lysate. Immediately prior to treatment, the labeled medium is removed. Cells are then washed and treated with the test article in unlabeled medium. At various time intervals after treatment, an aliquot of medium can be removed and counted for radioactivity using a liquid scintillation counter. With this method, Shirhatti and Krishna demonstrated that approximately 65–70% of the incorporated ^{14}C label was in the ATP pool; the remaining label was incorporated into the ADP and 5'-AMP pools. In the presence of toxic drugs, a marked decrease in cellular ATP levels with a concomitant increase in ^{14}C leakage into the medium was observed to correlate well with LDH leakage. Since the total [^{14}C]adenine uptake can be estimated from the disappearance of [^{14}C]adenine from the medium without the need to lyse the cells, this method is noninvasive. Thus, an advantage of this method is that multiple samples of medium can be taken from the same cultures at various time points after treatment.

MTT Assay

The primary function of mitochondria is to produce and maintain sufficient levels of ATP for the cell to carry out its energy-requiring activities. Therefore, the more active the cell, the more ATP is required, and subsequently mitochondria are more active and abundant. To produce ATP, mitochondria actively metabolize pyruvate, a product of glycolysis, that is coupled with coenzyme A to produce acetyl CoA in the matrix of the mitochondria. Acetyl CoA is also provided as a substrate to the mitochondria through amino acid metabolism and oxidation of fatty acids. Once in the mitochondria, regardless of its source, acetyl CoA is circulated through the tricarboxylic acid cycle (TCA cycle), where it reacts with various enzymes to produce a chain of substrates and release of electrons, resulting in the production of ATP. One of these enzymes, succinate dehydrogenase, is responsible for converting succinate to fumarate, which provides a pair of electrons (from the hydrogen atoms of the substrate) to be used in ATP production. Tetrazolium MTT (3-(4,5-dimethylthiazol-2-yl)-2 diphenyl tetrazolium bromide) is a pale yellow substrate that can also be cleaved by succinate dehydrogenase. Formazan, the product of this reaction, is a dark blue pigment that can be used as an indicator of mitochondrial function. Since the conversion takes place only in living cells, the amount of formazan produced correlates with the number of viable cells present. Mosmann used this reaction as a basis for the development of a rapid colorimetric assay for cell viability (56). Absorbance at 540 nm can be measured using a spectrophotometer.

Calcium Ions

Changes in homeostasis of Ca^{2+} can also occur as the result of cellular injury. Ca^{2+} ions are essential second messengers and regulators of critical enzyme functions (i.e., DNA endonucleases) and cell division. Calcium ions that normally enter the cell down an electrochemical gradient through voltage-dependent Ca^{2+} channels are taken up by the endoplasmic reticulum and mitochondria, and packaged. Ca^{2+} stores are then released from the cell by plasma membrane Ca^{2+} ATPase upon mediation by hormones, growth factors, and neurotransmitters. Although there is a sustained increase in calcium influx, the efficiency and sensitivity of the calcium ion pump are enhanced, enabling the calcium efflux to compensate for the increased influx (67). Thus, a rapid but transient increase in intracellular Ca^{2+} may be caused by receptor-mediated physiological agonists, such as bradykinin, that act on the cell surfaces (46,58). In contrast, slow, sustained increases are usually associated with irreversible cell damage (66). Cell damage results in an increase in intracellular free Ca^{2+} concentration from normal levels of approximately 10^{-7} M to micromolar levels through various mechanisms, including increased permeability of the cell plasma membrane to external Ca^{2+}, the release of internal stores of Ca^{2+}, damage to the calcium ion pump, or effects on critical cellular transport proteins.

Intracellular Ca^{2+} concentrations can be measured using aequorin, a Ca^{2+}-sensitive photoprotein. Cells are loaded with aequorin using a low Ca^{2+} centrifugation technique (58), then cultured in dishes placed over a sensitive photomultiplier tube. At various time points after treatment, the calcium ion concentration is measured by quantitating the light emitted from the aequorin-loaded cells. Alternative methodology involves the use of fluorescent imaging with fluorescent calcium chelators such as Quin-2, Fura-2, and Indo-1, which can localize and quantify intracellular calcium reserves. This methodology was used to associate sustained elevations of calcium ions with subsequent cell blebbing and loss of membrane permeability (18).

ASSAY VALIDATION

Validation of assays is necessary to demonstrate the relevance, reliability, and predictability of new methodology, prior to gaining acceptance and usage as replacements for traditional *in vivo* methods. In order to accurately assess the specificity and sensitivity of an assay, a wide variety of compounds with different mechanisms of action must be tested. Since lethality may be the end result of a variety of toxic mechanisms, a battery of *in vitro* tests with different end points should be more predictive than a single assay. Several factors should be considered when designing a validation study. First, the goals of the validation must be defined as a basis for the selection of appropriate *in vitro* and *in vivo* end points, treatment protocols, and test compounds. For example, if the goal is to validate the predictivity of an *in vitro* assay for determining acute *in vivo* lethality, it would be appropriate to select *in vitro* end points that measure basal cytotoxicity and are reflective of the *in vivo* mechanisms responsible for lethality (i.e., impaired basal cell functions and/or structures). Prior to defining the treatment protocol, it is advantageous to know the *in vivo* pharmacokinetics and metabolism of each test compound selected for validation. A continuous *in vitro* exposure has been shown to more closely approximate *in vivo* conditions where there is a slow rate of elimination (30). If the parent compound is metabolized to a more or less toxic species, then an exogenous metabolic activation system should be provided for cell systems other than hepatocytes.

The results of the *in vitro* tests should be compared to an appropriate parameter of *in vivo* lethality, such as LD_{50} values from an acute *in vivo* toxicity test. If an appropriate animal model is used that is not a good predictor of human toxicity, then the *in vitro* method developed against that model may be of limited value (12). When available, human data should be used from an appropriate database. Correlation of *in vivo* LD_{50} dose–response data to an *in vitro* IC_{50} (50% inhibitory concentration) response is generally done by linear regression analysis using the actual concentrations of the test agents or the rank order of their toxicity in each test system. The rank order of toxicity is preferable if the absolute values of the *in vitro* and *in vivo* end points differ by more than a factor of 1,000 (75). The correlation coefficient (r) of the line provides a measure of the strength of the relationship of the two test systems, where an r of 1 is indicative of a perfect positive correlation.

Several factors should be considered when evaluating the predictivity of the assay. Since the compound comes into direct contact with target cells in an *in vitro* assay, intravenous (IV) or intraperitoneal (IP) LD_{50} data, when available, should be more comparable than data from oral studies, in which the compound may have limited absorption and systemic bioavailability (31,62). Total cellular protein ID_{50} data from tests with 27 compounds believed to interfere with critical basal cell functions were compared with LD_{50} values (31). For 21 compounds having both rat oral and mouse IP data available, a weak but significant correlation ($r = 0.49$) was obtained using log oral LD_{50} values. The *in vivo/in vitro* correlation for these same compounds was improved ($r = 0.68$) by using mouse IP data. In addition, by removing three compounds that are metabolized to more or less toxic metabolites, the correlation was further improved to 0.82. The best correlations ($r = 0.94$ and 0.95) were obtained when compounds with similar mechanisms of action were compared using *in vivo* data from the more sensitive species. Thus, when a human database is not available, a better correlation may be obtained when LD_{50} data from the more sensitive species and route are used, and when compounds are grouped on the basis of their mechanism of toxicity.

Early Validation Studies

As early as 1954 Pomerat and Leake published a cytotoxicity study with 110 compounds tested on primary explants of fetal chicken cells (64). However, few studies prior to 1976 compared cytotoxicity *in vitro* with systemic *in vivo* toxicity using standardized procedures. For the most part, good correlation was found with small groups of related compounds (37).

In 1980, Ekwall presented a large-scale study with 205 drugs of various classes tested in HeLa cells using standardized procedures (20). Cytotoxicity was first assessed microscopically on the basis of the absence or scarcity of spindle-shaped cells at 24 hr, and metabolic inhibition was assessed after 7 days by evaluating pH changes in the growth medium apparent as color change of phenol red. Preliminary tests by the same author with a subsample of the 205 compounds were first performed to (a) compare the toxicity of a sample of 25 drugs in HeLa cells versus other cell systems (26) and (b) compare the toxicity of a random sample of 52 drugs with systemic LD_{50} toxicity values of mice and man (20). The first of these studies indicated that the relative levels of inhibitory toxicity showed similar differential sensitivities regardless of the cell system, indicating a qualitatively similar mechanism of action characteristic of basal cytotoxicity. In the second study, seven compounds were more toxic in humans as the result of target organ toxicity to specialized neuroreceptors not found *in vitro*, while the remaining compounds expressed similar *in vitro* and *in vivo* toxicities indicative of basal cytotoxicity. These studies showed that a tiered approach to assessing two end points improves the likelihood of detecting toxicity with at least one of the end points and provides useful mechanistic information for some compounds.

This same standardized test system was used to test a group of 29 plasticizers *in vitro* in HeLa cells (27). Seven of the compounds were also tested in other test systems with other cell types, including chick embryo cells, mouse L-cells, human diploid WI-38 cells, and mouse cerebellar explants. All tests had a similar rank order of toxicity in which cytotoxicity was correlated with increasing chain length of the alcohol groups until the point where solubility was inhibited. Data for 20 of the compounds were also shown to correlate well with rodent intraperitoneal LD_{50} values, suggesting similar mechanisms of lethality due to basal cytotoxicity. Data from this test system and another cell line were also compared to cytotoxicity (LDH release) data obtained with primary hepatocyte cultures to determine the value of using metabolically competent hepatocytes in general cytotoxicity screening (22). Of the 14 compounds that were hepatotoxic, the majority expressed similar toxicity with cell lines and liver cells, indicative of acute cytotoxicity not mediated by reactive metabolites. However, four of the hepatotoxic compounds, known to cause more specific metabolism-mediated hepatocellular damage, were shown to be more selectively cytotoxic to the hepatocytes.

When possible, large numbers of compounds of many different chemical classes should be used to validate a test system. A cytotoxicity study of 114 compounds was conducted (16) by measuring the protein content in HEP G_2 cells, a human-hepatoma-derived established cell line. A diverse array of compounds of various chemical classes were tested, including surfactants, alcohols, organic acids, and some of their salts, inorganic acids, and salts; heavy metal compounds; and miscellaneous compounds and solvents. Twenty-four hours after treatment, the cell membranes were lysed and the amount of protein was assayed by the Lowry method. The relative toxicity of each compound was determined as the concentration required to produce a 50% reduction in cell protein content (PI_{50}). Consistently low values were observed with very toxic compounds such as the heavy metals and organic amines. Subsets of the data showed good correlation when compared with data from other *in vitro* assays; however, the lack of adequate *in vivo* data precluded meaningful comparisons.

Multicenter Studies

Over the last decade, with the support of groups like FRAME (Fund for the Replacement of Animals in Medical Experiments), more thorough validations have been performed as multicenter programs involving several laboratories testing the same set of compounds, usually in a blind fashion. Multicenter testing not only facilitates the testing of larger numbers of compounds in a variety of assays but also enhances the credibility of the results. A multicenter approach allows for the evaluation of interlaboratory variability and circumvents the inherent bias of validations performed by the laboratory that first developed the technique. In addition, with more laboratories involved in selecting the compounds, a more diverse sample of compounds are generally tested.

FRAME

In 1982, FRAME established a multicenter research project aimed at developing, standardizing, and validating a cell culture method for assessing cytotoxicity. A large set of compounds was selected to include chemicals of different mechanisms of activity and with different degrees of toxicity, stability, volatility, and solubility. In addition, some of the compounds were known to be metabolically changed to more or less toxic metabolites (3). The group limited their testing to human BCL-D1 fibroblast-like cells, since results obtained in general cytotoxicity tests have been shown not to depend on the choice of cell type (68). After a 72-hr treatment period, total protein was assessed as the end point for measuring cytotoxicity using kenacid blue staining (51). This method, as previously described, is based on a direct relationship between protein content, cell number, and binding of the stain. Results from testing 50 chemicals, of diverse toxicities and mechanisms of action, were generally in close agreement among the four participating laboratories.

A subset of 30 of the FRAME compounds was also tested for cytotoxicity in a blind trial using the kenacid blue protein assay, the neutral red uptake assay, and a morphometric assay aimed at determining the highest tolerated dose (HTD) based on minimal morphological alterations (70). 3T3-L1 cells, a continuous fibroblast cell line derived from mouse embryos, were treated for 24 hr, then assessed for cytotoxicity by each of the three methods. When ranked in order of toxicity, a close correlation was observed between the relative cytotoxicities of chemicals tested by all three methods. Since an exogenous metabolic system was not provided, some of the chemicals known to require metabolic activation to a more toxic metabolite were less toxic *in vitro*.

In addition to developing and validating alternative *in vitro* test systems, FRAME manages an Alternative Test Validation Scheme in which sets of compounds are coded and supplied to research groups to validate new test methods blindly at a number of laboratories throughout the world. The ATP assay, as previously described, was validated in a test using 20 of the FRAME compounds (48). L929 mouse fibroblasts were treated for 4 hr, then ATP levels were determined using the luciferin–luciferase bioluminescent assay. ATP_{50} values were calculated as the concentrations reducing cellular ATP by 50%. The ranking of the test compounds by ATP_{50} values was similar to that obtained by cell death (CD_{50}). However, animal lethality data were not available at that time for comparison.

In vivo data may be derived from a variety of sources using different species, stains, routes of administration, and treatment protocols. Thus, one of the biggest problems with the FRAME study, as well as with other studies, was the unbiased selection and availability of *in vivo* toxicity data of sufficiently high quality and reproducibility. When possible, rat oral and mouse IP lethality data produced at one laboratory (Imperial Chemical Industries; ICI) were used to provide *in vivo* toxicity profiles for the FRAME validation compounds, 50 of which have been published (65). These data, along with additional data provided from the Registry of Toxic Effects of Chemical Substances (RTECS, compiled by NIOSH), were used to compare rat oral and mouse IP LD_{50} values to *in vitro* ID_{50} data (13) for 59 of the 150 compounds tested in the FRAME *in vitro* screen. Using linear regression analysis to compare log-transformed *in vitro* and *in vivo* data, correlation coefficients of 0.76 and 0.80 were obtained with the rat oral and mouse IP data, respectively (14). As was suggested by Fry et al. (30,31), the best correlations ($r = 0.81$) were obtained using LD_{50} data from the most sensitive species for each compound.

MEIC

A similar multicenter program was initiated in 1983 by the Scandinavian Society of Cell Toxicology under the title MEIC (Multicenter Evaluation of *In Vitro* Cytotoxicity). Whereas the main emphasis of the FRAME study has been to test the interlaboratory variability of methods, the MEIC study has concentrated on the predictivity of *in vitro* results compared to the *in vivo* response, and the relevance of the results to various types of human toxicity (7). The use of a battery of *in vitro* test systems with different cell types and end points should provide a higher predictive value. Initially, 50 reference compounds were selected, without bias, on the basis of known human and rodent acute lethality dosages and toxicokinetics (5). To date, more than 50 international laboratories have tested at least a portion of the compounds in over 50 *in vitro* test systems. The primary findings of a few of these studies will be reviewed.

As a preliminary validation study, Ekwall et al. (23,25) published the results of the first ten MEIC compounds tested in a battery of *in vitro* cytotoxicity assays, encompasssing four different cell systems (primary rat hepatocytes treated 1 or 24 hr, and 3T3 and HepG$_2$ firbroblasts treated 24 hr). Each cell system was evaluated for three different end points—intracellular LDH, total protein, and MTT. These results were combined with previously published data from the same compounds tested in the MIT-24 assay with HeLa cells and used to derive a multivariate partial least squares (PLS) model. As a means of predicting human lethality, the model was then compared with rodent LD$_{50}$ values from the RTECS. In general, mouse LD$_{50}$ values were more predictive of human lethality than rat values. Although the sample of compounds in this preliminary study was small, the collective prediction using the PLS model was shown to be as predictive of human lethality as the mouse LD$_{50}$ values.

The first ten MEIC compounds were also tested in rat hepatocytes for 24 or 48 hr (59). Cytotoxicity was assessed by measuring mitochondrial activity and cell number was assessed with the MTT and Coomassie blue dye assays, respectively. Good correlations with oral rat LD$_{50}$ data were obtained with both the MTT and Coomassie blue assays after a 24-hr treatment ($r^2 = 0.86$ and 0.83, respectively). Although the values obtained in this study were not tested for correlation with human data, the results from this study correlated better with rat LD$_{50}$ data than did the results of the preliminary study described above. In a more recent study, MTT data with cultured human hepatocytes was compared with data from primary rat hepatocytes and the nonhepatic 3T3 murine line using the first ten MEIC compounds (47). This study showed that acute toxicity in humans was most accurately predicted with cultured human hepatocytes than with either rat hepatocytes or mouse 3T3 cells, suggesting that when available, human hepatocytes should be included in *in vitro* test batteries.

A few recent studies have been published on the results from testing the first 20 MEIC compounds. In an attempt to estimate the effects of chronic exposure, long-term cytotoxicity was investigated with human embryonic lung (MRC-5) cells (17), which can be maintained in culture for more than 6 weeks without requiring subculture. Cytotoxicity was quantified by assaying total protein. PI$_{50}$ values obtained from cultures treated for 6 weeks were compared to those obtained with the human epithelial HepG$_2$ cell line treated for 24 hr with the same compounds. Although the PI$_{50}$ values at 6 weeks were substantially lower than the 24-hr values, with the exception of digoxin, good correlation was observed ($r^2 = 0.94$). The first 20 compounds were also tested for total protein and LDH release after a 24-hr exposure to Hep-2 human epithelial cells (86). LDH release was only slightly less sensitive than total protein for measuring cytotoxicity. In general, the data from this study were in good agreement with the other studies with these compounds.

Another study of the first 20 MEIC compounds evaluated metabolic and functional end points as well as viability. Primary cultured rat skeletal muscle cells were treated for 1 or 24 hr with each reference compound (39). Viability was assessed by changes in intracellular creatine kinase and total protein, and decreased energy metabolism was assayed as a reduction in glucose consumption. Effects on function were determined by assaying changes in spontaneous contractility, which reflects not only the structural integrity of the excitable cell membranes but also the functional abilities of electromechanical coupling and contraction. Decreased contractility after exposure for 1 or 24 hr was the most sensitive measure of critical biological activities or cytotoxicity in this study and was reflective of therapeutically intended or acute toxic effects observed *in vivo*.

Cell growth and morphology were assessed for 48 of the MEIC compounds in primary rat hepatocytes, Madin-Darby bovine kidney (MDBK) cells, and McCoy cells, a human epithelial line derived from synovial fluid (72). Hepatocytes were observed for morphological changes for 24 hr after a 4–6-hr treatment, while the cell lines were observed for growth and morphology at 72 hr post treatment. Cell viability was determined by trypan blue exclusion and LDH release. For each compound tested, average values from all three parameters were used to determine minimum cytotoxic concentrations (CT_{50} and CT_{100}), defined as follows. CT_{50} was the concentration that induced morphometric changes in 50% of the cells or 50% cell death and/or a 50–100% increase in hepatocyte LDH release. CT_{100} was the concentration that induced marked morphometric changes or >50% cell death along with >100% increases in hepatocyte LDH release. The log of these values were compared with oral log LD_{50} values for rats and mice using linear regression analysis. The correlations between LD_{50} values and CT_{50} values were $r = 0.77$, 0.80, and 0.83 for McCoy cells, hepatocytes, and MDBK cell, respectively. These results agreed with those of Ekwall and Johannson, who also demonstrated that cell type had little effect on the overall relative cytotoxicity values (26). An accurate *in vivo* LD_{50} dose was predicted for at least 75% of the compounds studied. Using an empirical approach, Shrivastava et al. (73) also showed that CT_{50} and CT_{100} values can be used to predict an *in vivo* maximum tolerated dose (MTD). *In vitro* CT_{50} and CT_{100} values for 25 compounds in each of the three cell systems were shown to have a greater than 80% correlation with actual *in vivo* results from MTD studies with dogs and rats.

Upon completion of the initial test phase with numerous test systems, the MEIC group will evaluate the relevance and effectiveness of each assay for predicting human lethality using toxicokinetic models. Multivariate modeling will be used to select tests and batteries of tests that may be useful as supplements or alternatives to animal testing. In the final phase of validation, the tests that best predict human toxicity will be evaluated for reliability by contract laboratories using coded compounds. This approach should minimize the costs and time of validation by selecting test systems on the basis of relevance to be subsequently tested for reliability (24).

French Multicenter Study

Over the past few years, the French Ministry for Research and Higher Education has established a multicenter study with the goal of setting up a model of acute *in vitro* toxicity that is predictive of acute *in vivo* toxicity (28). Four end points—LDH release, neutral red uptake, the MTT assay of mitochondria function, and total cellular protein content—are to be evaluated in primary cultures of rat hepatocytes treated with various compounds. Recently, the validity and predictability of this model were evaluated by comparing the IC_{50} cytotoxicity results for several compounds with IV LD_{50} values using multivariate analysis (62). The 30 compounds tested were selected from those used in the FRAME project. IC_{50} values were closely correlated for the four end points ($r > 0.97$). Values from the neutral red assay were the most sensitive indicators of *in vitro* cytotoxicity (lowest IC_{50} values), as were the IV or IP LD_{50} values *in vivo*. Linear regression between these two parameters for 25 of the compounds yielded a statistically significant ($p < 0.001$) correlation coefficient ($r = 0.877$). With the limited number of compounds tested in this study, the model had a predictability of 95% with a confidence interval of 75–100% at concentrations up to 1,500 µg/ml. Additional compounds must still be tested to reduce the confidence interval to an acceptable limit before the use of this model can be considered.

THE ROLE OF PHARMACOKINETICS AND SAR IN MODELING

Preliminary results from numerous *in vitro* assays indicate that these tests are relevant for predicting the human lethality of most chemicals, particularly those that interfere with critical basal functions. As would be expected, compounds that are not accurately predicted by *in vitro* tests often have specific metabolic or toxicokinetic requirements resulting in variations in the time that the compound is maintained at concentrations high enough to produce a toxic response. Although metabolism can be easily achieved *in vitro* with cultured hepatocytes or an exogenous microsome system, the rate of biotransformation *in vivo* is affected by factors such as species differences, sex differences, and the route of administration. These factors subsequently influence the degree and rate of uptake and distribution, which are difficult to fully simulate *in vitro*. Even *in vivo*, under controlled conditions using the same sex and species, there can be as much as a 25-fold variation in activity between individuals due to genetic variability, and within individuals over time due to age, diurnal variability, seasonal changes, illness, and nutritional status.

Pharmacokinetics

In classic pharmacokinetic testing, animals are administered the parent compound by the applicable route, then concentrations of the parent compound and its metabolites are determined at various time points in the blood and excreta. Rate constants for absorption, distribution, and elimination can be calculated to describe the transfer of compound between various tissue compartments, which depends on the rate of blood flow to the tissue and the rate of diffusion across cell membranes. The volume of distribution (V_d) can also be calculated as a measure of the fluid volume in the body (plasma, extracellular fluid, and intracellular fluid) available to contain all of the compound at the same concentration as in the plasma.

If a compound is extensively bound to plasma proteins, the volume of distribution is equivalent to that of the plasma volume alone for agents that are acidic, but not lipophilic bases such as propranolol. Many xenobiotics bind reversibly to plasma proteins (albumin, glycoproteins) at nonspecific sites that can become saturated. Bound compound is held to be essentially biologically inactive since it is not free to bind to active sites on tissue membranes or diffuse across membranes into cells. The volume of distribution can increase as the unbound fraction of the compound in the plasma increases by the relationship $V_d = V_p + V_T f_p / f_T$, where V_p is the plasma volume, V_T is the volume of other body tissue water, and f_p and f_T are the fractions of unbound compound in the plasma and tissue, respectively (32). When unbound plasma concentrations in plasma water and cell water concentrations of a nonionizable compound are plotted against time, the concentration of the drug in cell water is in equilibrium with that of the plasma water at the highest concentration of drug (34). Based on this relationship, the highest concentration of a nonionizable compound that is not actively transported across the cell membrane cannot be higher in the cell water than the highest concentration in the plasma water. In addition, once steady state is achieved, the range of concentrations of the unbound xenobiotic in plasma water would reflect the maximum range of concentrations of the xenobiotic in the cells exposed to the xenobiotic through passive diffusion. Thus, the concentrations of unbound compound in the plasma water, and the clearance rates and distribution volumes measured in terms of concentration in plasma water, are the appropriate parameters for comparisons with *in vitro* concentration–response curves (36).

The concentration of unbound (free) xenobiotic in the plasma water can be measured through ultrafiltration. Ultrafiltration partitions free compound from relatively small plasma volumes by applying a pressure gradient on plasma, thus forcing a protein-free ultrafiltrate through a semipermeable membrane using centrifugal force. The concentration of free compound can then be determined directly from the ultrafiltrate. However, ultrafiltration may be unsuitable for many compounds due to nonspecific binding of the drugs to the devices. In these cases, equilibrium dialysis may be more appropriate.

Physiological Pharmacokinetic Modeling

A physiologically based model has been described as an approach for comparing the time course of the concentration of a xenobiotic *in vivo* with its effective concentration *in vitro* (36). These types of models attempt to integrate basic physiological and biochemical information into a comprehensive model for predicting the distribution and disposition of a compound. Since the concentration of compound at the local site of a target tissue or organ may not necessarily reflect the concentration in the blood, an organ in its simplest form is assumed to consist of two pharmacokinetic compartments, the blood in the organ and the cells in the organ. By repeated dosing with an optimal interval between doses, the concentration of the free compound within the cells of each organ can be maintained in steady state with the concentration in the blood flowing through the capillaries of the organs, minimizing the range of concentrations of free compound in the cells. The total concentration of a xenobiotic in an organ (C_T) can then be used to relate the concentration of compound in the cells at any given time to the concentration in the capillaries at that time. C_T can be calculated using the formula $C_T = RC_{out}$, where the partition ratio (R) is estimated for the organ by measuring the compound and its metabolites in the plasma water obtained from the blood flowing through the organ at various times, then calculating the areas under the curves (AUC) for the organ and blood.

If the unbound compound exists in only one form and is passed into and out of the cells solely by passive diffusion, and assuming that the compound or its metabolites reach an immediate steady state between the two compartments, then the appropriate values can be substituted into rate formulas and physiologically based pharmacokinetic models as described by Gillette (35,36). However, most compounds are weak acids or bases that pass through cell membranes in their nonionized forms. Thus, the total concentration of unbound compound would depend on the pK_a of the compound and the pH values of the blood and cells. In addition, if the compound is eliminated from the cells by metabolism or active excretion, the calculations must be further modified. These modifications require knowledge of the clearance values of the compound into and out of the cell, as well as measurement of enzyme activities and their effects on the intracellular concentration of the compound. The formulas are further complicated if the compound is actively transported into cells, then metabolized and/or cleared by passive diffusion. These parameters are best studied using *in vitro* pharmacokinetic experiments with purified enzyme (33,34).

A well-integrated approach for *in vitro* extrapolation should encompass data from a variety of pharmacokinetic and toxicokinetic assays. The validation of physiologically based models requires large amounts of *in vitro* as well as *in vivo* data. Although these models require complex sets of equations, they can often be simplified to include only the target organs or the organs in which the compound has been shown to accumulate (2). Regardless of the complexity, the integration of *in vitro* data with pharmacokinetic models can greatly enhance the interpretation and the reliability of risk assessment using *in vitro* test systems. For example, combining cytokinetic data with *in vitro* lethality data improved the prediction of acute human toxicity in multivariate analysis with the first ten MEIC compounds (23).

Computer SAR Modeling

Over the last few decades there have been numerous attempts to apply the concepts of quantitative structure–activity relationships (QSAR) to predicting *in vivo* mammalian toxicity on the basis of chemical structure. QSARs are statistical models that have historically been based on empiricism. These models assume that the total magnitude of a compound's interaction with a biological receptor can be modeled as an additive combination of each functional group's physicochemical interactions (63). Numerous physicochemical parameters such as molecular weight, quantum mechanical index, and reactivity constants may be incorporated into the model. In addition, substituent interaction constants may be included such as the Hammett σ electrostatic constant, the Taft E_s steric constant, the Hansch π hydrophobic constant, and dispersive descriptors based on molar refractivity.

A comprehensive review of the methodology and use of QSAR is beyond the scope of this chapter. The interested reader should refer to Phillips et al. (63) for a thorough and critical review of the utility of QSAR for predicting *in vivo* lethality. In general, these authors concluded that QSAR is not yet useful for predicting LD_{50} values of unrelated compounds or when based on electronic or structural descriptors of the substituents. QSAR has had greater predictive success when using small groups of related compounds and with certain physicochemical properties of compounds, particularly hydrophobicity. The hydrophobicity of a compound may be expressed as the logarithm of the partition coefficient (1-octanol/water partition coefficient), which is determined from the distribution of the compound between two immiscible solvents (water and 1-octanol), one polar and the other nonpolar (40). Hydrophobicity, estimated by the 1-octanol/water partition coefficient, may be a more useful predictor of biological activity than the electronic characteristics of a compound, since hydrophobicity correlates well with the lipophilicity of the compound and, in turn, its ease of transport across biological membranes. For some classes of compounds, such as intercalators, the use of charged partial surface area (CPSA) descriptors may also be appropriate. CPSAs encode the surface area and partial charge of the compound simultaneously. A more recent approach has been to link the functional group contributions determined by traditional QSAR and the pharmacophore geometry based on the steric and electrostatic fields presented to the active site on an enzyme. X-ray crystallographic data can also be used to predict interactions between enzymes, substrates, and inhibitors.

In general, structure–activity data alone do not appear to be sufficient to successfully predict *in vivo* lethality. However, the integration of descriptors based on the biological mechanisms of lethality should improve the ability of QSARs to correlate the LD_{50} values using large groups of unrelated compounds. The COMPACT (Computer Optimized Molecular Parametric Analysis for Chemical Toxicity) system is one such system developed by Parke et al. (61) that uses integrated molecular modeling to predict the mechanism of chemical toxicity. Using prior knowledge of receptor interactions, the particular receptor with which a compound interacts, the metabolic fate of the compound, and, in turn, its toxicity can be predicted from the molecular and electronic structures of the chemical. Ultimately, an analysis of a chemical structure using COMPACT could be combined with other QSAR predictions in order to select a drug candidate with the least toxic potential and with maximal pharmacological activity, prior to a compound being synthesized (60).

APPROACHES FOR EVALUATING HUMAN RISK

Risk can be defined as the probability of a hazard or injury occurring in man, animal, or the environment under a given set of conditions. Although a compound may be very toxic, risk may be minimal if there is a poor likelihood of exposure. Thus, the assessment of risk requires not only toxicity data, but also knowledge of the physical state, concentration, route, and frequency of exposure, physicochemical properties, structure–activity relations to similar compounds of known activity, and pharmacokinetic data from a relevant route of exposure. Physicochemical properties such as the volatility, solubility, and reactivity of a compound can be used to estimate the general likelihood of exposure. Other parameters, including molecular weight, ionization, steric properties, lipophilicity and protein binding, can be used to estimate the risk of exposure of the target cells. An optimal approach to modeling risk is to include and integrate as many of these parameters as possible with *in vitro* pharmacokinetic, metabolism, and toxicity data (80).

The development of an integrative approach for predicting human risk from *in vitro* data, as well as physicochemical properties and pharmacokinetics, can be facilitated by computerized model systems that incorporate an assortment of these complex *in vivo* and *in vitro* parameters. An analogy model can be built on the basis that a model system should behave analogously to the system that it predicts. Thus, the more similar the model system is to the predicted system, the more likely it is to contain relevant information. However, due to ethical considerations, we must increasingly rely on *in vitro* cytotoxicity model systems and physicochemical modeling and less on human and animal models.

Hellberg et al. (42) described a reasonable approach to the development of prediction models for human toxicity that combines several different and complementary model systems primarily based on *in vitro* and physicochemical data, supplemented by a limited number of *in vivo* systems. Multivariate data analysis was than applied to analyze the data, since this method can be used with a large number of possible colinear variables. In contrast, multiple regression analysis, typically used in modeling, is limited to applications in which the number of test systems is small compared to the number of chemicals in the study and the results may not be reliable if test systems are correlated. Multivariate analysis can be employed in analogy modeling by using the projection method PLS (partial least squares modeling) with cross-validation as described by Wold et al. (82–84). The PLS method is based on correlation studies between different data sets (*in vitro*, physicochemical, etc.) with the aim of finding combinations between the parameters of each set, then correlating between the combinations to predict *in vivo* toxicity (62). The individual contribution of each assay to the overall prediction can also be evaluated. The PLS method has been shown to handle multivariate data with strong correlations among the *x*-variables, as is seen with related *in vitro* cytotoxicity test systems. Applying this model to the first ten MEIC compounds, Hellberg et al. (42) showed that this model was relevant for predicting human toxicity using cytotoxicity data combined with physicochemical data.

The toxicity associated with most compounds appears to be related to basal cytotoxicity produced by interference with vital cell structures and/or functions essential for the survival and reproduction of cells which should be detected by almost any dividing cell. However, since a variety of mechanisms can lead to systemic toxicity and lethality, no single assay can be expected to be reliably predictive of human lethality for all compounds. In addition, some compounds produce organ-specific toxicity because the compound is selectively concentrated in the target tissue. For many of these compounds, pharmacokinetic information can be integrated with a battery of *in vitro* data to model the *in vivo* response, as previously described. However, other compounds adversely effect organ-specific functions by noncytotoxic receptor-mediated mechanisms, which cannot be accurately predicted using poorly differentiated cell systems. Thus, it will be difficult to completely eliminate the need for animal testing, but the numbers of animals can be effectively reduced by combining results of *in vitro* tests with pharmacokinetic studies in animals and with computer models based on structure activity.

REFERENCES

1. Allen RD, Allen NS, Travis JL. Video-enhanced contrast, differential interference contrast (AVIC-DIC) microscopy: a new method capable of analyzing microtubule-related motility in the reticulopodial network of *Allogromia laticollaris*. *Cell Motil* 1981;1:291–302.
2. Balant LP, Gex-Fabry M. Review: physiological pharmacokinetic modelling. *Xenobiotica* 1990; 20(11):1241–1257.
3. Balls M, Horner SA. The FRAME interlaboratory programme on *in vitro* cytotoxicology. *Food Chem Toxicol* 1985;23(2):209–213.
4. Benford DJ, Reavy HJ, Hubbard SA. Metabolizing systems in cell culture cytotoxicity tests. *Xenobiotica* 1988;18(6):649–656.
5. Bernson V, Bondesson I, Ekwall B, Stenberg K, Walum E. A multicentre evaluation study of *in vitro* cytotoxicity. *ATLA* 1987;14:144–146.
6. Bohm N, Sprenger E. Fluorescence cytophotometry: a valuable method for the quantitative determination of nuclear feulgen-DNA. *Histochemie* 1968;16:100–118.
7. Bondesson I, Ekwall B, Hellberg S, Romert L, Stenberg K, Walum E. MEIC: a new international multicenter project to evaluate the relevance to human toxicity of *in vitro* cytotoxicity tests. *Cell Biol Toxicol* 1989;5:331–347.
8. Borenfreund E, Puerner JA. A simple quantitative procedure using monolayer cultures for cytotoxicity assays (HTD/NR-90). *J Tissue Culture Methods* 1984;65:55–63.
9. Borenfreund E, Puerner JA. Toxicity determined *in vitro* by morphological alterations and neutral red absorption. *Toxicol Lett* 1985;24:119–124.
10. Brugmans, N, Cassiman, JJ, Van der Heydt, L, Oosterlinck, AJJ, Vlietinck, R, and Van den Berghe, H. Quantification of the degree of cell spreading of human fibroblasts by semiautomated analyses of the cell perimeter. *Cytometry*, 1982; 3:262–268.

11. Bunting WL, Kiely JH, Owen CA, Jr. Tadiochromium-labelled lymphocytes in the rat. *Proc Soc Exp Biol* 1963;113:370–374.
12. Chamberlain M, Parish WE. Hazard and risk based on *in vitro* test data. *Toxicol In Vitro* 1990; 4(4/5):694–697.
13. Clothier RH, Hulme LM, Ahmed AB, Reeves HL, Smith M, Balls M. In vitro cytotoxicity of 150 chemicals to 3T3-L1 cells assessed by the FRAME kenacid blue method. *ATLA* 1988;16:84–95.
14. Clothier RH, Hulme LM, Smith M, Balls M. Comparison of the *in vitro* cytotoxicities and acute *in vivo* toxicities of 59 chemicals. *Molec Toxicol* 1989;1:571–577.
15. DeLuca MA, McElroy WD. *Bioluminescence and chemiluminescence.* New York: Academic Press, 1981:122.
16. Dierickx PJ. Cytotoxicity testing of 114 compounds by the determination of the protein content in Hep G2 cell cultures. *Toxicol In Vitro* 1989;3:189–193.
17. Dierickx PJ, Ekwall B. Long-term cytotoxicity testing of the first twenty MEIC chemicals by the determination of the protein content in human embryonic lung cells. *ATLA* 1992;20:285–289.
18. Duffy PA. Mechanisms of cell toxicity: I. Cell death. *Toxicol In Vitro* 1992;6(1):91–92.
19. Ekwall B. Toxicity to HeLa cells of 205 drugs as determined by the metabolic inhibition test supplemented by microscopy. *Toxicology* 1980;17:273–295.
20. Ekwall B. Preliminary studies on the validity of *in vitro* measurement of drug toxicity using HeLa cells: IV. Therapeutic effects and side effects of 50 drugs related to the HeLa toxicity of the therapeutic concentrations. *Toxicol Lett* 1981;7:359–366.
21. Ekwall B. Screening of toxic compounds in mammalian cell cultures. *Ann NY Acad Sci* 1983; 407:64–77.
22. Ekwall B, Acosta D. In vitro comparative toxicity of selected drugs and chemicals in HeLa cells, Chang liver cells, and rat hepatocytes. *Drug Chem Toxicol* 1982;5:219–231.
23. Ekwall B, Bondesson I, Castell JV, et al. Cytotoxicity evaluation of the first ten MEIC chemicals: acute lethal toxicity in man predicted by cytotoxicity in five cellular assays and by oral LD50 tests in rodents. *ATLA* 1989;17:83–100.
24. Ekwall B, Bondesson I, Hellberg S, Hogberg J, Romert L, Stenberg K, Walum E. Validation of *in vitro* cytotoxicity tests: past and present strategies. *ATLA* 1991;19(2):226–233.
25. Ekwall B, Gomez-Lechon MJ, Hellberg S, et al. Preliminary results from the Scandinavian multicentre evaluation of *in vitro* cytotoxicity (MEIC). *Toxicol In Vitro* 1990;4(4/5):688–691.
26. Ekwall B, Johannson A. Preliminary studies on the validity of *in vitro* measurement of drug toxicity using HeLa cells: I. Comparative *in vitro* toxicity of 27 drugs. *Toxicol Lett* 1980;5:299–307.
27. Ekwall B, Nordensten C, Albanus L. Toxicity of 29 plasticizers to HeLa cells in the MIT-24 system. *Toxicology* 1982;24:199–210.
28. Fautrel A, Chesne C, Guillouzo A, et al. A multicentre study of acute *in vitro* cytotoxicity in rat liver cells: validation of *in vitro* cytotoxicity tests. *Toxicol In Vitro* 1991;5:543–547.
29. Fedoroff, S. Proposed usage of animal tissue culture terms. *In Vitro* 1966;2:155–159.
30. Fry JR, Garle MJ, Hammond AH. Choice of acute toxicity measures for comparison of *in vitro/in vivo* toxicity. *ATLA* 1988;16:175–179.
31. Fry JR, Garle MJ, Hammond AH, Hatfield A. Correlation of acute lethal potency with *in vitro* cytotoxicity. *Toxicol In Vitro* 1990;4(3):175–178.
32. Gillette JR. Factors affecting drug metabolism. *Ann NY Acad Sci* 1971;179:43–66.
33. Gillette JR. Problems in correlating *in vitro* and *in vivo* studies of drug metabolism. In: Benet LZ, Levy G, Ferraiolo BL, eds. *Pharmacokinetics: a modern view.* New York: Plenum, 1984:235–252.
34. Gillette JR. Solvable and unsolvable problems in extrapolating toxicological data between animal species and strains. In: Mitchell JR, Horning G, eds. *Drug metabolism and drug toxicity.* New York: Raven, 1984:237–260.
35. Gillette JR. Pharmacokinetics of biological activation and in activation of foreign compounds. In: Anders MW, ed. *Bioactivation of foreign compounds.* New York: Academic Press, 1985.
36. Gillette JR. On the role of pharmacokinetics in integrating results from *in vivo* and *in vitro* studies. *Food Chem Toxicol* 1986;24(6/7):711–720.
37. Goto Y, Dujovne CA, Shoeman DW, Arakawa K. Liver cell culture toxicity of general anaesthetics. *Toxicol Appl Pharmacol* 1976;36:121–130.
38. Gratzner HG. Monoclonal antibody to 5-bromo- and 5-iododeoxyuridine: a new reagent for detection of DNA replication. *Science* 1982;218:474.
39. Gulden M, Finger J. Effects of the first twenty MEIC reference chemicals on viability, glucose consumption and spontaneous contractility of primary cultured rat skeletal muscle cells. *ATLA* 1992;20:222–225.

40. Hansch C, Maloney PP, Fujita T, Muir RM. *Nature* 1962;194:178–180.
41. Hayflick L, Moorhead PS. The serial cultivation of human diploid cell strains. *Exp Cell Res* 1961;25:585.
42. Hellberg S, Eriksson L, Jonsson J, et al. Analogy models for prediction of human toxicity. *ATLA* 1990;18:103–116.
43. Holm G, Perlmann P. Quantitative studies on phytohaemagglutinin-induced cytotoxicity by human lymphocytes against homologous cells in tissue culture. *Immunology* 1967;12:525–536.
44. Horner SA, Fry JR, Clothier RH, Balls M. A comparison of two cytotoxicity assays for the detection of metabolism-mediated toxicity *in vitro*: a study with cyclophosphamide. *Xenobiotica* 1985;15: 681–686.
45. Ivett JL, Tice RR. Average generation time: a new method of analysis and quantitation of cellular proliferation kinetics. *Environ Mutagen* 1982;4:358.
46. Jackson TR, Hallam J, Downes CP, Hanley MR. Receptor coupled events in bradykinin action: rapid production of inositol phosphates and regulation of cytosolic Ca^{2+} in a neural cell line. *EMBO J* 1987;6:49–54.
47. Jover R, Ponsoda X, Castell JV, Gomez-Lechon MJ. Evaluation of the cytotoxicity of ten chemicals on human cultured hepatocytes: predictability of human toxicity and comparison with rodent cell culture systems. *Toxicol In Vitro* 1992;6(1):47–52.
48. Kemp RB, Cross DM, Meredith RWJ. Adenosine triphosphate as an indicator of cellular toxicity *in vitro*. *Food Chem Toxicol* 1986;24(6/7):465–466.
49. Kemp RB, Cross DM, Meredith RWJ. Comparison of cell death and adenosine triphosphate content as indicators of acute toxicity *in vitro*. *Xenobiotica* 1988;18(6):633–639.
50. Khochbin S, Chabanas A, Albert P, Albert J, Lawrence J-J. Application of bromodeoxyuridine incorporation measurements to the determination of cell distribution within the S phase of the cell cycle. *Cytometry* 1988;9:499–503.
51. Knox P, Uphill PF, Fry JR, Benford J, Balls M. The FRAME multicentre project on *in vitro* cytotoxicology. *Food Chem Toxicol* 1986;24(6/7):457–463.
52. Laughton G. Quantification of attached cells in microtiter plates based on Coomassie brilliant blue G-250 staining of total cellular protein. *Anal Biochem* 1983;140:417–423.
53. Litterst CL, Lichtenstein EP. Effects and interactions of environmental chemicals on human cells in tissue culture. *Arch Environ Health* 1971;22:454.
54. Lowry OH, Rosebrough NJ, Farr AL, Randall RJ. Protein measurement with the Folin phenol reagent. *J Biol Chem* 1951;193:265–271.
55. Maile W, Lindl T, Weiss DG. New methods for cytotoxicity testing: quantitative video microscopy of intracellular motion and mitochondria-specific fluorescence. *Mol Toxicol* 1987;1:427–437.
56. Mosmann T. Rapid colorimetric assay for cellular growth and survival: application of proliferation and cytotoxicity assays. *J Immunol Methods* 1983;65:55–63.
57. Nagele RG, Lee H. A new method for the preparation of "double-fixed" quick-frozen, freeze-substituted cells for whole-cell transmission electron microscopy. *J Microsc* 1987;148:89–95.
58. Olson R, Santone K, Medler D, Oakes SG, Abraham R, Powis G. An increase in intracellular free Ca^{2+} associated with serum free growth stimulation of Swiss 3T3 fibroblasts by epidermal growth factor in the presence of bradykinin. *Biol Chem* 1988;263:18,030–18,035.
59. Otoguro K, Komiyama K, Omura S, Tyson CA. An *in vitro* cytotoxicity assay using rat hepatocytes and MTT and Coomassie blue dye as indicators. *ATLA* 1991;19:352–360.
60. Parke DV, Ioannides C, Lewis DFV. Computer modelling and *in vitro* tests in the safety evaluation of chemicals-strategic applications. *Toxicol In Vitro* 1990;4(4/5):680–685.
61. Parke DV, Lewis DFV, Ioannides C. Current procedures for the evaluation of chemical safety. In: Richardson ML, ed. *Risk assessment of chemicals in the environment*. London: Royal Society of Chemistry, 1988:45–72.
62. Peloux A-F, Federici C, Bichet N, Gouy D, Cano J-P. Hepatocytes in primary culture: an alternative to LD50 testing? Validation of a predictive model by multivariate analysis. *ATLA* 1992;20:8–26.
63. Phillips JC, Gibson WB, Yam J, Alden CL, Hard GC. Survey of the QSAR and *in vitro* approaches for developing non-animal methods to supersede the *in vivo* LD_{50} test. *Food Chem Toxicol* 1990;28(5):375–398.
64. Pomerat CM, Leake CD. Short term cultures for drug assays: general considerations. *Ann NY Acad Sci* 1954;58:1110–1124.
65. Purchase IFH, Farrar DG, Whitaker IA. Toxicology profiles on substances used in the FRAME cytotoxicology research project. *ATLA* 1987;14:184–242.
66. Putney JW. Calcium-mobilizing receptors. *Trends Pharmacol Sci* 1987;8:481–486.

67. Rasmussen H. The cycling of calcium as an intracellular messenger. *Sci Am* 1989;261(4):66–73.
68. Reinhardt CA, Pelli DA, Zbinden G. Interpretation of cell toxicity data for estimation of potential irritation. *Food Chem Toxicol* 1985;23:247.
69. Richards GP, Bemis JA, Sample JD. A simple planimetric method to quantify cytotoxicity in cell culture monolayers. *J Virol Methods* 1988;20:33–38.
70. Riddell RJ, Clothier RH, Balls M. An evaluation of three *in vitro* cytotoxicity assays. *Food Chem Toxicol* 1986;24(6/7):469–471.
71. Shirhatti V, Krishna G. A simple and sensitive method for monitoring drug-induced cell injury in cultured cells. *Anal Biochem* 147:410–418.
72. Shrivastava R, Delomenie C, Chevalier A, John G, Ekwall B, Walum E, Massingham R. Comparison of *in vivo* acute lethal potency and *in vitro* cytotoxicity of 48 chemicals. *Cell Biol Toxicol* 1992;8(2):157–170.
73. Shrivastava R, John GW, Rispat G, Chevalier A, Massingham R. Can the *in vivo* maximum tolerated dose be predicted using *in vitro* techniques? A working hypothesis. *ATLA* 1991;19:393–402.
74. Sorenson EMB. Validation of a morphometric analysis procedure using indomethacin-induced alterations in cultured hepatocytes. *Toxicol Lett* 1989;45:101–110.
75. Stark DM, Shopsis C, Borenfreund E, Babich H. Progress and problems in evaluating and validating alternative assays in toxicology. *Food Chem Toxicol* 1986;24(6/7):449–455.
76. Stoker M, O'Neill C, Berryman S, Waxman V. Anchorage and growth regulation in normal and virus-transformed cells. *Int J Cancer* 1968;3:683.
77. Takasugi M. An improved fluorochromatic cytotoxic test. *Transplant* 1971;12:148–151.
78. Toplin I. A tissue culture cytotoxicity test for large-scale cancer chemotherapy screening. *Cancer Res* 1959;19:959–965.
79. Walker PMB. The mitotic index and interphase processes. *J Exp Biol* 1954;31:8.
80. Walum E, Balls M, Bianchi V, et al. ECITTS: an integrated approach to the application of *in vitro* test systems to the hazard assessment of chemicals. *ATLA* 1992;20:406–428.
81. Westphal C, Horler H, Pentz S, Frosch D. A new method for cell culture on an electron-transparent melamine foil suitable for successive LM, TEM and SEM studies of whole cells. *J Microsc* 1988;150:225–231.
82. Wold S, Albano S, Dunn WJ 3rd, et al. Multivariate data analysis in chemistry. In: Kawalski BR, ed. *Chemometrics: mathematics and statistics in chemistry*. Dordrecht: D. Reidel, 1984;17–96.
83. Wold S, Dunn WJ 3rd. Multivariate quantitative structure-activity relationships (QSAR): conditions for their applicability. *J Chem Inform Comp Sci* 1983;23:6–13.
84. Wold S, Ruhe A, Wold H, Dunn WJ 3rd. The colinearity problem in linear regression: the partial least squares (PLS) approach to generalized inverses. *SIAM J Stat Comput* 1984;5:735–743.
85. Yuhas JM, Toya RE, Pazmino NH. Neuraminidase and cell viability: failure to detect cytotoxic effects with dye-exclusion techniques. *JNCI* 1974;53(2):465–468.
86. Zanetti C, Angelis ID, Stammati A-L, Zucco L. Evaluation of toxicity testing of 20 MEIC chemicals on Hep-2 cells using two viability endpoints. *ATLA* 1992;20:120–125.

In Vitro Toxicology,
edited by Shayne Cox Gad.
Raven Press, Ltd., New York, © 1994.

6

Pyrogenicity and Muscle Irritation

Shayne Cox Gad

Toxicology, SYNERGEN, Boulder, Colorado 80301

Pyrogenicity and muscle irritation are product hazard end points of concern in those parts of the health care industry where the body surface is penetrated and the product is introduced into the region of the blood vessels ("fluid path") and/or into the muscles. This generally encompasses many medical devices (syringes, catheters, and so on) and biologicals and pharmaceuticals which are administered parenterally.

Pyrogenicity is the induction of a febrile (fever) response by the parenteral (usually IV or IM) administration of exogenous material, usually bacterial endotoxins. Pyrogenicity is usually associated with microbiological contamination of a final formulation or product but is now increasingly of concern because of the increase in interest in biosynthetically produced materials. Generally, ensuring the sterility of product and process will guard against pyrogenicity. Pyrogenicity testing is performed extensively in the medical device industry. If a device is to be introduced directly or indirectly into the fluid path, it is required that it be evaluated for pyrogenic potential.

Muscle irritation is the local inflammation, pain, and damage that result from the parenteral injection of pharmaceuticals into a muscle mass. It is due to a range of physicochemical factors as well as chemical/biological interactions, and is particularly of concern with antibiotics.

PYROGENICITY

Both *in vivo* and *in vitro* tests are currently in use. The *in vitro* test is preferred except for those cases in which it may not be employed.

In Vivo

The *United States Pharmacopeia* specifies a pyrogen test using rabbits as a model. This test is the standard for limiting risks of a febrile reaction to an acceptable level, and involves measuring the rise in body temperature in a group of three rabbits for 3 hr after injection of 10 ml of test solution.

Apparatus and Diluents

Render the syringes, needles, and glassware free from pyrogens by heating at 250°F for not less than 30 min or by any other suitable method. Treat all diluents and solutions for washing and rinsing of devices or parenteral injection assemblies in a manner that will ensure that they are sterile and pyrogen-free. Periodically perform control pyrogen tests on representative portions of the diluents and solutions for washing or rinsing of the apparatus.

Temperature Recording

Use an accurate temperature-sensing device such as a clinical thermometer, or thermistor probes or similar probes that have been calibrated to ensure an accuracy of ±0.1°C and have been tested to determine that a maximum reading is reached in less than 5 min. Insert the temperature-sensing probe into the rectum of the test rabbit to a depth of not less than 7.5 cm and, after a period of time (not less than that previously determined as sufficient), record the rabbit's temperature.

Test Animals

Use healthy, mature rabbits. House the rabbits individually in an area of uniform temperature between 20°C and 23°C and free from disturbances likely to excite them. The temperature should vary no more than ±3°C from the selected temperature. Before using a rabbit for the first time in a pyrogen test, condition it not more than 7 days before use by a sham test that includes all of the steps described under Procedure, except injection. Do not use a rabbit for pyrogen testing more frequently than once every 48 hr, or prior to 2 weeks following a maximum rise in its temperature of 0.6°C or more while being subjected to the pyrogen test, or after it has been given a test specimen that was adjusted to be pyrogenic.

Procedure

Perform the test in a separate area designated solely for pyrogen testing and under environmental conditions similar to those under which the animals are housed and free from disturbance likely to excite them. Withhold all food from the rabbits used during the period of the test. Access to water is allowed at all times, but may be restricted during the test. If rectal-temperature-measuring probes remain inserted throughout the testing period, restrain the rabbits with light-fitting Elizabethan collars that allow the rabbits to assume a natural testing posture. Not more than 30 min prior to the injection of the test dose, determine the "control temperature" of each of the test dose animals, allowing for later determination of any temperature increase resulting from the injection of a test solution. In any one group of test rabbits, use only those rabbits whose control temperatures do not vary by more than 1°C from each other, and do not use any rabbit with a temperature exceeding 39.8°C.

Unless otherwise specified in the individual protocol, inject into an ear vein of each of three rabbits 10 ml of the test solution per kg of body weight, completing each injection within 10 min after the start of administration. The test solution is either the product, constituted if necessary as directed on the label, or the material under test. For pyrogen testing of devices or injection assemblies, use washings or rinsings of the surfaces that come in contact with the parenterally administered material or with the injection site or internal tissues of the patient. Ensure that all test solutions are protected from contamination. Perform the injection after warming the test solution to a temperature of 37 ± 2°C. Record the temperature at 1, 2, and 3 hr after the injection.

Test Interpretation and Continuation

Consider any temperature decrease as zero rise. If no rabbit shows an individual rise in temperature of 0.6°C or more above its respective control temperature, and if the sum of the three individual maximum temperature rises does not exceed 1.4°C, the product meets the requirements for the absence of pyrogens. If any rabbit shows an individual temperature rise of 0.6°C or more, or if the sum of the three individual maximum temperature rises exceeds 1.4°C, continue the test using five other rabbits. If not more than three of the eight rabbits show individual rises in temperature of 0.6°C or more, and if the sum of eight individual maximum temperature rises does not exceed 3.7°C, the material under examination meets the requirements for the absence of pyrogens.

In Vitro

Pyrogenicity (or bacterial endotoxin testing) is one of the great success stories for *in vitro* testing. Some 15 years ago, the limulus amebocyte lysate (LAL) test was developed, validated, and accepted as an *in vitro* alternative (2,15) to the rabbit test. An *in vitro* test for estimating the concentration of bacterial endotoxins that may be present in or on the sample of the article(s) to which the test is applied uses LAL that has been obtained from aqueous extracts of the circulating amebocytes of the horseshoe crab, *Limulus polyphemus*, and that has been prepared and characterized for use as an LAL reagent for gel–clot formation. The test's limitation is that it detects only the pyrogens of Gram-negative bacteria. This is generally not significant since most environmental contaminants that gain entrance to sterile products are Gram-negative (3).

Where the test is conducted as a limit test, the specimen is determined to be positive or negative to the test judged against the endotoxin concentration specified in the individual monograph. Where the test is conducted as an assay of the concentration of endotoxin, with calculation of confidence limits of the result obtained, the specimen is judged to comply with the requirements if the result does not exceed (a) the concentration limit specified in the individual monograph, and (b) the specified confidence limits for the assay. In either case the determination of the reaction end point is made with parallel dilutions of redefined endotoxin units.

Since LAL reagents have also been formulated to be used for turbidimetric (including kinetic) assays or colorimetric readings, such tests may be used if shown to comply with the requirements for alternative methods. These tests require the establishment of a standard regression curve and the endotoxin content of the test material is determined by interpolation from the curve. The procedures include incubation for a preselected time of reacting endotoxin and control solutions with LAL reagent and reading the spectrophotometric light absorbance at suitable wavelengths. In the case of the turbidimetric procedure the reading is made immediately at the end of the incubation period. In the kinetic assays, the absorbance is measured throughout the reaction period and rate values are determined from those readings. In the colorimetric procedure the reaction is arrested at the end of the preselected time by the addition of an appropriate amount of acetic acid solution prior to the readings. A possible advantage in the mathematical treatment of results, if the test is otherwise validated and the assay suitably designed, could be the confidence interval and limits of potency from the internal evidence of each assay itself.

Reference Standard and Control Standard Endotoxins

The reference standard endotoxin (RSE) is the USP Endotoxin Reference Standard, which has a defined potency of 10,000 USP endotoxin units (EU) per vial. Constitute the entire contents of one vial of the RSE with 5 ml of LAL reagent water, vortex for not less than 20 min, and use this concentrate for making appropriate serial dilutions. Preserve the concentrate in a refrigerator, for making subsequent dilutions, for not more than 14 days. Allow it to reach room temperature, if applicable, and vortex it vigorously for not less than 5 min before use. Vortex each dilution for not less than 1 min before proceeding to make the next dilution. Do not use stored dilutions. A control standard endotoxin (CSE) is an endotoxin preparation other than the RSE that has been standardized against the RSE. If a CSE is a preparation not already adequately characterized, its evaluation should include characterizing parameters both for endotoxin quality and performance (such as reaction in the rabbit), and for suitability of the material to serve as a reference (such as uniformity and stability). Detailed procedures for its weighing and/or constitution and use to ensure consistency in performance should also be included. Standardization of CSE against the RSE using an LAL reagent for the gel–clot procedure may be effected by assaying a minimum of four vials of the CSE or four corresponding aliquots, where applicable, of the bulk CSE and one vial of the RSE, as directed under Test Procedure, but using four replicate reaction tubes at each level of the dilution series for the RSE and four replicate reaction tubes similarly for each vial or aliquot of the CSE. If the dilutions for the four vials or aliquots of the CSE cannot all be accommodated with the dilutions for the one vial of the RSE on the same rack for incubation, additional racks may be used for accommodating some of the replicate dilutions for the CSE, but all of the racks containing the dilutions of the RSE and CSE are incubated as a block. However, in such cases, the replicate dilution series from the one vial of the RSE are accommodated together on a single rack and the replicate dilution series from any one of the four vials or aliquots of the CSE are not divided between racks. The antilog of the difference between the mean log 10 end point of the RSE and the mean log 10 end point of the CSE is the standardized potency of the CSE, which is then converted to and expressed in units/ng under stated drying conditions for the CSE, or units per container, whichever is appropriate. Standardize each new lot of CSE prior to use in the test. Calibration of a CSE in terms of the RSE must be with the specific lot of LAL reagent and the test procedure with which it is to be used. Subsequent lots of LAL reagent from the same source and with similar characteristics need only checking of the potency ratio. The inclusion of one or more dilution series made from the RSE when the CSE is used for testing will enable observation of whether or not the relative potency shown by the latter remains within the determined confidence limits. A large lot of a CSE may, however, be characterized by a collaborative assay of a suitable design to provide a representative relative potency and the within-laboratory and between-laboratory variance.

A suitable CSE has a potency of not less than 2 EU/ng and not more than 50 EU/ng, where in bulk form, under adopted uniform drying conditions, e.g., to a particular low moisture content and other specified conditions of use, and a potency within a corresponding range where filled in vials of a homogeneous lot.

Preparatory Testing

Use an LAL reagent of confirmed label or determined sensitivity. In addition, where there is to be a change in lot of CSE, LAL reagent, or another reagent, conduct tests of a prior satisfactory lot of CSE, LAL, and/or other reagent in parallel on changeover. Treat any containers or utensils employed so as to destroy extraneous surface endotoxins that may be present, such as by heating in an oven at 250°F or above for sufficient time.

The validity of test results for bacterial endotoxins requires an adequate demonstration that specimens of the article, or of solutions, washings, or extracts thereof to which the test is to be applied, do not of themselves inhibit or enhance the reaction or otherwise interfere with the test. Validation is accomplished by testing untreated specimens or appropriate dilutions thereof, concomitantly with and without known and demonstrable added amounts of RSE or a CSE, and comparing the results obtained. Appropriate negative controls are included. Validation must be repeated if the LAL reagent source or the method of manufacture or formulations of the article is changed.

Test for Confirmation of Labeled LAL Reagent Sensitivity

Confirm the labeled sensitivity of the particular LAL reagent with the RSE (or CSE) using not less than four replicate vials, under conditions shown to achieve an acceptable variability of the test, *viz.*, the antilog of the geometric mean log 10 lysate gel–clot sensitivity is within 0.5 to 2.0, where the labeled sensitivity is in EU/ml. The RSE (or CSE) concentrations selected to confirm the LAL reagent label potency should bracket the stated sensitivity of the LAL reagent. Confirm the labeled sensitivity of each new lot of LAL reagent prior to use in the test.

Inhibition or Enhancement Test

Conduct assays, with standard endotoxin, of untreated specimens in which there is no endogenous endotoxin detectable, and of the same specimens to which endotoxin has been added, as directed under Test Procedure, but use not less than four replicate reaction tubes at each level of the dilution series for each untreated specimen and for each specimen to which endotoxin has been added. Record the end points (E, in units/ml) observed in the replicates. Take the logarithms (e) of the end points, and compute the geometric means of the log end points for the RSE (or CSE) for the untreated specimens and for specimens containing endotoxin by the formula antilog, e/f, where e is the sum of the log end points of the dilution series used and f is the number of replicate end points in each case. Compute the amount of endotoxin in the specimen to which endotoxin has been added. The test is valid for the article if this result is within twofold of the known added amount of endotoxin. Alternatively, if the test has been appropriately set up, the test is valid for the article if the geometric mean end-point dilution for the specimen to which endotoxin has been added is within one twofold dilution of the corresponding geometric mean endpoint dilution of the standard endotoxin.

Repeat the test for inhibition or enhancement using specimens diluted by a factor not exceeding that given by the formula, x/y, (see Maximum Valid Dilution, below). Use the least dilution sufficient to overcome the inhibition or enhancement of the known added endotoxin for subsequent assays of endotoxin in test specimens.

If endogenous endotoxin is detectable in the untreated specimens under the conditions of the test, the article is unsuitable for the inhibition or enhancement test, or it may be rendered suitable by removing the endotoxin present by ultrafiltration or by appropriate dilution. Dilute the untreated specimen (as constituted, where applicable, for administration or use) to a level not exceeding the maximum valid dilution, at which no endotoxin is detectable. Repeat the test for inhibition or enhancement using the specimens at those dilutions.

Test Procedure

In preparing for and applying the test, observe precautions in handling the specimens in order to avoid gross microbial contamination. Washings or rinsings of devices must be with LAL reagent water in volumes appropriate to their use and, where applicable, of the surface area which comes into contact with body tissues or fluids. Use such washings or rinsings if the extracting fluid has been in contact with the relevant pathway or surface for not less than 1 hr at controlled room temperature (15–30°C). Such extracts may be combined, where appropriate.

For validating the test for an article, for endotoxin limit tests or assays, or for special purposes where so specified, testing of specimens is conducted quantitatively to determine response end points for gel–clot readings. Usually graded strengths of the specimen and standard endotoxin are made by multifold dilutions. Select dilutions so that they correspond to a geometric series in which each step is greater than the next lower by a constant ratio. Do not store diluted endotoxin, because of loss of activity by absorption. In the absence of supporting data to the contrary, negative and positive controls are incorporated into the test.

Use not less than two replicate reaction tubes at each level of the dilution series for each specimen under test. Whether the test is employed as a limit test or as a quantitative assay, a standard endotoxin dilution series involving not less than two replicate reaction tubes is conducted in parallel. A set of standard endotoxin dilution series is included for each block of tubes, which may consist of a number of racks for incubation together, provided the environmental conditions within blocks are uniform.

Preparation

Since the form and amount per container of standard endotoxin and of LAL reagent may vary, constitution and/or dilution of contents should be as directed in the labeling. The pH of the test mixture of the specimen and the LAL reagent is in the range of 6.0–7.5 unless specifically directed otherwise in the individual monograph. The pH may be adjusted by the addition of sterile, endotoxin-free sodium hydroxide or hydrochloric acid or suitable buffers to the specimen prior to testing.

Maximum Valid Dilution

The maximum valid dilution (MVD) is appropriate to injections or to solutions for parenteral administration in the form constituted or diluted for administration, or, where applicable, to the amount of drug by weight if the volume of the dosage form for administration could be varied. Where the endotoxin limit concentration is specified in the individual monograph in terms of volume (in EU/ml), divide the limit by γ, which is the labeled sensitivity (in EU/ml) of the lysate employed in the assay, to obtain the MVD factor. Where the endotoxin limit concentration is specified in the individual monograph in terms of weight or of units of active drug (in EU/mg or in EU/unit), multiply the limit by the concentration (in mg/ml or in units/ml) of the drug in the solution tested or of the drug constituted according to the label instructions, whichever is applicable, and divide the product of the multiplication by γ to obtain the MVD factor. The MVD factor so obtained is the limit dilution factor for the preparation for the test to be valid.

Procedure

To 10×75-mm test tubes add aliquots of the appropriately constituted LAL reagent and the specified volumes of specimens, endotoxin standard, negative controls, and a positive product control consisting of the article, or of solutions, washings, or extracts thereof, to which the RSE (or a standardized CSE) has been added at a concentration of endotoxin of 2 for LAL reagent (see under Test for confirmation of labeled LAL reagent sensitivity). Swirl each gently to mix and place in an incubating device such as water bath or heating block, accurately recording the time at which the tubes are so placed. Incubate each tube, undisturbed, for 60 ± 2 min at $37 \pm 1°C$, and carefully remove it for observation. A positive reaction is characterized by the formation of a firm gel that remains when inverted through 180 degrees. Record such a result as a positive ($+$). A negative result is characterized by the absence of such a gel or by the formation of a viscous gel that does not maintain its integrity. Record such a result as a negative ($-$). Handle the tubes with care, and avoid subjecting them to unwanted vibrations, or false-negative observations may result. The test is invalid if the positive product control or the endotoxin standard does not show the end-point concentration to be within $\pm$ twofold dilutions from the label claim sensitivity of the LAL reagent or if any negative control shows a gel–clot end point.

Calculation and Interpretation

Calculate the concentration of endotoxin (in units/ml or in units/g or mg) in or on the article under test by the formula: pS/U, where S is the antilog of the geometric mean log 10 of the end points, expressed in EU/ml for the standard endotoxin; U is the antilog of e/f, where e is the log 10 of the end-point dilution factors, expressed in decimal fractions, and f is the number of replicate reaction tubes read at the endpoint level for the specimen under test; and p is the correction factor for those cases where a specimen of the article cannot be taken directly into test but is processed as an extract, solution, or washing.

Where the test is conducted as an assay with sufficient replication to provide a suitable number of independent results, calculate for each replicate assay the concentration of endotoxin in or on the article under test from the antilog of the geometric mean log end-point ratios. Calculate the mean and the confidence limits from the replicate logarithmic values of all the obtained assay results by a suitable statistical method.

Interpretation

The article meets the requirements of the test if the concentration of endotoxin does not exceed that specified in the individual monograph, and the confidence limits of the assay do not exceed those specified.

IRRITATION OF PARENTERALLY ADMINISTERED AGENTS

Intramuscular (IM) and intravenous (IV) injection of parenteral formulations of pharmaceuticals can produce a range of discomfort resulting in pain, irritation, and/or damage to muscular or vascular tissue. These are normally evaluated for prospective formulations before use in humans by histopathological evaluation of damage in intact animal models, usually the rabbit (4,5,11). Attempts have been made to make this *in vivo* methodology both more objective and quantitative based on measuring the creatinine phosphokinase released in the tissue surrounding the injection site (4,12). Currently, a protocol utilizing a cultured rat skeletal muscle cell line (L6) as a model has been evaluated in an interlaboratory validation program among 11 pharmaceutical company laboratories. This methodology (17) measures creatine kinase levels in media after exposure of the cells to the formulation of interest, and predicts *in vivo* IM damage based on this end point. It is reported to give excellent rank-correlated results across a range of antibiotics (16). The current multilaboratory evaluation covers a broader structural range of compounds and has shown a good quantitative correlation (with *in vivo* results) for antibiotics and a fair correlation for a broader range of parenteral drug products. Likewise, Kato et al. (7) have proposed a model which uses cultured rat primary skeletal muscle fibers. Damage is evaluated by the release of creatinine phosphokinase. An evaluation using six parenterally administered antibodies (rashing their EC_{50} values) showed good relative correlation with *in vivo* results.

Another proposed *in vitro* assay for muscle irritancy for injectable formulations is the red blood cell hemolysis assay (1). Water-soluble formulations are gently mixed in a 1:2 ratio with freshly collected human blood for 5 sec, then mixed with a 5% w/v dextrose solution and centrifuged for 5 min. The percent red blood cell survival is then determined by measuring differential absorbance at 540 nm, and this is compared against values for known irritants and nonirritants. Against a very small group of compounds (four), this is reported to be an accurate predictor of muscle irritation.

REFERENCES

1. Brown S, Templeton L, Prater DA, Potter CJ. Use of an *in vitro* hemolysis test to predict tissue irritancy in an intramuscular formulation. *J Parenter Sci Technol* 1989;43:117–120.
2. Cooper JF. Principles and applications of the limulus test for pyrogen in parenteral drugs. *Bull Parenter Drug Assoc* 1975;3:122–130.
3. Devleeschouwer MJ, Cornil MF, Dony J. Studies on the sensitivity and specificity of the limulus amebocyte lysate test and rabbit *pyrogen* assays. *Appl Environ Microbiol* 1985;50:1509–1511.
4. Gad SC, Chengelis CP. *Acute toxicity: principles and methods.* Caldwell, NJ: Telford Press, 1988.
5. Gray JF. Pathological evaluation of injection injury. In: Robinson J, ed. *Sustained and controlled release drug delivery systems.* New York: Marcel Dekker, 1978:351–405.
6. Hoover D, Gardner J, Timmerman T, Klepfer A, Laska D, White S, McGrath J, Buening M, Williams P. Comparison of *in vitro* and *in vivo* models to assess venous irritation of parenteral antibiotics. *Fundam Appl Toxicol* 1990;14:578–597.
7. Kato I, Harihara A, Mizushima Y. An in vitro method for assessing muscle irritation of antibotics using rat primary cultured skeletal muscle fibers. *Toxicol Appl Pharmacol* 1992;117:194–199.
8. Laska DA, Williams PD, Reboulet JT, Morris RM. The L6 muscle cell line as a tool to evaluate parental products for irritation. *J Parenter Sci Technol* 1991;45(2):77–82.
9. Meltzer HY, Morozak S, Bozer M. Effect of intramuscular injections on serum creatinine phospho-kinase activity. *Am J Med Sci* 1970;259:42–48.
10. Nelson AA, Price CW, Welch H. Muscle irritation following the injection of various penicillin preparations in rabbits. *J Am Pharm Assoc* 1949;38:237–239.
11. Shintani S, Yarmazaki M, Nakarmura M, Nakazama I. A new method to determine the irritation of drugs after intramuscular injection in rabbits. *Toxicol Appl Pharmacol* 1967;11:293–301.
12. Sidell FR, Calver DL, Kaminskis A. Serum creatine phosphokinase activity after intramuscular injection. *JAMA* 1974;228:1884–1887.
13. United States Pharmacopeia. Bacterial endotoxins test. USP XXII—The United States Pharmacopeia. Rockville, MD: USP Convention, 1990:1493–1495.
14. United States Pharmacopeia. Pyrogen test. USP XXII—The United States Pharmacopeia. Rockville, MD: USP Convention, 1990:1515.
15. Weary M, Baker B. Utilization of the limulus amebocyte lysate test for pyrogen testing of large-volume parenterals, administration sets and medical devices. *Bull Parenter Drug Assoc* 1977; 31:127–133.
16. Williams PD, Masters BG, Evans LD, Laska DA, Hattendorf GH. An *in vitro* model for assessing muscle irritation due to parenteral antibiotics. *Fundam Appl Toxicol* 1987;9:10–17.
17. Young MF, Trobetta LD, Sophia JV. Correlative *in vitro* and *in vivo* study of skeletal muscle irritancy. *Toxicologist* 1986;6(1):1225.

In Vitro Toxicology,
edited by Shayne Cox Gad.
Raven Press, Ltd., New York, © 1994.

7

In Vitro Assays for Developmental Toxicity

Stephen G. Whittaker and Elaine M. Faustman

*Department of Environmental Health, University of Washington,
Seattle, Washington 98195*

The observation that the conceptus is uniquely sensitive to the action of certain chemical and physical agents has served to fuel the considerable interest in developmental toxicology. A classic example of one such chemical is thalidomide. This sedative/hypnotic drug elicits congenital malformations in humans at dosages considerably lower than those required to induce overt toxicity in the mothers. Other drugs prescribed for human use that are proven teratogens include diethylstilbesterol and certain synthetic retinoids.

As reported by Warburton and Fraser (1), the frequency of early spontaneous abortion in humans is at least 15% of all recognized pregnancies. Approximately 3% of liveborns have major congenital malformations; birth defects account for 20% of postnatal deaths (reviewed in ref. 2). It has been estimated that there are no known causal associations for 55–70% of birth defects. Thus, crucial questions are raised. First, what fraction of miscarriages and abnormalities reflects intrinsic properties of the human reproductive process? Second, what is the contribution of external factors, such as environmental and industrial exposure, to this high frequency of fetal wastage?

Recognizing the need to determine adverse effects of reproduction and development, a series of toxicological safety evaluation protocols were developed in the mid-1960s. Consisting of three experimental segments, this approach is the current method by which rats and/or rabbits are used to detect potential hazard to human reproduction and development. The Segment II protocol is generally recognized as the most powerful experimental component, since the test agent is administered to pregnant females throughout the period of embryonic development. However, these standard *in vivo* tests are expensive and require extensive facilities and considerable technical expertise (3,4). There are between 50,000 and 70,000 chemicals currently in the marketplace, existing either as untested drugs, industrial by-products, or environmental pollutants (5). Furthermore, an additional 700–1000 of such agents are introduced each year. Clearly, the screening of this many agents is totally impractical using the standard assays for *in vivo* teratogenicity.

In vitro tests for developmental toxicity have been proposed as a means by which chemicals of concern may be prioritized for further *in vivo* screening. The aim is to reduce the use of animals in teratology testing and increase the rate of screening. The combination of *in vivo* and *in vitro* methods may yield optimal information on the spectrum of effects on the developing conceptus. For example, such short-term assays are useful in structure–activity analyses, in which the relative potencies of structurally related agents may be assessed. Additionally, the mechanisms underlying the developmental toxicity of chemical and physical agents may be readily studied in such assays.

There are two major factors that contribute to the difficulties associated with designing *in vitro* test systems for teratogenicity. The first is that the mechanisms of teratogenicity are poorly understood. Second, the process of development includes a very complex sequence of proliferation and differentiation processes. There is no unifying "somatic mutation theory" for the process of teratogenicity. Consequently, *in vitro* systems have been proposed that monitor a variety of end points, including cell death, altered cell–cell interactions, cell migration, reduced biosynthesis, altered cellular, biochemical and morphological differentiation, mechanical disruption, and growth inhibition. Two major philosophical approaches have been taken to design these *in vitro* testing systems for teratogenicity (6). The first approach has modeled such systems after "like" events, where processes such as regeneration, reaggregation, and cell–cell communication are monitored as a model process which has characteristics similar to those of the *in vivo* developmental process. Examples of these assays include the mouse ovarian tumor cell assay (7) and the hydra assay (8). The second approach to *in vitro* testing for teratogenicity is to design systems which allow the investigator to examine limited aspects of embryogenesis ("windows" of development). Examples of this approach include monitoring chondrogenesis in limb bud cultures and monitoring early organogenesis in rodent postimplantation cultures. In these approaches either limited time periods during gestation are monitored or limited organ system processes are observed *in vitro*.

The systems currently under development for *in vitro* developmental toxicity screening are summarized in Table 1. It should be emphasized that successful application of *in vitro* techniques is critically dependent upon the reliability of the test procedures. The assays should be reproducible between laboratories, possess readily quantifiable end points that are relevant to *in vivo* systems, and exhibit sensitivity (i.e., few false-negatives) and specificity (i.e., few false-positives).

This review specifically aims to summarize the current approaches under development for screening for developmental toxicants *in vitro*. Particular emphasis is placed on the end points monitored, sensitivity, specificity, and, where available, validation data.

TABLE 1. *Summary of developmental toxicity assays*

Intact embryo/fetus	**Cell culture**
Mammals	*Primary cell cultures*
Preimplantation	Drosophila embryo cells
Postimplantation	Chick embryo neural retina cells
Other vertebrates	Neural cells
Chick	*Established cell lines*
Fish	Mouse ovarian tumor cells
Frog	Neuroblastoma cells
Invertebrates	Embryonal stem cells
Insects	Vaccinia-infected cell lines
Hydra	Cell–cell communication
	Teratocarcinoma cell lines
	Human embryonic palatal mesenchyme cells
Intact organ culture	
Limb bud	
Palatal shelves	

PRIMARY CELL CULTURE

Nonmammalian Species

Drosophila Embryo Cell Culture

Primary cultures of embryonic drosophila cells have been proposed by the author as an *in vitro* teratogen screening system (9–11). These cultures differentiate into several cell types: Neuroblasts form neurons and organize into ganglia, and myoblasts form myotubes. Differentiation is quantitated using an automated image analyzer; a positive response is indicated by a statistically significant reduction in the number of myotubes or ganglia compared to controls. Over 150 chemicals (including both teratogens and nonteratogens and structurally related compounds) have been tested. A low false-negative rate (<10%) was observed (12,13). A microsomal monooxygenase fraction from either rats or drosophila has been added to these cultures, and an enhancement of the effect of cyclophosphamide was observed (14).

Chick Embryo Neural Cell Culture

The chick neural cell culture technique (15) has been proposed as a teratogen screen by Daston and Yonker (16). Neural retinas derived from day-6 chick embryos are dissociated into single cells and incubated in the presence of test chemical for 24 h. After several days in culture, cells differentiate to form tissue layers that are comparable to those in the intact retina. The following end points may be quantifiably assessed: number and size of aggregated cells, protein content, histology, and protein expression. Daston et al. (17) reported the testing of 17 substances with this system; accuracy was 94% compared to mammalian *in vivo* data.

Mammalian Species

Limb Bud Cells

Single cell suspensions derived from both rodent and avian embryonic limb buds can be cultured via trypsinization and plating at high cell density. The attached cells proliferate and differentiate into chondrocytes over a 5- to 6-day culture period (18–23).

Several differentiation-specific processes can be monitored *in vitro*, including cell aggregation, cell condensation, and cellular differentiation into cartilagenous tissue (6). General cytotoxicity can be monitored via staining with the vital dye, neutral red. Differentiation can be quantified using the cartilage-specific stain, alcian blue, or by monitoring $^{35}SO_4^{2-}$ incorporation into proteoglycans. Effects of test compounds on differentiation are quantitatively expressed as inhibition of alcian blue staining or radiolabel incorporation.

The teratogenic potency of a number of chemicals was assessed in a validation study involving 25 test chemicals by determining the concentration of compound that reduces alcian blue staining to 50% of concurrent control values (or IC_{50}) (18,19,21,24–26). These laboratories reported that the IC_{50} values of teratogens are similar to the doses required to elicit teratogenicity *in vivo*. Kistler (27) determined the *in vitro* activity of 25 retinoids in the limb bud cell culture system and concluded that this system may be useful as a preliminary screen to select nonteratogenic retinoids.

This system is sensitive to teratogens that perturb differentiation-specific processes, in addition to those that inhibit overall cell growth and proliferation. The extensive validation studies using both limb bud and neuronal cells will be discussed in detail in the next section (25).

Guntakatta et al. (20) employed double radiolabeling techniques in which limb bud cells are cultured in the presence of [^{3}H]thymidine (labels DNA) and $^{35}SO_4^{2-}$ (incorporated into sulfated proteoglycans). This assay was designed to monitor specific disruption of extracellular matrix protein and glycoprotein synthesis which leads to reduction in cartilage proteoglycan. Thus, a $^3H/^{35}S$ ratio of >1 indicates specific inhibition of proteoglycan synthesis, suggesting teratogenic potential. Nineteen of 22 known mouse teratogens inhibited proteoglycan or DNA synthesis; five nonteratogens failed to elicit selective inhibition. The overall predictive accuracy of the limb bud cell system was approximately 89%, and the false-negative rate was approximately 15%. No false-positives were observed.

Neural Cells

Neural crest and midbrain neural cells have been successfully cultured and undergo differentiation *in vitro* (18,28). Neural crest cells are derived from explanted segments of neural tube and are dissociated, trypsinized, and plated. In the presence of fetal bovine serum, these cells differentiate into pigment-containing melanocytes after 6 days in culture (18,29). If horse serum is present, they differentiate into neuron-like cells. The effects of 14 known teratogens and nonteratogens have been monitored in this *in vitro* system. Alterations in the growth and differentiation of these cells included detachment of cells, vacuolation, altered melanocyte or neuronal morphology, and inhibition of differentiation. A positive relationship between teratogenicity *in vivo* and alterations in these cultures was noted (18,29).

The use of micromass cultures derived from embryonic midbrains has been developed and extensively characterized in the laboratory of Oliver Flint while at ICI Pharmaceuticals (25,28,30). Neuronal cell cultures are established by trypsinizing embryonic midbrain (mesencephalon) tissues, preparing single cell suspensions, and plating at high cell density. Biochemical and morphological differentiation of neuronal cell foci occurs after 5 days of culture. This differentiation is monitored by staining the cultures with hematoxylin and quantitating differentiation by automated image analysis. Flint has verified that the foci observed in these cultures are primarily neuronal cells by selective silver-staining techniques, reaction of monoclonal antibodies directed against neuronal ganglioside markers, and radiolabeled neurotransmitter uptake (28). Additionally, our laboratory is actively investigating the presence of several differentiation-specific and cytoskeletal markers in midbrain cultures. Our immunohistochemical analysis confirms the presence of differentiated cells that possess neuron-specific markers, such as GQ ganglioside, neural cell adhesion molecule (NCAM), microtubule-associated protein 2 (MAP2), MAP 5, neuron-specific enolase, and acetylated tubulin (31). Using differentiation-related expression of the protooncogene *src* and neurofilament protein, Sweeney and Faustman (32,33) were able to show dose-related decreases in protein expression. Such markers of neuronal differentiation may prove to be useful indicators of chemical alterations. Ribeiro and Faustman (34,35) conducted cell-cycle analyses on the micromass cultures and demonstrated the utility of examining alterations in cellular kinetics in identifying chemical induced perturbations of these cells.

In an extensive validation effort, Flint and Orton (25) evaluated the responses of midbrain and limb bud cell cultures to 46 compounds (27 teratogens and 19 nonteratogens) in a blind trial. A complete monooxygenase system was successfully included in these cultures to provide metabolizing enzymes. Inhibition of differentiation (i.e., alcian blue staining) was monitored as an indicator of potential teratogenicity; concentrations of test compounds inhibiting differentiation to 50% of control values were determined. Of 27 teratogens, 25 inhibited either neuronal or limb bud differentiation. Only two false-negatives were observed: 2,4-dichlorophenoxyacetic acid and thalidomide. If cell density was reduced, thalidomide did cause inhibition of limb bud differentiation. Eleven percent (2/19) of the nonteratogens inhibited neuronal or limb differentiation. Glutethimide (structurally related to thalidomide) and dimenhydrinate (both nonteratogens *in vivo*) inhibited differentiation in both cultures. If inhibition of differentiation in one cell type alone was examined, then predictability went from 90% (both assays) to 85% for neuronal cells and 82% for limb bud cells. Flint and co-workers have examined a series of structurally related teratogenic and nonteratogenic compounds. The accuracy of the assay was sufficient to differentiate among the developmental toxicity of three pairs of structurally related compounds. The contribution of the exogenous monooxygenase system and metabolism by the differentiating cultures themselves is under further investigation (36–39).

Based on the utility of the micromass assay for identifying developmental toxicants, this system was recognized by the European Federation of Pharmaceutical Industries as having promising potential.

ESTABLISHED CELL LINES

Mouse Ovarian Tumor Cells

This assay relies on the assumption that teratogens that interfere with embryonic cell interactions also inhibit lectin-mediated attachment of cells. Mice are inoculated with ascitic mouse ovarian tumor cells one week before the experiment is performed. Approximately 12 hr before use, the cells are radioactively labeled by intraperitoneal injection with [³H]thymidine. Cells are then harvested, exposed to test chemical, and allowed to sediment on concanavalin-A-coated polyethylene disks. The amount of radioactivity associated with the disks after washing indicates the extent of cell attachment. Inhibition of attachment at noncytotoxic concentrations has been used by the authors to indicate a potential teratogen. In a validation effort involving 102 test agents, 60 of the 74 teratogens (81%) inhibited cell attachment; 21 of the 28 nonteratogens (75%) were noninhibitory (40,41). Nineteen percent of the teratogens tested (14/74) did not specifically inhibit attachment, possibly reflecting effects on DNA replication or mitosis. Refer to the following section for combined validation results with the palatal mesenchymal cell assay.

Thalidomide was scored as a positive in this system when a complete system for monooxygenation was included (42). Braun et al. (42) investigated the relationship between attachment inhibition and *in vivo* teratogenicity. For 54 of the 60 inhibitory teratogens, they found a significant correlation between the inhibitory *in vitro* dose and the lowest reported *in vivo* teratogenic dose.

Human Embryonic Palatal Mesenchymal Cells

A line of human embryonic palatal mesenchymal (HEPM) cells derived from a day-55 human abortus has been extensively characterized and proposed as a screening assay for teratogens (43–46). The HEPM cells consist of undifferentiated fibroblast-like diploid cells with a stable chromosomal complement, high plating efficiency (>90%), and a cell-cycle transit time of approximately 2 hr.

The theory underlying this assay is that teratogens will cause growth inhibition of these rapidly proliferating embryonic cells. Dose–response curves for cell growth inhibition are generated and an IC_{50} value is established. Growth inhibition is assayed by determining cell number as a percentage of control in the presence of the test compound. Growth inhibition below a test chemical concentration of 1 mM was postulated to reflect potential teratogenicity. Thirty-five teratogenic and 20 nonteratogenic compounds were tested in a series of validation assessments. The test compounds were compiled from agents suggested by the Environmental Protection Agency (EPA) consensus workshop (47) and included most of the false-negatives from the mouse ovarian tumor (MOT) assay validation studies (7,40). The HEPM assay correctly identified 23 of the 35 (66%) teratogens as true-positives in this assay and identified 12 of the 20 (60%) nonteratogens as true-negatives. Combining the results from the tumor cell assay of Braun et al. (7,40) and the HEPM assay yields an overall predictability of 90%; the rate of false-negatives is 3%. Incorporation of an exogenous metabolic activation system in the HEPM assay yielded concentration-dependent inhibition of growth by cyclophosphamide. The inhibitory concentrations were comparable to those observed in the whole-embryo culture system.

The NIEHS (through the National Toxicology Program) evaluated the MOT assay (7) and the HEPM assay (44,45). This evaluation study used 44 coded compounds (30 animal teratogens and 14 nonteratogens). These agents were tested in each assay in two different laboratories (47–49). The optimal combined MOT/HEPM assay is approximately 70% accurate and has a greater than 80% sensitivity value (50,51). These assay results agreed with *in vivo* teratogenicity data for 60–70% of test chemicals, depending on the assay used. Draus et al. (24) compared the effects of some 20 compounds in the HEPM growth inhibition assay and the mouse limb bud assay. Using rat liver S9 systems when metabolic activation was required, preliminary results suggest that the mouse limb bud assay may be a more sensitive assay.

Neuroblastoma Cells

Mummery et al. (52) proposed using differentiating murine neuroblastoma cells in culture as predictors of teratogenicity. Such cells differentiate into neurites in culture under specific culture conditions; both growth inhibition and stimulation of differentiation can be monitored in the presence of test chemicals. Thirty-nine teratogens and 18 nonteratogens were tested for their ability to induce differentiation and inhibit growth. Eighty-six percent of the test compounds were correctly identified as teratogens. The authors contend that the proportions of both false-negatives (10%) and false-positives (22%) were comparable to other *in vitro* teratogenicity screening systems.

Embryonal Stem Cells

Laschinski et al. (53) describe an *in vitro* developmental toxicity screen using embryonal stem cells (ESCs) derived from mouse blastocysts. The concentration of test chemical that elicits cytotoxicity in these pluripotent euploid cells is compared to corresponding data from day-14 mouse embryo fibroblasts. The authors determined that the embryonal stem cells showed a higher sensitivity to known teratogens than did fibroblast cultures. Thus, an A/D ratio is calculated, where A corresponds to the differentiated fibroblasts and D is represented by the undifferentiated embryonal stem cells. Comparing the *in vitro* ESC results with *in vivo* teratogenicity data from mice revealed a 31% false-negative rate (i.e., 5 of 16 chemicals tested). However, the authors stress the need to incorporate exogenous biotransformation systems in the assay.

Vaccinia-Infected Cell Lines

The ability of primate-derived cell cultures to suppress infection by vaccinia virus has been proposed as a teratogen-screening test (54). Vaccinia-infected monolayers are exposed to the test compound. After a 24- to 46-hr incubation at 37°C, the number of active viruses released from infected cells is determined by counting plaques. Infected monolayers that are either untreated or treated with solvent alone serve as controls. The rationale underlying this system is that viruses will only reproduce if they infect actively proliferating cells. Furthermore, virion replication involves a complex sequence of genetic and molecular events that are postulated to reflect differentiation-like processes. In validation studies, vaccinia-WR-infected BSC 40 cell monolayers were exposed to 42 teratogens and nine nonteratogens. Thirty-three of the 42 (79%) teratogens tested inhibited virus proliferation, and eight of the nine (89%) nonteratogens were noninhibitory. Six of the 42 (14%) teratogens were false-negatives, and three teratogens stimulated the virus. One out of nine (11%) nonteratogens was a false-positive. The assay was sensitive to two agents known to require metabolic activation. Qualitative comparisons between the RD_{50} (dose producing 50% inhibition/stimulation compared to a control infected culture) and the lowest reported teratogenic dose *in vivo* suggested a linear correlation ($r = 0.98$). To determine whether this viral assay detects differentiation-specific effects rather than general growth inhibition, the cytotoxic effects of each teratogen at the RD_{50} were assayed on uninfected cell cultures. Only six of the 42 teratogens were positive for cytotoxicity. The viral end point was considerably more reliable than any of these cytotoxicity end points in predicting teratogenicity, suggesting that the assay is monitoring specific rather than general effects.

The teratogens used in this assay were separated into (a) "molecular teratogens," agents that acted on DNA information, storage, and transfer, and (b) "morphogenetic teratogens," which interfered with cytoplasmic metabolism and with cytoskeleton and surface recognition. The highest correlation to *in vivo* results was seen with the "molecular teratogens"; however, 82% of the "morphogenetic teratogens" were also correctly assigned.

Cell–Cell Communication Assay

Inhibition of intercellular communication during critical periods of organogenesis has been proposed as the mechanism of action for certain teratogens. Inhibition of gap-junction-mediated communication is monitored using the metabolic cooperation assay (55–57). This system involves assaying the recovery of a few (usually 100) 6-thioguanine-resistant cells (HGPRT$^-$) in the presence of an excess (usually 4×10^5 cells) of 6-thioguanine-sensitive cells (HGPRT$^+$). Under control conditions, a phosphorylated 6-thioguanine product from HGPRT$^+$ cells is transferred via gap junctions to HGPRT$^-$ cells. Incorporation of this phosphorylated product into cellular DNA results in the death of both cell populations. However, inhibition of cell–cell communication results in the recovery of HGPRT$^-$ cells. Such assays are interpreted as positive only when chemical concentrations that elicit rescue of HGPRT$^-$ cells are neither cytostatic nor cytotoxic. Originally proposed as an assay for tumor promoters, it is evident that many other critical biological processes are mediated via cell–cell communication (56,57). A series of compounds with varying teratogenic potential have been tested (58–63), including a series of ethylene glycol derivatives, diphenylhydantoin, warfarin, phorbol esters, phenoxyacetic acid derivatives, retinoids, and nonteratogens such as saccharin and ascorbic acid. Known teratogens were shown to inhibit metabolic cooperation at concentrations equivalent to those effective in *in vivo* teratogenicity studies; the nonteratogens saccharin and ascorbic acid failed to inhibit metabolic cooperation over these concentration ranges.

Since a variety of well-established nonteratogenic tumor promoters inhibit metabolic cooperation *in vitro*, the use of this system as a screen for teratogens is still uncertain (60). Some teratogens may elicit developmental toxicity primarily through inhibition of cell–cell communication. Recent modifications of the metabolic cooperation assay such as monitoring intercellular communication in human cell lines, such as HEPM cells, may maximize the information obtainable from a single assay (64).

Teratocarcinoma Cell Lines

Hulme et al. (65) described the use of a differentiating teratocarcinoma cell line as an *in vitro* developmental toxicity screen. Originally derived from a mouse testicular teratocarcinoma, these cells can be stimulated to differentiate by retinoic acid treatment. Differentiation is monitored by determining synthesis of laminin. Thus the effects of test agents on differentiation in undifferentiated, differentiating, and differentiated cells may be determined. Only six chemicals have been tested thus far in this system, so its utility is unknown at this time. One potential confounding aspect of this system is that retinoic acid, itself an *in vivo* teratogen, is required to stimulate differentiation.

WHOLE-ANIMAL SYSTEMS

Nonmammalian Systems

Chick

The chick embryo has been extensively utilized in developmental toxicity studies. Chemically induced perturbation of development is readily amenable to analysis following injection of test agent into the subgerminal yolk or chorioallantoic vessels. Embryos or chicks (in egg hatchability studies) are subsequently examined for structural and skeletal abnormalities.

In 1967 the World Health Organization recommended against the use of this *in ovo* system because of its nonmammalian pharmacokinetics and high, nonspecific sensitivity. Subsequently, considerable effort has been expended in characterizing and standardizing the chick embryotoxicity screening test (CHEST) (66–72). Modifications of the *in ovo* system have facilitated the simultaneous screening of genotoxicity and embryotoxicity (73,74). Jelinek et al. (67) reported the testing of 130 substances for their ability to cause death, malformations, and growth retardation *in ovo*. The lower portion of the embryotoxicity dose–response curve was determined for 117 out of the test agents. Of the 13 "nonembryotoxic" agents, four had solubility limitations and nine reached 'unrealistic' amounts. Numerous agents requiring metabolic activation were detected as positive in this system. However, the absence of maternal metabolism and drug distribution, in addition to differences in the functional properties of the membranes surrounding the chick embryo, represent severe disadvantages (5). Clearly, this system requires extensive review and validation to assess its utility.

Fish

A variety of fish systems have been utilized in the study of reproductive and developmental toxicity (75–77). Fish embryos represent a simple vertebrate system in which the embryo can be manipulated and monitored throughout the entire developmental period. Fish species utilized for such studies include Japanese medaka, zebra fish, rainbow trout, and fathead minnows. Assays can be performed in static systems (in which eggs are placed in deep Petri dishes) or in flow-through systems (in which water is continually circulated) (75). Alternatively, embryos may be microinjected with test agent (78). End points such as hatchability, larval mortality, and teratogenicity may be monitored, and a standardized morphological scoring system has been developed (79). Exogenous monooxygenase systems may be added to the fish system. Additionally, endogenous piscine monooxygenase systems may be induced (78,80,81).

Several compounds have been tested for developmental toxicity in these fish systems, including metals (75,76,82), pesticides (75,83), carcinogens (84–88), and complex mixtures (78). Birge et al. (76) tested 34 inorganic elements and 25 organic compounds in multiple fish and amphibian populations. These investigators reported that the rainbow trout was generally the most sensitive species to teratogenic effects when compared to goldfish, largemouth bass, sunfish, and amphibians. However, channel catfish embryos were more sensitive to mercury than were rainbow trout embryos. Although a variety of malformation types were observed, upwards of 80–90% of the gross anomalies identified in fish embryos following exposure to either inorganic or organic toxicants affected the skeletal system. Further characterization of dose–exposure-time relationships is required before this response can be generalized.

Frog

Utilized extensively as a model system for developmental biology, *Xenopus laevis* has only recently been used for teratological screening (76,89–93). The frog embryo teratogenesis assay, *Xenopus* (FETAX), monitors effects on the blastula stage through hatching to swimming tadpoles. Critical end points include: swimming behavior, lethality, no observable effect concentrations, developmental stage attained, growth, motility, pigmentation, and gross anatomical observations.

An embryonic teratogenic index (TI) is determined by dividing the concentration of chemical that causes 50% abnormal surviving tadpoles (EC_{50}) by the concentration that kills 50% of the embryos (LC_{50}) (90). TI values of ≥ 1.0 indicate teratogenic potential; TI values < 1.0 indicate embryotoxicity or co-effective teratogenicity. Dumont and Epler (89) tested 34 known teratogens and six nonteratogens; only three false-negatives were observed, but the false-positive rate was higher. Exposure of FETAX blastulae to 5-azacytidine and methotrexate yielded positive results; pseudoepedrine was moderately positive; amaranth and aspartame were negative (94). Ethanol and caffeine are weak and moderate teratogens, respectively, in the FETAX assay; 5-fluorouracil is a strong teratogen (95). FETAX has been used for studies with mixtures of toxicants (96).

Sabourin et al. (93) compared the efficacy of the frog system with the hydra and planaria systems for four known mammalian teratogens. The frog embryo system offered several advantages over the other systems because of its numerous end points and was distinctly more sensitive than the planarian assay. However, since the FETAX assay is run for only 96 hr, late developmental effects such as limb dismorphogenesis are not monitored.

Insects

The *Drosophila melanogaster* screen involves deposition of eggs onto a nutrient medium containing test chemical (97). The developing fly feeds on this medium; exposure is throughout the metamorphosis period from egg through third instar to pupa formation. Numerous morphological abnormalities and distinct abnormality patterns are seen in adult flies. Advantages to this system include the capacity to absorb, circulate, metabolize, and excrete chemicals (98). However, it is impossible to precisely define the chemical concentrations to which the eggs are exposed. Several chemicals and physical treatments [heat (99)] have been used to induce abnormalities in drosophila. However, most compounds tested have been water-soluble (97). An NTP validation study is currently underway.

Cricket embryos have been examined as an invertebrate teratology model (100). End points such as number of compound eyes are monitored after exposure to a variety of individual compounds, as well as to complex organic mixtures.

Hydra

The hydra reaggregation and differentiation assay evaluates the effects of test chemicals on adult hydra, as well as on an "artificial hydra embryo" (8,101,102). Adult hydra are exposed to a test substance, and the minimal toxic concentration is determined. Subsequently, dissociated hydra cells are allowed to reform adult, free-standing hydra. The "embryo" is exposed to test chemical during this process of whole-body regeneration. The dose of the test compound causing toxicity in the adult hydra (A) is then compared to the dose causing developmental toxicity in the "embryo" (D) by generating an A/D ratio. An A/D ratio greater than 1 has been used by the authors to identify compounds that are selectively more toxic to the developing organism and has been proposed as a method to identify teratogenic hazard. Thalidomide and vinblastine yielded A/D ratios of 60 and 30, respectively (101). However, most substances yield ratios near unity, suggesting lack of selective developmental toxicity. A modification of the hydra assay compares the effects of test substances on intact adult polyps with effects on the regenerating isolated adult digestive system (103). Thus, effects on re-differentiation versus reorganization can be investigated.

The utility of this assay is suggested by the authors from the observation that of 30 agents tested, close agreement of the A/D ratio in the *in vitro* assay to *in vivo* A/D ratios in mammals was observed (93,101,104,105). Structure–activity relationships for a series of glycols and glycol ethers were examined in the hydra assay, and a series of predictions of their potential *in vivo* teratogenicity was suggested (106). However, Welsch (59) cautions that *in vivo* studies with glycol ethers show dramatically different A/D ratio for such compounds compared to the A/D ratios observed in the hydra assay. Other investigators have also questioned the utility of A/D ratio for hazard prediction (107,108). Clearly, an extensive validation effort is required to critically determine the utility of this assay.

Other Invertebrates

Several other invertebrates have been proposed for teratogenicity testing, including planaria (93,109,110), sea urchin embryos (111–114), and brine shrimp larvae

(115,116). However, none of these systems have been sufficiently well characterized or validated.

Mammalian Whole Embryos

Preimplantation Embryos

The preimplantation stage represents a critical period in embryonic development because the organism consists of relatively few pluripotent cells. Consequently, the preimplantation embryo is a potentially sensitive target for developmental toxicants.

Fertilized eggs of mice, rats, and rabbits are readily cultured from the one-cell stage through blastocyst stages (6,117–123). A variety of experimental manipulations are possible, including (a) treatment *in vivo* followed by culturing *in vitro*, (b) culturing in serum from treated rodents, or (c) treatment *in vitro* followed by reimplantation into foster dams (117,120–126). End points monitored in preimplantation embryo culture can include lethality, morphological alterations, growth retardation, micronucleus formation, sister chromatid exchange, and biochemical changes such as oxygen utilization, nucleic acid synthesis, specific protein synthesis, and isozyme pattern changes (117,120,122,126,127). Since cytochrome P450 monooxygenases have been detected in preimplantation mouse embryos (128), it may be possible to detect both direct- and indirect-acting agents in these cultures. Although the effects of chemical agents on preimplantation embryos depend on the number of affected cells (129), exposure to mutagens early in development has been shown to yield abnormalities (6,125,130–132). However, the primary effect of exposure during preimplantation is lethality and growth retardation (6,121,122). Agents tested in the preimplantation embryo culture system include cancer chemotherapeutic compounds (133,134), hormones (135), polycyclic aromatic hydrocarbons (136), metals (127), miscellaneous therapeutic agents (137,138), ethylene oxide (131), and radiation (127).

Postimplantation Embryos

The whole-embryo culture technique has been utilized extensively as an *in vitro* screen for developmental toxicants (139–149). Rat or mouse embryos are explanted from the uterus at early somite stages, placed into culture medium, and maintained in culture from 24 hr to 4 days. During this period of early organogenesis, embryonic growth and development can be supported over most of this postimplantation embryonic phase, up to 72 hr (142,149,150). Modifications of the culture technique have allowed extension of the culture period (151–156), but the success rate is relatively low and impractical for routine teratogenicity testing.

The end points routinely monitored in whole-embryo culture include viability, gross and histological abnormalities, growth, and macromolecular content. Although several morphological scoring systems have been developed in attempts to standardize, quantitate, and objectively evaluate the extensive embryonic development that occurs in postimplantation culture (157–159), further efforts are required before general embryotoxicity and specific teratogenic effects can be distinguished (4).

Chemicals requiring metabolic activation can be assessed in this system by inclusion of exogenous biotransformation systems (postmitochondrial supernatant or microsomes) (139,160–163), co-cultivation with hepatocytes (164,165), or culture in the presence of serum from treated humans and monkeys for embryo culture medium (166,167). However, Juchau et al. (168,169) reported that cultured rat conceptuses contain cytochrome P450 in sufficient quantities to elicit biotransformation. Both Ferrari et al. (170) and Flynn et al. (171) reported that sera from women with a history of chronic spontaneous abortion affects *in vitro* development of postimplantation embryos when used as an embryo culture medium.

Agents that have been tested in the postimplantation culture system include: vitamins and antimetabolites (172,173), metals (174–176), ethanol and its metabolites (177,178), caffeine (179), salicylates (180–183), cyclophosphamide and its metabolites (160,184–187), hydroxyurea (188), chlorambucil (189), DES and E2 (190,191), retinoic acid and its derivatives (192–195), solvents (196), saccharin (197), immunosuppressive agents (198), miscellaneous cancer chemotherapeutic agents (199,200), antibiotics (201), diphenylhydantoin (202), thalidomide (203), urethane (204), valproic acid (202,205), hyperthermia (206–208), fungal toxins (209–212), ethylating and methylating agents (213,214), aromatic amines and their metabolites (162,163,168,215–218), glycol ethers (219), nitroheterocyclic compounds (220), and substituted phenols (221). Bechter et al. (192) showed excellent qualitative and quantitative correlations between whole-embryo culture and *in vivo* teratogenicity for five structurally related retinoids.

However, carefully controlled validation studies using this culture system are rare. The majority of the studies referred to above have focused primarily on mechanistic teratology and assessments of structure–activity relationships. Schmid (140) tested 38 chemicals in this system, including 19 known *in vivo* teratogens and 19 compounds reported to have no adverse effects on *in utero* development, and reported good agreement of *in vivo* and *in vitro* results. Similarly, Sadler et al. (222) compared the *in vivo* and *in vitro* results for four compounds and reported concordance with *in vivo* responses for these agents. However, *in vivo* pharmacokinetic considerations are essential when using this system as a screen for developmental toxicants (222). Thus, this system is useful for the screening of close structural analogues when data for *in vivo* developmental toxicity of related compounds exist (223).

ORGAN CULTURE

Limb Buds

Originally applied in the laboratories of Shepard and Kochhar, the limb bud culture system is one of the most well-characterized organ culture systems. Rodent limbs are excised from embryos at approximately 10–11 days (33–45 somite stage, mouse). Morphological differentiation *in vitro* is highly consistent, reproducible, and complex (6,149). At the 10- to 11-day stage, the limb buds are largely undifferentiated, containing only blastema and surrounding epithelium but with minimal collagen or glycosaminoglycans. After 7 days in culture, these explants develop cartilaginous bone structures representing scapula, humerus, ulna, radius, and hand skeleton (226). The following developmental end points can be monitored: cell proliferation, differential growth, nucleic acid and protein content, morphogenetic cell death, size and shape of limb parts, chondrogenesis, and collagen or proteoglycan biosynthesis (227).

Concentration–response relationships for abnormal development have been established using quantitative assessments of limb development. Neubert (6) described a scoring system for morphogenetic differentiation which assigns a score to each bone rudiment and digit. Thus, a statistical analysis of treatment effects in addition to the detection of gross abnormalities may be performed (149).

Numerous *in vivo* teratogens induce abnormal development in limb buds *in vitro*. These agents include antimetabolites (228), alkylating agents (227,229–234), thalidomide derivatives (235), pesticides (236), analgesics and antirheumatics (237), caffeine (238), sulfonamides (239), and vitamins and derivatives (227).

The main advantage of organ culture is that complex interactions of different mechanisms can be studied in the developing organ. However, this is a laborious technique and lacks complete metabolic activation, although exogenous biotransformation systems have been incorporated into the system (229,240).

Palatal Shelves

Both Shiota et al. (241) and Buckalew and Abbott (242) described a technique for the cultivation of explanted palates from mouse fetuses by a suspension culture technique. The palates of day-12 fetuses close within 72 hr of culture, and those of day-13 fetuses within 48 hr. Both groups report that the *in vitro* fusion of palatal shelves accurately mimics *in vivo* development. Abbott (243) examined the responses of embryonic palates to retinoic acid, dexamethasone, and TCDD. The resultant data were difficult to interpret; it was determined that cofactors were essential in the response of this defined system to teratogens.

CONCLUSIONS

The need to prioritize substances according to their developmental toxicity hazard potential has been the driving force behind the development of *in vitro* test systems. Clearly, the standard multisegment *in vivo* teratology tests cannot be applied to the many thousands of untested substances to which humans are exposed.

The *in vitro* systems of most use are those that allow determinations of specific effects on development. Assays in which generalized cytotoxicity can be distinguished from differentiation-specific effects are also of considerable utility. Examples of this latter class of assay are whole-embryo culture, limb bud organ culture, and primary cell cultures of limb buds and neural tissue.

As stated in the introductory paragraphs of this chapter, such assays are useful only when test procedures are proven to be reliable in the hands of investigators other than those of the originator. Despite the large number of reviews (4–6,108, 120,139,146,223,244–249) and conferences (250–254) held on the topic of *in vitro* developmental toxicity test validation, the utility of many of the *in vitro* assays described in this review is unknown, since the required extensive interlaboratory validation efforts have not been performed. The problems associated with validation of short-term assays in general are delineated earlier in this book, and many of those principles apply here. Issues specific for *in vitro* developmental toxicity assays are as follows: (a) Selection of chemicals is problematic since the assignment of potential developmental toxicity is usually not a simple + or − call but is dose-dependent; (b) there are very few human teratogens identified and minimal good segment II studies for comparative evaluation of the true human teratogens; and (c) which *in vitro* end points/alterations should be used to label the test chemicals as developmental toxicants or teratogens?

In vitro systems do appear to be useful for prioritizing chemicals or determining gradients of chemical potencies. A powerful use is in the testing of structurally related compounds with different teratogenic potencies. Currently, there is a lack of organized studies in which the same agents (>100) are tested in several systems.

To conclude, the use of *in vitro* systems as predictors of animal or human teratogenicity is questionable at the present without the necessary validation experiments. However, reliable and validated assays hold great promise as prescreens for prioritizing chemicals for subsequent testing in pregnant animals. Additionally, they are of considerable utility in the elucidation of mechanisms of actions of teratogens.

ACKNOWLEDGMENTS

Appreciation is expressed for the valuable editorial and secretarial assistance of Zamyat Kirby and Azure Morgan Skye and for support by NIH ES-03157 and ES-07032.

REFERENCES

1. Warburton D, Fraser FC. Spontaneous abortion risks in man: data from reproductive histories collected in a medical genetics unit. *Hum Genet* 1964;16:1–12.
2. Manson JM, Wise LD. Teratogens. In: Amdur MO, Doull J, Klaassen CD, eds. *Casarett and Doull's toxicology*. New York: Pergamon Press, 1991;226–254.
3. Palmer AK. The design of subprimate animal studies. In: Wilson JG, Fraser FC, eds. *Handbook of teratology*, vol 4. New York: Plenum Press, 1978;215–253.
4. Brown NA, Freeman SJ. Alternative tests for teratogenicity. *ATLA* 1984;12:7–23.
5. Peters PWJ, Piersma AH. *In vitro* embryotoxicity and teratogenicity studies. *Toxicol In Vitro* 1990;4:570–576.

6. Neubert D. The use of culture techniques in studies on prenatal toxicity. *Pharmacol Ther* 1982; 18:397–434.
7. Braun AG, Emerson DJ, Nichinson BB. Teratogenic drugs inhibit tumor cell attachment to lectin-coated surfaces. *Nature* 1979;282:507–509.
8. Johnson EM, Goman RM, Gabel GEG, George ME. The *Hydra attenuata* system for detection of teratogenic hazards. *Teratogenesis Carcinog Mutagen* 1982;2:263–276.
9. Bournias-Vardiabasis N, Teplitz RL. Use of drosophila embryo cell cultures as an *in vitro* teratogen assay. *Teratogenesis Carcinog Mutagen* 1982;2:333–341.
10. Bournias-Vardiabasis N, Teplitz RL, Chernoff GF, Seecof RL. Detection of teratogens in the drosophila embryonic cell culture test: assay of 100 chemicals. *Teratology* 1983;28:109–122.
11. Buzin CH, Bournias-Vardiabasis N. Teratogens induce a subset of small heat shock proteins in drosophila primary embryonic cell cultures. *Proc Natl Acad Sci USA* 1984;81:4075–4079.
12. Bournias-Vardiabasis N. Letter to the editor—alternative tests for teratogens. *Reprod Toxicol: A Med Lett* 1985;4:10.
13. Bournias-Vardiabasis N, Buzin CH, Reilly JG. The effect of 5-azacytidine and cytidine analogs on *Drosophila melanogaster* cells in culture, *Roux's Arch Dev Biol* 1983;192:299–302.
14. Bournias-Vardiabasis N, Flores J. Drug metabolizing enzymes in *Drosophila melanogaster*: teratogenicity of cyclophosphamide *in vitro*. *Teratogenesis Carcinog Mutagen* 1983;3:255–262.
15. Moscona A. Rotation-mediated histogenetic aggregation of associated cells. *Exp Cell Res* 1961;22:455–475.
16. Daston GP, Yonker JE. Chick embryo retina cell culture as an *in vitro* teratogen screen. *Toxicologist* 1987;7:141.
17. Daston GP, Yonker JE, Baines D, Poynter JI. Chick embryo cell culture: teratogen screen and mechanistic probe. *Toxicologist* 1988;8:114.
18. Wilk AL, Greenberg JH, Horigan EA, Pratt RM, Martin GR. Detection of teratogenic compounds using differentiating embryonic cells in culture. *In Vitro* 1980;16:269–276.
19. Hassell JR, Horigan EA. Chondrogenesis: a model developmental system for measuring teratogenic potential of compounds. *Teratogenesis Carcinog Mutagen* 1982;2:325–331.
20. Guntakatta M, Matthews EJ, Rundell JO. Development of a mouse embryo limb bud cell culture system for the estimation of chemical teratogenic potential. *Teratogenesis Carcinog Mutagen* 1984;4:349–364.
21. Kistler A. Inhibition of chondrogenesis by retinoids: limb bud cell cultures as a test system to measure the teratogenic potential of compounds? *Concepts Toxicol* 1985;3:86–100.
22. Ede DA, Flint OP, Wilby OK, Colquhoun P. The development of precartilage condensations in limb bud mesenchyme *in vitro* and *in vivo*. In: Ede DA, Hinchliffe JR, Balls M, eds. *Vertebrate limb and somite morphogenesis*. New York: Cambridge University Press, 1977;161–179.
23. Solursh M, Jansen KL, Singley CT, Linsenmayer TF, Reiter RS. Two distinct regulatory steps in cartilage differentiation. *Dev Biol* 1982;94:311–325.
24. Draus MA, Kennedy EM, Tait JD, Farrow MG. A comparison of two *in vitro* assays for the evaluation of teratogenic potential. *Environ Mutagen* 1984;6:460.
25. Flint OP, Orton TC. An *in vitro* assay for teratogens with cultures of rat embryo midbrain and limb bud cells. *Toxicol Appl Pharmacol* 1984;76:383–395.
26. Uphill PF, Wilkins SR, Allen JA. *In vitro* micromass teratogen test: results from a blind trial of 25 compounds. *Toxicol In Vitro* 1990;4:623–626.
27. Kistler A. Limb bud cell cultures for estimating the teratogenic potential of compounds. Validation of the test system with retinoids. *Arch Toxicol* 1987;60:403–414.
28. Flint OP. A micromass culture method for rat embryonic neural cells. *J Cell Sci* 1983;61:247–262.
29. Greenberg JH. Detection of teratogens by differentiating embryonic neural crest cells in culture: evaluation as a screening system. *Teratogenesis Carcinog Mutagen* 1982;2:319–323.
30. Flint OP, Boyle FT. An *in vitro* test for its application in the selection of nonteratogenic triazole antifungals. *Concepts Toxicol* 1985;3:29–35.
31. Wroble JT, Whittaker SG, Faustman EM. Characterization of differentiation-specific and cytoskeletal markers in micromass cultures. *Toxicologist* 1992;12.
32. Sweeney C, Faustman EM. Expression of differentiated characteristics in rodent embryo central nervous system cell cultures: effects of teratogen exposure. *Teratology* 1990;39:484.
33. Sweeney C, Faustman EM. Differentiation-related expression of proto-oncogene *src* in CNS micromass cultures: effects of chemical exposure. *Toxicologist* 1990;10:28.
34. Ribeiro PL, Faustman EM. Chemically induced growth inhibition and cell cycle perturbations in cultures of differentiating rodent embryonic cells. *Toxicol Appl Pharmacol* 1990;104:200–211.

35. Ribeiro PL, Faustman EM. Embryonic micromass limb bud and midbrain cultures: different cell cycle kinetics during differentiation *in vitro*. *Toxicol In Vitro* 1990;4:602–608.

36. Brown LP, Flint OP, Orton TC, Gibson GG. *In vitro* metabolism of teratogens by differentiating rat embryo cells. *Food Chem Toxic* 1986;24:737–742.

37. Brown LP, Flint OP, Orton TC, Gibson GG. Metabolism of teratogens by differentiating rat embryo cells. *Teratology* 1986;33:52A.

38. Brown LP, Flint OP, Orton TC, Gibson GG. Chemical teratogenesis: testing methods and the role of metabolism. *Drug Metab Rev* 1986;17:221–260.

30. Brown LP, Foster JR, Orton TC, Flint OP, Gibson GG. Inducibility and functionality of rat embryonic/foetal cytochrome P-450: a study of differentiating limb-bud and mid-brain cells *in vitro*. *Toxicol In Vitro* 1989;3:253–260.

40. Braun AG, Buckner CA, Emerson DF, Nichinson BB. Quantitative correspondence between the *in vivo* and *in vitro* activity of teratogenic agents. *Proc Natl Acad Sci USA* 1982;79:2056–2060.

41. Braun AG, Nichinson BB, Horowicz PS. Inhibition of tumor cell attachment to concanavalin A-coated surfaces as an assay for teratogenic agents: approaches to validation. *Teratogenesis Carcinog Mutagen* 1982;2:342–354.

42. Braun AG, Harding FA, Weinreb SL. Teratogenic drugs inhibit tumor cell attachment to lectin-coated surfaces P-450. *Toxicol Appl Pharmacol* 1986;82:175–179.

43. Yoneda T, Pratt RM. Mesenchymal cells from the human embryonic palate are highly responsive to EGF. *Science* 1981;213:565.

44. Pratt RM, Grove RI, Willis WD. Prescreening for environmental teratogens using cultured mesenchymal cells from the human embryonic palate. *Teratogenesis Carcinog Mutagen* 1982;2:313–318.

45. Pratt RM, Willis WD. *In vitro* screening assay for teratogens using growth inhibition of human embryonic cells. *Proc Natl Acad Sci USA* 1985;82:5791–5794.

46. Welsch F, Stedman DB, Willis WD, Pratt RM. Karyotype, growth, and cell cycle analysis of human embryonic palatal mesenchymal cells: relevance to the use of these cells in an *in vitro* teratogenicity screening assay. *Teratogenesis Carcinog Mutagen* 1986;383–392.

47. Smith MK, Kimmel GL, Kochhar DM, Shepard TN, Spielberg SP, Wilson JG. A selection of candidate compounds for *in vitro* teratogenesis test validation. *Teratogenesis Carcinog Mutagen* 1983;3:461–480.

48. Yang LL, Steele VE, Lamb JC, IV, et al. Evaluation and validation of two *in vitro* teratology systems: results from the first twelve coded compounds. *Environ Mutagen* 1986;8:94.

49. Steele VE, Elmore EL, Lamb JC, IV, et al. Validation of two short-term *in vitro* assays to identify potential teratogens. *Teratology* 1986;33:61C.

50. National Toxicology Program, NIEHS. Evaluation of two *in vitro* teratology testing systems. NTP-86-372, December 2, 1986.

51. Steele VE, Morrissey RE, Elmore EL, et al. Evaluation of two *in vitro* assays to screen for potential developmental toxicants. *Fund Appl Toxicol* 1988;11:673–684.

52. Mummery CL, Van Den Brink CE, Van Der Saag PT, De Laat SW. A short-term screening test for teratogens using differentiating neuroblastoma cells *in vitro*. *Teratology* 1984;29:271–279.

53. Laschinski G, Vogel R, Spielmann H. Cytotoxicity test using blastocyst-derived euploid embryonal stem cells: a new approach to *in vitro* teratogenesis testing. *Reprod Toxicol* 1991;5:57–64.

54. Keller SJ, Smith MK. Animal virus screens for potential teratogens. I. Poxvirus morphogenesis. *Teratogenesis Carcinog Mutagen* 1982;2:361–374.

55. Trosko JE, Chang C-C, Netzloff M. The role of inhibited cell–cell communication in teratogenesis. *Teratogenesis Carcinog Mutagen* 1982;2:31–45.

56. Trosko JE, Chang CC. Role of intracellular communication in tumor promotion. In: Slaga TJ, ed. *Mechanisms of tumor promotion*, vol IV. Boca Raton, FL: CRC Press, 1984;119–145.

57. Loch-Caruso R, Trosko JE. Inhibited intercellular communication as a mechanistic link between teratogenesis and carcinogenesis. *CRC Crit Rev Toxicol* 1985;16:157–183.

58. Loch-Caruso R, Trosko JE, Corcos IA. Interruption of cell–cell communication in Chinese hamster V79 cells by various alkyl glycol ethers: implications for teratogenicity. *Environ Health Perspect* 1984;57:119–123.

59. Welsch F. The applicability of *in vitro* methods to teratogenicity testing and to studies on the mechanism of action of chemical teratogens. *CIIT Activities* 1986;6:1,3–7.

60. Welsch F, Stedman DB. Inhibition of metabolic cooperation between Chinese hamster V79 cells by structurally diverse teratogens. *Teratogenesis Carcinog Mutagen* 1984;4:285–301.

61. Rubinstein C, Jone C, Trosko JE, Chang CC. Inhibition of intercellular communication in cultures

of Chinese hamster V79 cells by 2,4-dichlorophenoxyacetic acid and 2,4,5-trichlorophenoxyacetic acid. *Fund Appl Toxicol* 1984;4:731–739.

62. Davidson JS, Baumgarten IM, Harley EH. Effects of 12-*O*-tetradecanoylphorbol-13-acetate and retinoids on intercellular junctional communication measured with a citrulline incorporation assay. *Carcinogenesis* 1985;6:645–650.

63. Chen TH, Kavanagh TJ, Chang CC, Trosko JE. Inhibition of metabolic cooperation in Chinese hamster V79 cells by various organic solvents and simple compounds. *Cell Biol Toxicol* 1984; 1:155–171.

64. Welsch F, Stedman DB, Carson JL. Effects of a teratogen on [^{3}H]-uridine nucleotide transfer between human embryonal cells and on gap junctions. *Exp Cell Res* 1985;159:91–102.

65. Hulme LM, Atkinson KA, Clothier RH, Balls M. The potential usefulness of a differentiating carcinoma cell line in *in vitro* toxicity testing. *Toxicol In Vitro* 1990;4:589–592.

66. Jelinek R. Use of chick embryo in screening for embryotoxicity. *Teratogenesis Carcinog Mutagen* 1982;2:255–261.

67. Jelinek R, Peterka M, Rychter A. Chick embryotoxicity screening test—130 substances tested. *Ind J Exp Biol* 1985;23:588–595.

68. Schowing J. Chick embryos as experimental material for teratogenic investigations. *Concepts Toxicol* 1985;3:58–73.

69. Summerbell D, Hornbruch A. The chick embryo: a standard against which to judge *in vitro* systems. In: Neubert D, Merker H-J, eds. *Culture techniques*. New York: Walter de Gruyter, 1981;529–538.

70. Gebhardt DOE. The use of the chick embryo in applied teratology. In: Woollam DHM, ed. *Advances in teratology*. London: Academic Press, 1972;97–111.

71. Vesely D, Vesela D, Jelinek R. Nineteen mycotoxins tested on chick embryos. *Toxicol Lett* 1982;13:239–245.

72. Fisher M, Schoenwolf GC. The use of early chick embryos in experimental embryology and teratology: improvements in standard procedures. *Teratology* 1983;27:65–72.

73. Muscarella DE, Keown JF, Bloom SE. Evaluation of the genotoxic and embryotoxic potential of chlorpyrifos and its metabolites *in vivo* and *in vitro*. *Environ Mutagen* 1984;6:13–23.

74. Bloom SE. Sister chromatid exchange studies in the chick embryo and neonate: actions of mutagens in a developing system. *Basic Life Sci* 1984;29:509–533.

75. Birge WJ, Black JA, Ramey BA. The reproductive toxicology of aquatic contaminants. In: Saxena J, Fisher F, eds. *Hazard assessment of chemicals: current developments*, vol 1. New York: Academic Press, 1981;59–115.

76. Birge WJ, Black JA, Westerman AG, Ramey BA. Fish and amphibian embryos—a model system for evaluating teratogenicity. *Fundam Appl Toxicol* 1983;3:237–242.

77. Cameron IL, Lawrence WC, Lum JB. Medaka eggs as a model system for screening potential teratogens. *Prog Clin Biol Res* 1985;163C:239–243.

78. Medcalfe CD, Sonstegard RA. Oil refinery effluents: evidence of cocarcinogenic activity in the trout embryo microinjection assay. *J Natl Cancer Inst* 1985;75:1091– 1097.

79. Shi M, Faustman EM. Development and characterization of a morphological scoring system for medaka (*Oryzias latipes*) embryo development. *Aquatic Toxicol* 1989;15:127–140.

80. Binder RL, Stegeman JJ. Microsomal electron transport and xenobiotic monooxygenase activities during the embryonic period of development in the killifish, *Fundulus heteroclitus*. *Toxicol Appl Pharmacol* 1984;73:432–443.

81. Binder RL, Stegeman JJ, Lech JJ. Induction of cytochrome P-450-dependent monooxygenase systems in embryos and eleutheroembryos of the killifish, *Fundulus heteroclitus*. *Chem–Biol Interact* 1985;55:185–202.

82. Hiraoka Y, Ishiasawa S, Kamada T, Okuda H. Acute toxicity of 14 different kinds of metals affecting medaka fry. *Hiroshima J Med Sci* 1985;34:327–330.

83. Schreiweis DO, Murray GJ. Cardiovascular malformations in *Oryzias latipes* embryos treated with 2,4,5-trichlorophenoxyacetic acid (2,4,5-T). *Teratology* 1976;14:287–290.

84. Hendricks JD, Wales JH, Sinnhuber RO, Nixon JE, Loveland PM, Scanlan RA. Rainbow trout (*Salmo gairdneri*) embryos: a sensitive animal model for experimental carcinogenesis. *Fed Proc* 1980;39:3222–3229.

85. Hendricks JD, Scanlan RA, Williams JL, Sinnhuber RO, Grieco MP. Carcinogenicity of *N*-methyl-*N*'-nitro-*N*-nitroso-guanidine to the livers and kidneys of rainbow trout (*Salmo gairdneri*) exposed as embryos. *J Natl Cancer Inst* 1980;64:1511–1519.

86. Ishikawa T, Masahito P, Takayama S. Usefulness of the medaka, *Oryzias latipes*, as a test animal:

DNA repair processes in medaka exposed to carcinogens. *Natl Cancer Inst Monogr* 1984;65:35–43.

87. Solomon FP, Faustman EM. Developmental toxicity of four model alkylating agents on Japanese medaka fish (*Oryzias latipes*) embryos. *Environ Toxicol Chem* 1987;6:747–753.

88. Faustman-Watts E, Solomon F. Examination of a candidate test compound and structural homolog in two *in vitro* teratogenicity test systems. *Teratology* 1985;31:33A.

89. Dumont JN, Epler RG. Validation studies on the FETAX teratogenesis assay (frog embryos). *Teratology* 1984;29:27A.

90. Dumont JN, Schultz TW, Buchanan MV, Kao GL. Frog embryo teratogenesis assay: *Xenopus* (FETAX)—a short-term assay applicable to complex environmental mixtures. In: Waters MD, Sandhu SS, Lewtas J, Claxton L, Chernoff N, Nesnow S, eds. *Short-term bioassays in the analysis of complex environmental mixtures III*. New York: Plenum Press, 1983;393–405.

91. Dumont JN, Schultz TW, Epler RG. The response of the FETAX model to mammalian teratogens. *Teratology* 1983;27:39A.

92. Dumpert K, Zietz E. Platanna (*Xenopus laevis*) as a test organism for determining the embryotoxic effects of environmental chemicals. *Ecotoxicol Environ Safety* 1984;8:55–74.

93. Sabourin TD, Faulk RT, Gross LB. The efficacy of three non-mammalian test systems in the identification of chemical teratogens. *J Appl Toxicol* 1985;5:227–233.

94. Bantle JA, Fort DJ, Rayburn JR, DeYoung DJ, Bush SJ. Further validation of FETAX: evaluation of the developmental toxicity of five known mammalian teratogens and non-teratogens. *Drug Chem Toxicol* 1990;13:267–282.

95. Dawson DA, Bantle JA. Development of a reconstituted water medium and preliminary validation of the frog embryo teratogenesis assay—*Xenopus* (FETAX). *J Appl Toxicol* 1987;7:237–244.

96. Dawson DA, Wilke TS. Evaluation of the frog embryo teratogenesis assay: *Xenopus* (FETAX) as a model system for mixture toxicity hazard assessment. *Environ Toxicol Chem* 1991;10:941–948.

97. Schuler RL, Hardin BD, Niemeier RW. Drosophila as a tool for the rapid assessment of chemicals for teratogenicity. *Teratogenesis Carcinog Mutagen* 1982;2:293–301.

98. Wilson JG. Survey of *in vitro* systems: their potential use in teratogenicity screening. In: Wilson JG, Fraser FC, eds. *Handbook of teratology*, vol 4. New York: Plenum Press, 1978;135–153.

99. Eberlein S. Stage specific embryonic defects following heat shock in drosophila. *Dev Genet* 1986;6:179–197.

100. Walton BT. Use of the cricket embryo (*Acheta domesticus*) as an invertebrate teratology model. *Fundam Appl Toxicol* 1983;3:233–236.

101. Johnson EM, Gabel BEG. An artificial embryo for detection of abnormal developmental biology. *Fundam Appl Toxicol* 1983;3:243–249.

102. Johnson EM, Christian MS. The hydra assay for detecting and ranking developmental hazards. *Concepts Toxicol* 1985;3:107–113.

103. Wilby OK, Newall DR, Tesh JM. A hydra assay as a pre-screen for teratogenic potential. *Am Coll Toxicol Proc* 1985; Poster 6.

104. Johnson EM. A subvertebrate system for rapid determination of potential teratogenic hazards. *J Environ Pathol Toxicol* 1980;4:153–156.

105. Wiger R, Stottum A. *In vitro* testing for developmental toxicity using the *Hydra attenuata* assay. *NIPH ANN* 1982;8:43–47.

106. Johnson EM, Gabel BEG, Larson J. Developmental toxicity and structure/activity correlates of glycols and glycol ethers. *Environ Health Perspect* 1984;57:135–139.

107. Rogers JM. Comparison of maternal and fetal toxic dose responses in mammals. *Teratogenesis Carcinog Mutagen* 1987;7:297–306.

108. Daston GP, D'Amato RA. *In vitro* techniques in teratology. *Toxicol Ind Health* 1989;5:555–585.

109. Best JB, Morita M, Ragin J, Best J Jr. Acute toxic responses of the freshwater planarian, *Dugesia clorotocephela*, to methylmercury. *Bull Environ Contam Toxicol* 1981;27:49–54.

110. Best JB, Morita M. Planarians as a model system for *in vitro* teratogenesis studies. *Teratogenesis Carcinog Mutagen* 1982;2:277–291.

111. Nacci D, Jackim E, Walsh R. Comparative evaluation of three rapid marine toxicity tests: sea urchin early embryo growth test, sea urchin sperm cell toxicity test and microtox. *Environ Toxicol Chem* 1986;5:521–525.

112. Jackim E, Nacci D. Improved sea urchin DNA-based embryo growth toxicity test. *Environ Toxicol Chem* 1986;5:561–565.

113. Hose JE. Potential uses of sea urchin embryos for identifying toxic chemicals: description of a

bioassay incorporating cytologic, cytogenetic and embryological endpoints. *J Appl Toxicol* 1985; 5:245–254.

114. Hinkley RE, Jr, Wright BD. Comparative effects of halothane, enflurane, and methoxyflurane on the incidence of abnormal development using sea urchin gametes as an *in vitro* model system. *Anesth Analg* 1985;64:1005–1009.

115. Kerster HW, Schaeffer DJ. Brine shrimp (*Artemia salina*) nauplii as a teratogen test system. *Ecotoxicol Environ Safety* 1983;7:342–349.

116. Sleet RB, Brendel K. Homogeneous populations of *Artemia nauplii* and their potential use for *in vitro* testing in developmental toxicology. *Teratogenesis Carcinog Mutagen* 1985;5:41–54.

117. Eibs H-G, Spielmann H. Preimplantation embryos, part II: culture and transplantation. In: Neubert D, Merker H-J, Kwasigroch TE, eds. *Methods in prenatal toxicology: evaluation of embryonic effects in experimental animals*, Stuttgart: Georg Thieme Publishers, 1977;221–230.

118. Spielmann H, Eibs HG. Recent progress in teratology: a survey of methods for the study of drug action during the preimplantation period. *Arzneimittelforschung* 1978;28:1733–1742.

119. Spielmann H, Druger C, Vogel R. Embryotoxicity testing during the preimplantation period. *Concepts Toxicol* 1985;3:22–28.

120. Spielmann N, Kruger C, Tenschert B, Vogel R. Studies in the embryotoxic risk of drug treatment during the preimplantation period in the mouse. *Drug Res* 1986;36:219–223.

121. Fabro S, Mclachlan JA, Dies NM. Chemical exposure of embryos during the preimplantation stages of pregnancy: mortality rate and intrauterine development. *Am J Obstet Gynecol* 1984;929–938.

122. Biggers JD, Borland RM. Physiological aspects of growth and development of the preimplantation mammalian embryo. *Annu Rev Physiol* 1976;38:95–119.

123. Iannaccone PM. Long-term effects of exposure to methylnitrosourea on blastocysts following transfer to surrogate female mice. *Cancer Res* 1984;44:2785–2789.

124. Bossert NL, Iannaccone PM. Midgestational abnormalities associated with *in vitro* preimplantation *N*-methyl-*N*-nitrosourea exposure with subsequent transfer to surrogate mothers. *Proc Natl Acad Sci USA* 1985;82:8757–8761.

125. Vogel R, Kruger C, Granata I, Spielmann N. Development and sister chromatid exchange of mouse morulae and blastocysts cultured in rat serum containing active metabolites of cyclophosphamide. *Toxicol Lett* 1985;28:23–28.

126. Muller W-U, Streffer C. Risk to preimplantation mouse embryos of combinations of heavy metals and radiation. *Int J Radiat Biol* 1987;51:997–1006.

127. Filler R, Lew K. Developmental onset of mixed-function oxidase activity in preimplantation mouse embryos. *Proc Natl Acad Sci USA* 1981;78:6991–6995.

128. Austin CR. Embryo transfer and sensitivity to teratogenesis. *Nature* 1973;244:333–334.

129. Iannacone PM, Tsao TY, Stols L. Effects on mouse blastocysts of *in vitro* exposure to methylnitrosourea and 3-methylcholanthrene. *Cancer Res* 1982;42:864–868.

130. Rutledge JC, Generoso WM. Fetal pathology produced by ethylene oxide treatment of the murine zygote. *Teratology* 1989;39:563–572.

131. Generoso WM, Rutledge JC, Aronson J. Developmental anomalies: mutational consequence of mouse zygote exposure. *Banbury Rep* 1990;34:311–319.

132. Spielmann H, Jacob-Muller U, Eibs HG, Beckord W. Investigations on cyclophosphamide treatment during the preimplantation period. I. Differential sensitivity of preimplantation mouse embryos to maternal cyclophosphamide treatment. *Teratology* 1981;23:1–5.

133. Vogel R, Spielmann N. Increased sister-chromatid exchange frequency in preimplantation mouse embryos after maternal cyclophosphamide treatment before implantation. *Toxicol Lett* 1986;32:81–88.

134. Eibs H-G, Spielmann H, Hagele M. Effects of sex steroid treatment during the preimplantation period on the development of mouse embryos *in vivo* and *in vitro*. In: Neubert D, Merker H-J, Nau H, Langman J, eds. *Role of pharmacokinetics in prenatal and perinatal toxicology*. Stuttgart: Georg Thieme Publishers, 1978;435–438.

135. Pedersen RA. Benzo(*a*)pyrene metabolism in early mouse embryos. In: Neubert D, Merker HJ, eds. *Culture techniques: applicability for studies on prenatal differentiation and toxicity*. Berlin: Walter de Gruyter, 1981;447–454.

136. Lutwak-Mann C, Hay MF, New DAT. Action of various agents on rabbit blastocysts *in vivo* and *in vitro*. *J Reprod Fertil* 1969;18:235–257.

137. Spielmann H, Eibs HG, Jacob-Muller U. *In vivo* and *in vitro* studies on the effects of cyclo-

phosphamide treatment before implantation in the mouse and rat. In: Neubert D, Merker HJ, Nau H, Langman J, eds. *Role of pharmacokinetics in prenatal and perinatal toxicology.* Stuttgart: Georg Thieme Publishers, 1978;422–433.

138. Shepard TH, Fantel AG, Mirkes PE, et al. Teratology testing: I. Development and status of short-term prescreens. II. Biotransformation of teratogens as studied in whole embryo culture. *Prog Clin Biol Res* 1983;135:147–164.

139. Schmid BP. Teratogenicity testing of new drugs with the postimplantation embryo culture system. *Concepts Toxicol* 1985;3:46–57.

140. Schmid BP. Action sites of known *in vivo* teratogens in extracorporeally exposed rat embryos. *Concepts Toxicol* 1985;3:74–85.

141. Sadler TW. The role of mammalian embryo culture in developmental biology and teratology. In: Kalter H, ed. *Issues and reviews in teratology,* vol 3. New York: Plenum Press, 1985;273–294.

142. Sadler TW, Horton WE, Warner CW. Whole embryo culture: a screening technique for teratogens? *Teratogenesis Carcinog Mutagen* 1982;2:243–253.

143. Sadler TW, Horton WE Jr, Hunter ES. Mammalian embryos in culture: a new approach to investigating normal and abnormal developmental mechanisms. *Prog Clin Biol Res* 1985;171:227–240.

144. Fantel AG. Culture of whole rodent embryos in teratogen screening. *Teratogenesis Carcinog Mutagen* 1982;2:231–242.

145. Kochhar DM. The use of *in vitro* procedures in teratology. *Teratology* 1975;11:273–288.

146. Kochhar DM. *In vitro* testing of teratogenic agents using mammalian embryos. *Teratogenesis Carcinog Mutagen* 1980;1:63–74.

147. Kitchin KT, Schmid BP, Sanyal MK. Rodent whole-embryo culture as a teratogen screening method. *Methods Find Exp Clin Pharmacol* 1986;8:291–301.

148. Brown NA, Fabro SE. The *in vitro* approach to teratogenicity testing. In: Snell K, ed. *Developmental toxicology.* New York: Praeger, 1982;31–57.

149. New DAT. Whole-embryo culture and the study of mammalian embryos during organogenesis. *Biol Rev* 1978;53:81–122.

150. Chen LT, Hsu YC. Development of mouse embryos *in vitro*: Preimplantation to the limb bud stage. *Science* 1982;218:66–68.

151. Eto K, Takakubo F. Improved development of rat embryos in culture during the period of craniofacial morphogenesis. *J Craniofacial Genet Dev Biol* 1985;5:351–355.

152. Priscott PK, Yeoh GCT, Oliver IT. The culture of 12- and 13-day rat embryos using continuous and noncontinuous gassing of rotating bottles. *J Exp Zool* 1984;230:247–253.

153. Wee EL, Wolfson LG, Zimmermann EF. Palate shelf movement in mouse embryo culture: evidence for skeletal and smooth muscle contractility. *Dev Biol* 1976;48:91–103.

154. Tarlatzis BC, Sanyal MK, Biggers WJ, Naftolin F. Continuous culture of the postimplantation rat conceptus. *Biol Reprod* 1984;31:415–426.

155. Sanyal MK, Naftolin F. *In vitro* development of the mammalian embryo. *J Exp Zool* 1983;228: 235–251.

156. Sadler TW, Warner CW. Use of whole embryo culture for evaluating toxicity and teratogenicity. *Pharmacol Rev* 1984;36:1455–1505.

157. Klug S, Lewandowski C, Neubert D. Modification and standardization of the culture of early postimplantation embryos for toxicological studies. *Arch Toxicol* 1985;58:84–88.

158. Brown NA, Fabro S. Quantitation of rat embryonic development *in vitro*: a morphological scoring system. *Teratology* 1981;24:65–78.

159. Fantel AG, Greenaway JC, Juchau MR, Shepard TH. Teratogenic bioactivation of cyclophosphamide *in vitro*. *Life Sci* 1979;25:67–72.

160. Kitchin KT, Sanyal MK, Schmid BP. A coupled microsomal-activating/embryo culture system: toxicity of reduced-nicotinamide adenine dinucleotide phosphate (NADPH). *Biochem Pharmacol* 1981;30:985–992.

161. Faustman-Watts E, Greenaway JC, Namkung MJ, Fantel AG, Juchau MR. Teratogenicity *in vitro* of 2-acetylaminofluorene: role of biotransformation in the rat. *Teratology* 1983;27:19–28.

162. Faustman-Watts EM, Namkung MJ, Greenaway JC, Juchau MR. Analysis of metabolites of 2-acetylamino-fluorene generated in an embryo culture system: relationship of biotransformation to teratogenicity *in vitro*. *Biochem Pharmacol* 1985;34:2953–2959.

163. Brown NA, Kram D. Intact human and rodent hepatic cells used for bioactivation in an embryo culture system. *Teratology* 1982;25:30A.

164. Oglesby LA, Ebron MT, Beyer PE, Carver BD, Kavlock RJ. Co-culture of rat embryos and hepatocytes: *in vitro* detection of a proteratogen. *Teratogenesis Carcinogen Mutagen* 1986;6:129–138.

165. Chatot CL, Klein NW, Pierro LJ. Successful culture of rat embryos on human serum: use in the detection of teratogens. *Science* 1980;207:471–473.
166. Brinster RL. Teratogen testing using preimplantation mammalian embryos. In: Shepard TH, Miller JR, Marois M, eds. *Methods for detection of environmental agents that produce congenital defects.* New York: Elsevier, 1975;113–124.
167. Klein NW, Chatot CL, Plenefisch JD, Carey SW. Human serum teratogenicity studies using *in vitro* cultures of rat embryos. In: Waters MD, Sandhu SS, Lewtas J, Claxton L, Chernoff N, Nesnow S, eds. *Short-term bioassays in the analysis of complex environmental mixtures III.* New York: Plenum Press, 1983;407–415.
168. Juchau MR, Giachelli CM, Fantel AG, Greenaway JC, Shepard TN, Faustman-Watts EM. Effects of 3-methylcholanthrene and phenobarbital on the capacity of embryos to bioactivate teratogens during organogenesis. *Toxicol Appl Pharmacol* 1985;80:137–146.
169. Juchau MR, Harris C, Stark KL, et al. Cytochrome P450-dependent bioactivation of pro-dysmorphogens in cultured conceptuses. *Reprod Toxicol* 1991;5:259–263.
170. Ferrari DA, Gilles PA, Klein NW. Sera teratogenicity to cultured rat embryos in women with histories of spontaneous abortion. *Teratology* 1991;43:460.
171. Flynn TJ, Scialli AR, Gibson RR. Cultured organogenesis-staged rat embryos as biomarkers for nutritional factors in human reproductive failure. *Teratology* 1991;43:468.
172. Horton WE Jr, Sadler TW. Mitochondrial alterations in embryos exposed to β-hydroxybutyrate in whole embryo culture. *Anat Rec* 1985;213:94–101.
173. Turbow MM, Chamberlain JG. Direct effects of 6-aminonicotinamide on the developing rat embryo *in vitro* and *in vivo*. *Teratology* 1968;1:103–108.
174. Kitchin KT, Ebron MT, Svendsgaard D. *In vitro* study of embryotoxic and dysmorphogenic effects of mercuric chloride and methylmercury chloride in the rat. *Food Chem Toxicol* 1984;22:31–37.
175. Klein NW, Vogler MA, Chatot C, Pierro LJ. The use of cultured rat embryos to evaluate the teratogenic activity of serum: cadmium and cyclophosphamide. *Teratology* 1980;21:199–208.
176. Warner CW, Sadler T, Tulis S, Smith M. Zinc amelioration of cadmium induced teratogenesis *in vitro*. *Teratology* 1984;30:47–53.
177. Brown NA, Goulding EH, Fabro S. Ethanol embryotoxicity: direct effects on mammalian embryos *in vitro*. *Science* 1979;206:573–575.
178. Campbell MA, Fantel AG. Teratogenicity of acetyldehyde *in vitro*: relevance to the fetal alcohol syndrome. *Life Sci* 1983;32:2641–2647.
179. Schmid BP, Attenon P, Cicurel L. *In vitro* exposure of rat embryos to caffeine and its metabolites. *Teratology* 1986;33:57A.
180. Greenaway JC, Shepard TH, Fantel AG, Juchau MR. Sodium salicylate teratogenicity *in vitro*. *Teratology* 1982;26:167–171.
181. Greenaway JC, Bark DN, Juchau MR. Embryotoxic effects of salicylates: role of biotransformation. *Toxicol Appl Pharmacol* 1984;74:141–149.
182. Cicurel L, Schmid B. *In vitro* teratogenicity of acetylsalicylic acid on rat embryos: studies with various culture conditions. *Methods Findings Exp Clin Pharmacol* 1986;8:227–232.
183. McGarrity C, Samani NJ, Beck F. The *in vivo* and *in vitro* action of sodium salicylate on rat embryos. *J Anat* 1978;127:646.
184. Greenaway JC, Fantel AG, Shepard TN, Juchau MR. The *in vitro* teratogenicity of cyclophosphamide in rat embryos. *Teratology* 1982;25:335–343.
185. Kitchin KT, Schmid BP, Sanyal MK. Teratogenicity of cyclophosphamide in a coupled microsomal activating/embryo culture system. *Biochem Pharmacol* 1981;30:59–64.
186. Mirkes PE, Greenaway JC, Shepard TH. A kinetic analysis of rat embryo response to cyclophosphamide exposure *in vitro*. *Teratology* 1983;28:249–256.
187. Mirkes PE, Greenaway JC, Hilton J, Brundrett R. Morphological and biochemical aspects of monofunctional phosphoramide mustard teratogenicity in rat embryos cultured *in vitro*. *Teratology* 1985;32:241–249.
188. Kochhar DM. Assessment of teratogenic response in cultured postimplantation mouse embryos: effects of hydroxyurea. In: Neubert D, Merker HJ, eds. *New approaches to the evaluation of abnormal embryonic development.* Stuttgart: Thieme-Edition Publishing, 1975;250–277.
189. Mirkes PE, Greenaway JC. Teratogenicity of chlorambucil in rat embryos *in vitro*. *Teratology* 1982;26:135–143.
190. Beyer BK, Juchau MR. Cytochrome P-450 dependent embryotoxicity of estradiol 17. *Teratology* 1986;33:45C.
191. Beyer BK, Greenaway JC, Juchau MR. DES-induced embryotoxicity *in vitro*. *Teratology* 1985;31:45A.

192. Bechter R, Terlouw GDC, Tsuchiya M, Tsuchiya T, Kistler A. Teratogenicity of arotinoids (retinoids): comparison of the whole embryo culture system with the *in vivo* mouse model and the limb bud cell culture assay. Submitted, 1991.
193. Goulding EN, Pratt RM. Isotretinoin teratogenicity in mouse whole embryo culture. *J Craniofacial Genet Dev Biol* 1986;6:99–112.
194. Morriss GM, Steele CE. Comparison of the effects of retinol and retinoic acid on postimplantation rat embryos *in vitro*. *Teratology* 1977;15:109–120.
195. Webster WS, Johnston MC, Lammer EJ, Sulik KK. Isotretinoin embryopathy and the cranial neural crest: an *in vivo* and *in vitro* study. *J Craniofacial Gen Dev Biol* 1986;6:211–222.
196. Kitchin KT, Ebron MT. Further development of rodent whole embryo culture: solvent toxicity and water insoluble compound delivery system. *Toxicology* 1984;30:45–57.
197. Kitchin KT, Ebron MT. Studies of saccharin and cyclohexylamine in a coupled microsomal activating/embryo culture system. *Food Chem Toxicol* 1983;21:537–541.
198. Schmid BP. Monitoring of organ formation in rat embryos after *in vitro* exposure to azathioprine, mercaptopurine, methotrexate or cyclosporin A. *Toxicology* 1984;31:9–21.
199. Svoboda KK, O'Shea KS. Optic vesicle defects induced by vincristine sulfate: an *in vivo* and *in vitro* study in the mouse embryo. *Teratology* 1984;29:223–239.
200. Naruse I, Shoji R. Whole embryo culture as a primary screening system for teratogens—effects of vinblastine on rat embryos *in vitro*. *Proc Jpn Acad* 1986;62B:31–34.
201. Greenaway JC, Fantel AG. Enhancement of rifampin teratogenicity in cultured rat embryos. *Toxicol Appl Pharmacol* 1983;69:81–88.
202. Bruckner A, Lee YJ, O'Shea KS, Henneberry RC. Teratogenic effects of valproic acid and diphenylhydantoin on mouse embryos in culture. *Teratology* 1983;27:29–42.
203. Tesh JM, Newall DR. Teratogenic effects of thalidomide on rat embryos *in vitro*. *Teratology* 1985;31:68A.
204. Itoh A, Matsumoto N. Organ-specific susceptibility to clastogenic effect of urethane, a trial of application of whole embryo culture to testing system for clastogen. *J Toxicol Sci* 1984;9:175–192.
205. Kao J, Brown NA, Schmid B, Goulding EN, Fabro S. Teratogenicity of valproic acid: *in vivo* and *in vitro* teratogenicity. *Teratogenesis Carcinog Mutagen* 1981;1:367–382.
206. Crockroft DL, New DAT. Abnormalities induced in cultured rat embryos by hyperthermia. *Teratology* 1978;17:277–284.
207. Hirsekorn JM. The effects of hyperthermia on the developing central nervous system in the mouse embryo. *Anat Rec* 1980;196:79A.
208. Mirkes PE. Effects of acute exposure to elevated temperatures on rat embryo growth and development *in vitro*. *Teratology* 1985;32:259–266.
209. Fantel AG, Greenaway JC, Shepard TH, Juchau MR, Selleck SB. The teratogenicity of cytochalasin D and its inhibition by drug metabolism. *Teratology* 1981;23:223–231.
210. Geissler FT, Faustman-Watts E. Teratogenicity of aflatoxin B_1: role of biotransformation. *Toxicologist* 1985;5:187.
211. Geissler F, Faustman EM. Developmental toxicity of aflatoxin B_1 in the rodent embryo *in vitro*: contribution of exogenous biotransformation systems to toxicity. *Teratology* 1987;37:101–111.
212. Geissler FT, Eaton D, Faustman-Watts E. Investigation of the role of endogenous embryonic biotransformation in mycotoxin-induced dysmorphogenesis. *Teratology* 1986;33:45A.
213. Faustman E, Little S, Kirby Z, Mirkes P. Detection of DNA damage in rodent embryos exposed to alkylating agents *in vitro*: correlations with developmental toxicity. *Toxicologist* 1986;6:96.
214. Faustman E, Kirby Z, Gage D, Varnum M. *In vitro* developmental toxicity of five direct-acting alkylating agents in rodent embryos: structure–activity patterns. *Teratology* 1989;40:199–210.
215. Faustman-Watts EM, Greenaway JC, Namkung MJ, Fantel AG, Juchau MR. Teratogenicity *in vitro* of two deacetylated metabolites of *N*-hydroxy-2-acetylaminofluorene. *Toxicol Appl Pharmacol* 1984;76:161–171.
216. Faustman-Watts EM, Yang HYL, Namkung MJ, Greenaway JC, Fantel AG, Juchau MR. Mutagenic, cytotoxic and teratogenic effects of 2-acetylaminofluorene and reactive metabolites *in vitro*. *Teratogenesis Carcinog Mutagen* 1984;4:273–283.
217. Faustman-Watts EM, Fiachelli CM, Juchau MR. Carbon monoxide inhibits monooxygenation by the conceptus and embryotoxic effects of proteratogens *in vitro*. *Toxicol Appl Pharmacol* 1986;83:590–595.
218. Faustman-Watts E, Namkung M, Juchau M. Modulation of the embryotoxicity *in vitro* of reactive metabolites of 2-acetylaminofluorene by reduced glutathione, ascorbate and via sulfation. *Toxicol Appl Pharmacol* 1986;86:400–410.

219. Rawlings SJ, Shuker DEG, Webb M, Brown NA. The teratogenic potential of alkoxy acids in post-implantation rat embryo culture: structure–activity relationships. *Toxicol Lett* 1985;28:49–58.
220. Greenaway JC, Fantel AG, Juchau MR. On the capacity of nitroheterocyclic compounds to elicit an unusual axial asymmetry in cultured rat embryos. *Toxicol Appl Pharmacol* 1986;82:307–315.
221. Kavlock RJ, Oglesby LA, Hall LL, et al. *In vivo* and *in vitro* structure–dosimetry–activity relationships of substituted phenols in developmental toxicity assays. *Reprod Toxicol* 1991;5:255–258.
222. Sadler TW, Warner CW, Tulis SA, Smith MK, Doerger J. Factors determining the *in vitro* response of rodent embryos to teratogens. *Concepts Toxicol* 1985;3:36–45.
223. Welsch F. Short-term methods of assessing developmental toxicity hazard. *Issues Rev Toxicol* 1990;5:115–153.
224. Shepard TH, Bass GL. Organ culture of limb buds from riboflavin-deficient and normal rat embryos in normal and riboflavin-deficient media. *Teratology* 1970;3:163–168.
225. Kochhar DM. Effect of azetidine-2-carboxylic acid, a proline analog, on chondrogenesis in cultured limb buds. In: Bass R, Beck F, Merker H-J, Neubert D, Randham B, eds. *Metabolic pathways in mammalian embryos during organogenesis and its modification by drugs.* Stuttgart: Georg Thieme, 1970;475–482.
226. Bass R, Bochert G, Merker H-J, Neubert D. Some aspects of teratogenesis and mutagenesis in mammalian embryos. *J Toxicol Environ Health* 1977;2:1353–1374.
227. Kochhar DM. Embryonic limb bud organ culture in assessment of teratogenicity of environmental agents. *Teratogenesis Carcinog Mutagen* 1982;2:303–312.
228. Neubert D, Lessmollmann U, Hinz N, Dillmann I, Fuchs G. Interference of 6-mercaptopurine riboside, 6-methylmercaptopurine riboside and azathioprine with the morphogenetic differentiation of mouse extremities *in vivo* and in organ culture. *Naunyn Schmiedebergs Arch Pharmacol* 1977;298:93–105.
229. Manson JM, Simons R. *In vitro* metabolism of cyclophosphamide in limb bud culture. *Teratology* 1979;19:149–158.
230. Stahlmann R, Bluth U, Neubert D. Effects of some "indirectly" alkylating agents on differentiation of limb buds in organ culture. In: Neubert D, Merker H-J, eds. *Culture techniques.* New York: Walter de Gruyter, 1981;207–222.
231. Stahlmann R, Bluth U, Wiessler M, Neubert D. Interference of acetoxyalkyl-nitrosamines with limb bud differentiation in organ culture. *Arch Toxicol* 1983;54:109–129.
232. Bochert G, Platzek T, Wiessler M. Comparison of effects on limb development *in vivo* and *in vitro* using methyl(acetoxymethyl) nitrosamine. In: Neubert D, Merker HJ, eds. *Culture techniques.* New York: Walter de Gruyter, 1981;223–235.
233. Bochert G, Platzek T, Blankenburg G, Wiessler M, Neubert D. Embryotoxicity induced by alkylating agents: left-sided preponderance of paw malformations induced by acetoxymethyl-methylnitrosamine in mice. *Arch Toxicol* 1985;56:139–150.
234. Sadler TW, Kochhar DM. Chlorambucil-induced cell death in embryonic mouse limb buds. *Toxicol Appl Pharmacol* 1976;37:237–256.
235. Neubert D, Tapken S, Baumann I. Influence of potential thalidomide metabolites and hydrolysis products on limb development in organ culture and on the activity of proline hydroxylase—further data on our hypothesis on the thalidomide embryopathy. In: Neubert D, Merker HJ, Nau N, Langman J, eds. *Role of pharmacokinetics in prenatal and perinatal toxicology,* Stuttgart: Georg Thieme, 1978;359–382.
236. Welsch F, Baumann I, Neubert D. Effects of methyl-parathion and methyl-paraoxon on morphogenetic differentiation of mouse limb buds in organ culture. In: Neubert D, Merker HJ, Nau H, Langman J, eds. *Role of pharmacokinetics in prenatal and perinatal toxicology.* Stuttgart: Georg Thieme, 1978;351–358.
237. Flint OP. The effects of sodium salicylate, cytosine arabinoside, and eserine sulphate on rat limb buds in culture. In: Merker H-J, Nau H, Neubert D, eds. *Teratology of the limbs.* New York: Walter de Gruyter, 1980;325–338.
238. Schreiner CM, Zimmerman EF, Wee EL, Scott WJ Jr. Caffeine effects on cyclic AMP levels in the mouse embryonic limb and palate *in vitro*. *Teratology* 1986;34:21–27.
239. Kawanishi N, Fallon JT, Holmes LB. Effects of acetazolamide on limb chondrogenesis *in vitro* of the day 10.5 mouse embryo. *Teratology* 1985;32:28B.
240. Kastner M, Blankenburg G, Neubert D. Isolated and reconstituted monooxygenases as supplement for organ culture. *Teratology* 1985;32:24A–25A.
241. Shiota K, Kosazuma T, Klug S, Neubert D. Development of the fetal mouse palate in suspension organ culture. *Acta Anat* 1990;137:59–64.

242. Buckalew AR, Abbott BD. A new procedure for serum-free palatal culture. *Teratology* 1991; 43:461.
243. Abbott BD. Responses of embryonic palates to selected teratogens in serum-free organ culture. *Teratology* 1991;43:461.
244. Neubert D. Toxicity studies with cellular models of differentiation. *Xenobiotica* 1985;15:649–660.
245. Johnson EM, Christian MS. When is a teratology study not an evaluation of teratogenicity? *J Am Coll Toxicol* 1984;3:431–434.
246. Neubert D, Blankenburg C, Lewandowski C, Klug S. Misinterpretations of results and creation of "artifacts" in studies on developmental toxicity using systems simpler than *in vitro* systems. *Prog Clin Biol Res* 1985;171:241–266.
247. Faustman EM. Short-term tests for teratogens. *Mutation Res* 1988;205:355–384.
248. Fabro S, Brown NA, Scialli AR. Alternative tests for teratogens. *Reprod Toxicol: A Med Lett* 1984;3:21–24.
249. Johnson EM. A review of advances in prescreening for teratogenic hazards. *Prog Drug Res* 1985;29:121–154.
250. Homburger F, Marquis J. Third international conference on safety evaluation and regulation and joint American–Swiss seminar on alternative embryotoxicity and teratogenicity tests. *J Am Coll Toxicol* 1985;4:185–191.
251. Kimmel GL, Smith K, Kochhar DM, Pratt RM. Proceedings of the consensus workshop on *in vitro* teratogenesis testing. *Teratogenesis Carcinog Mutagen* 1981;2:i–v.
252. Neubert D, Merker H-J, eds. *Culture techniques: applicability for studies in prenatal differentiation and toxicity.* New York: Walter de Gruyter, 1981.
253. Picard JJ. Proceedings, *in vitro* culture of post-implantation rodent embryos. *Reprod Toxicol* 1991;5:221–222.
254. Schwetz B. *Interpretation of segment II developmental toxicity studies: identification of criteria for short-term test validation.* Research Triangle Park, NC: NIEHS, 1991.

In Vitro Toxicology,
edited by Shayne Cox Gad.
Raven Press, Ltd., New York, 1994.

8

Neurotoxicology *In Vitro*

Phillip G. Nelson and Douglas E. Brenneman

Laboratory of Developmental Neurobiology, National Institute of Child Health and Human Development, National Institutes of Health, Bethesda, Maryland 20892

In vitro systems have taken their place as major tools in neuroscience. Over the past two decades, the number of specific preparations and the problems that can be addressed have multiplied, so that today essentially a complete array of neurobiological systems at the molecular, cellular, and system level is represented in the tissue culture arena. This review will briefly summarize some examples of neurobiological studies presently in progress as illustrative of possible uses in neurotoxicological applications. A number of systems will be presented with regard to toxicological utility and problems and prospects for neurotoxicology screening and analytic work discussed. In particular, some examples dealing with the difficult problem of correlation between *in vivo* and *in vitro* observations will be presented.

IN VITRO SYSTEMS IN NEUROSCIENCE

Striking advances in the methodologies involved in preparing dissociated cell cultures from the central nervous system (CNS) have been made in the past few years. Essentially any region of the vertebrate and indeed mammalian CNS can be maintained successfully for periods of many days, weeks, or months. Selected cell types can be identified by a number of techniques and isolation of homogeneous populations of neurons accomplished by the separation of identified cells or selective maintenance of desired cell types. We are approaching the realization of the goal implicit in the dissociated cell culture approach, of being able to study specific cell types in isolation and in controlled combinations, so that interaction among the cells of the nervous system can be analyzed in some detail. The mechanism involved in such cellular interactions can be expected to play a central role in the regulation of nervous system development. Morphological, neurochemical, and physiological methods similarly have shown a remarkable increase in power and precision in the past few years. The conjunction between analytic capabilities and tissue culture preparations has resulted in considerable progress in cellular neuroscience. Patch-clamp analysis of a variety of membrane ionic channels and receptors has been carried out in peripheral and central neurons and glial cells. Excitatory and inhibitory receptors have been characterized pharmacologically, and the relationship between pharmacological and synaptic receptors has been studied (1,2). Intracellular changes in calcium ion concentration have been measured using a variety of techniques under a variety of experimental conditions (3). A number of trophic factors important for development of the nervous system have been identified and purified, and their genes have been cloned (4–5a). We will deal with some of the techniques that have been successful in preparing cultured neurons and glia to maximize their experimental usefulness, and we will describe some of the experimental methods recently applied to cultured neural material and give some detailed account of studies that illustrate the new approaches to important questions.

CULTURES OF SPECIFIC CELL TYPES

Glia

In 1980, McCarthy and DeVellis (6) developed a procedure for preparing nearly pure populations of astroglia and oligodendroglia from the postnatal rat cerebral cortex. Their relatively simple and reliable technique has been used in a number of laboratories, with minor variations in subsequent years. The method is based on the principle that the different cell types within the complex tissue of the brain have a number of intrinsic properties that can be utilized to produce an enriched population under appropriately designed culture conditions. These authors list cellular adhesiveness, culture medium requirements, developmental time-course, and growth patterns as particularly useful properties to exploit for purposes of cell separation. Appropriate criteria for judging the success of any cell purification scheme are essential, and these authors used ultrastructural properties, marker enzymes, and pharmacological responsiveness as means of identifying the cell types that they were trying to isolate. We will describe this method in some detail because it exemplifies a number of considerations pertinent to the general problem of establishing pure culture of known types.

Postnatal (1–2 days) rats were chosen because it was established easily that with a conventional dissociation procedure and culture medium containing a relatively high (15%) fetal calf serum concentration, essentially no neurons survived. Thus, a preparation was obtained that contained primarily astroglia and oligodendroglia, and the purification problem became that of selectively growing these two types of cells. It was noted that the mixed culture became a strictly layered or stratified structure at a specific time (9–10 days) after establishment of the culture. The morphological appearance suggested that this stratification, in fact, represented a separation of the two cell types into (a) a bed layer of astrocytes attached to the culture dish and (b) a layer of oligodendroglia growing on top of the astrocytes. The astrocytes were quite tightly adherent to the surface of the culture flask, with the oligodendrocytes less well attached to the astrocytes, and the authors were able to design a method of mechanically shaking the oligodendrocytes free while leaving the astrocytes still attached to the flask. This differential adhesiveness, combined with the fact that the astrocytes were more active mitotically, allowed (with another cycle of plating, separation, and replating) the preparation of cultures >98% pure for one or the other cell type.

Clearly, it is essential in any purification procedure to have means of assessing the degree of purification that is obtained. There was no doubt that the two cell populations prepared by the method of McCarthy and De Vellis (6) were different by light-microscopic criteria, but, in addition, fine structural, pharmacological, and enzyme marker studies established satisfactorily that the cell types had properties characteristic of astrocytes and oligodendrocytes. The presence of numerous intermediate filaments and a paucity of microtubules characterized the astrocyte population, whereas the converse was true for the oligodendrocytes. Astrocytes, but not oligodendrocytes, exhibited characteristic morphologic response to cAMP or brain extracts. Cyclic nucleotide phosphohydrolase (CNPase) appears to be localized in myelin and oligodendrocytes *in vivo* and, appropriately, could be detected readily in the purified oligodendrocyte cultures, but was undetectable in the astrocyte preparations. Glycerol phosphate dehydrogenase (GPDH) is an oligodendrocyte marker which is induced markedly *in vivo* by hydrocortisone. A low level of this enzyme was detected in the astrocyte culture, and this was induced approximately threefold by hydrocortisone. A tenfold higher level was measured in the oligodendrocyte cultures, and this was induced 16-fold further by hydrocortisone. Changes in cAMP levels produced by several pharmacological agents (α- and β-adrenergic agonists or antagonists, adenosine, and prostaglandin E) were different for the two types of purified cell cultures, in accordance with their presumptive cell type. Subsequent studies with immunocytochemical staining for the astroglial antigen, glial fibrillary acidic protein (GFAP) (7), has corroborated fully these findings.

Thus, a relatively simple method provided a well-validated, fairly large-scale separation of purified populations of two important cellular components of the mammalian CNS. A large number of studies have been done subsequently using these preparations to characterize these cells further and to analyze their interaction with other cells. Some representative studies will be described below.

A step fundamental to the understanding of the function of glial cells was to characterize the receptors on their surface membranes. The β-adrenergic receptors on different classes of cells from the CNS in cell cultures have been studied quantitatively using a combination of immunocytochemical and autoradiographic techniques (7). Most of these receptors were located on astroglia having a flat polygonal morphology. Fibroblasts and process-bearing GFAP-positive cells had a much lower level of β-adrenergic receptors and neurons, and oligodendroglia had essentially none. The importance of culture conditions and care in documenting the types of cells present in the cultures in interpreting receptor binding data is emphasized in these studies. Meningeal fibroblasts express β_2- while astrocytes express β_1-adrenergic receptors, and the relative dominance of the cultures by these cell types must be ascertained (e.g., by combined immunocytochemistry for fibronectin and

GFAP). Nominally minor changes in culture methodology can affect the mix of cell types that one obtains.

Purified glial cultures have been used effectively to study the second messenger systems to which glial receptors are coupled. Perhaps, not surprisingly, both cyclic nucleotide and phospholipid systems can be regulated in these cells by a broad variety of catecholaminergic, cholinergic, and peptidergic agonists (8). Altered levels of cAMP resulted from catecholamine and from peptidergic stimulation, and this was accompanied by an altered state of phosphorylation of GFAP and glial filaments (9). A transition from a polygonal to a process-bearing morphology occurred with these treatments, but further analysis indicated that no causal role of intermediate filament protein phosphorylation could be established with regard to the morphological change.

Astroglia cells have proven to be highly useful "feeder layers" for low-density neuronal cultures and, as noted below, synthesize and secrete powerful neurotrophic materials. The glia respond to a number of agonists with large changes in intracellular calcium (10,11), and these changes appear to propagate in waves through populations of the glia. Thus it is clear that, rather than being passive support cells, glial cells play an active dynamic role in nervous system development and function.

Neurons

The situation regarding glial lineage, purification, and identification is complicated, and this is even more true for neurons; in addition, the strategies for dealing with neuronal identification and separation are correspondingly complex.

Dodd and Jessell (12) have taken an immunocytochemical approach to the identification of subsets of spinal sensory neurons from dorsal root ganglia (DRG). They have used antibodies directed against intracellular peptides (substance P and somatostatin) and a sensory-neuron-specific enzyme (fluoride-resistant acid phosphatase). These three markers serve to distinguish three nonoverlapping populations of small DRG neurons which have a distinctive laminar projection pattern in the dorsal horn of the spinal cord. In addition, a number of complex surface-membrane carbohydrate-containing structures have been shown to identify subsets of sensory ganglion neurons and their distinctive axonal projection patterns within the spinal cord. The working assumption is that these surface glycoconjugates may be involved in the establishment of the specific connections characteristic of different functional types of sensory neurons. At least some aspects of this surface-membrane carbohydrate structure specificity is retained in culture; however, some antibodies that labeled adult DRG neurons failed to label cultured neurons, and, in general, antibodies against the carbohydrates labeled a lower proportion of cultured neurons than neurons in mature DRGs. These anticarbohydrate antibodies do provide powerful tools for identifying, and potentially isolating, functionally meaningful populations of DRG neurons, and at least some of these marker molecules are expressed *in vitro*.

Immunohistochemical methods have been utilized extensively in identifying different types of central neurons as well. This technique can be used in conjunction with autoradiographic studies of transmitter uptake. Inhibitory neurons utilizing gamma-aminobutyric acid (GABA) have been identified in this way by Neale et al. (13). A high degree of concordance was found between neurons that take up GABA and those that express glutamic acid decarboxylase, an enzyme involved in the production of GABA. Many other molecular neuronal phenotypes can be identified and are essential in analyzing experiments done with the complex mixtures of cell types that occur in typical dissociated cell cultures from the CNS (14).

A series of experiments illustrating the utility of some of these methodologies has been done by Brenneman and his colleagues (15,16). These workers are interested in the role of electrical activity in neurons in regulating development of the nervous system. Extensive experimentation *in vivo* had established that electrical activity does exert a critical developmental influence on neuronal survival and synaptic connections. The cell culture methodology is advantageous in investigating the mechanics involved in this activity–development coupling.

It was straightforward to establish that, *in vitro*, electrical activity does indeed have a major impact on neuronal survival; blockade of electrical activity with the specific voltage-dependent sodium channel blocker, tetrodotoxin (TTX), results in a substantial decrement in the number of surviving neurons. This sensitivity to action potential blockade occurs over a restricted developmental time window (from about 1 week to 3 weeks *in vitro* for cultures prepared from approximately 2-week-old mouse embryos). Furthermore, some cell types (e.g., DRG or GABAergic neurons) are unaffected, whereas other neuronal types do not survive tetrodotoxin exposure.

The hypothesis was tested that neuropeptides might be involved in the activity-dependent regulation of neuronal survival. The experiment was to add putative trophically active peptides to cultures blocked with TTX to see if these peptides could reverse the effects of TTX. One peptide, vasoactive intestinal peptide (VIP), proved to be effective in this regard at extraordinarily low concentrations (10^{-10} M, or even less). Using a variety of techniques, it was then possible to show the following:

1. VIP-containing neurons exist in the cultures, since 1–2% of the neurons showed VIP-like immunoreactivity.
2. VIP is released in an activity-dependent manner, since radioimmunoassay demonstrated VIP in the culture medium from control cultures, but no VIP was detectable from TTX-blocked cultures.
3. VIP does not appear to act directly on neurons. Cultures grown in a defined medium containing no fetal bovine or horse serum had a relatively enriched number of neurons with a relatively lower number of glial cells. Neurons in these cultures exposed to TTX are not rescued by VIP.
4. Glial cells possess VIP receptors.
5. Glial cells produce a trophic material that promotes neuronal survival, and the secretion of this material by glia is increased substantially by VIP treatment at concentrations like those described above.

A number of other closely related peptides (e.g., PHI, secretin) do not have the survival-promoting activity of VIP (17). Antibodies to VIP or VIP-blocking peptide fragments (VIP10-28) have a deleterious effect on neuronal survival indistinguishable from TTX.

Taken together, these findings led to a developmental schema of the following sort. Electrically active, VIP-containing neurons release VIP, which interacts with VIP receptors on glial cells. These activated glial cells elaborate a proteinaceous factor which acts on neurons as a trophic material promoting their survival. An attractive feature of this scheme is that it would seem to serve as a paradigm for much more extensive and general neuron–glial–neuron interactions that might be involved in developmental regulation and maintenance of neuronal integrity. As noted above, glial cells have an extraordinarily rich complement of receptors on their surface, giving them potential responsiveness to a broad array of neurotransmitters.

These developmental studies involved the utilization of a relatively complex culture system with several types of neurons and background cells. Identification of specific cell types was essential for these studies, and the ability to grow pure glial preparations and enriched neuronal populations was a key feature.

The development of a powerful antagonist for VIP has allowed a test of whether VIP plays a role in the development of the nervous system *in vivo* (18). When the antagonist is injected into rat pups or into the ventricle of older animals, substantial behavioral deficits and neuronal dysgeneses were produced. Such whole-animal validation of results obtained with tissue culture preparations is a crucial step in mechanistic understanding of developmental or neurotoxicological processes. Other examples where this has been accomplished in developmental neuroscience include cholinergic induction in the autonomic nervous system (5,19,20) and regulation of motoneuron number in the spinal cord (21–23).

Preparations of central neuronal cultures have been developed which, while not providing purified cell populations, do represent useful experimental preparations for a variety of biochemical, morphological, and physiological studies. These include cell cultures prepared from (a) the ventral or dorsal horn of the spinal cord, (b) the hippocampus, (c) the cerebral cortex, (d) granule cells from the cerebellum, (e) the brain stem, and (f) the basal nuclei from the forebrain (see ref. 24 for an excellent review).

An effective means of identifying certain populations of neurons has been developed and is being used in several laboratories, both for identification and for separation and purification of the neurons (24–26). The method relies on knowing the axonal projection pattern of the population of interest. Marker molecules are injected into the region to which the axons project, are taken up by the axonal endings, and are transported retrogradely to the cell bodies of the neurons. Insofar as a population of neurons in a given brain region are the only ones in that region that project to the injection site, this method serves to identify that population of neurons. This method has been used to label spinal motoneurons, since all and only the spinal cord neurons whose axons terminated in muscle would be motoneurons and labeled by materials injected into skeletal muscle. Similarly, however, cerebral cortical neurons which project to the pyramidal tract or to a subcortical structure, the superior colliculus, have been labeled by suitably injected retrogradely transported marker molecules (27).

PHYSIOLOGICAL STUDIES

Dissociated cell cultures of the CNS have been particularly useful in allowing rigorous biophysical characterization of membrane mechanisms involved in synaptic and pharmacological responses of neurons. Neurons from nearly every region of the mammalian central neurons have been available for a level of analysis far beyond that which can be attained *in vivo*. Recent progress in our understanding of excitatory amino acid responses exemplify this work; an excellent comprehensive review is available (1).

A large body of physiological and pharmacological experimentation *in vivo* had indicated that at least two and possibly three different amino acid receptors were involved in fast excitatory responses of central neurons. Considerable uncertainty has been attached to the interpretation of the membrane mechanisms involved in the different responses, however. In particular, it was unclear whether the response to glutamate involved an increase or decrease of membrane conductance and what ions contributed to the response. Tissue culture methods allowed the application of voltage-clamp techniques to the analysis of this problem, in conjunction with alteration in the ionic composition of extracellular and intracellular solutions in contact with the neuronal membrane. Known concentrations of the receptor agonists and antagonists are crucial for these experiments.

Glutamate has been shown to be a mixed excitatory agonist, activating receptors of both the *N*-methyl-D-aspartate (NMDA) and non-NMDA (kainate and/or quisqualate or K/Q preferring) type. Activation of K/Q-preferring receptor results in a voltage-independent increase in membrane conductance to monovalent cations; the reversal potential for this response is about 0 mV. Divalent cations have little effect on these responses. The response to NMDA receptor activation, by contrast, is markedly voltage-dependent in physiological solutions, and a region of negative slope conductance occurs between about -60 and -20 mV. This negative slope region is dependent on the presence of Mg^{2+} ions in the external medium; in 0 Mg^{2+} solutions the response to NMDA is nearly voltage-independent. The reversal potential of the NMDA response is also about 0 mV in physiological solutions. The conductance increase elicited by NMDA-type agonists has been shown to involve monovalent cations and also Ca^{2+} ions. In fact, the conductance increase of Ca^{2+} is quite large. Direct demonstration of an increase in cytoplasmic Ca^{2+} as a result of NMDA receptor activation has been possible using Ca^{2+}-sensitive dyes and optical detection methods (28,29).

Numerous experiments have shown that non-NMDA receptors were involved in excitatory interactions both *in vivo* and *in vitro*, and patch recording methods have demonstrated clearly a major contribution of NMDA receptors in excitatory synaptic potentials in both hippocampal and spinal cord cultures (30). The NMDA component of synaptic currents has a much longer time course than does the non-NMDA component. Persistent activation of the NMDA receptor is probably responsible for this prolonged synaptic current. Raising external Ca^{2+} from 1 to 20 mM results in a shift in the reversal potential of the NMDA-mediated component of the synaptic current from 0 mV to +10 mV, whereas the non-NMDA reversal potential is unaffected. This indicates that, as with the pharmacological responses, synaptically activated NMDA conductance involves channels through which Ca^{2+} ions as well as monovalent cations can move. In the presence of external Mg^{2+} ions, this conductance displays the same strong voltage dependence as do the pharmacological NMDA responses.

The dissociated neuronal cell culture system has been used in a variety of pharmacological studies directed at understanding the mechanism of action of anticonvulsant and other neuroactive compounds (31). Recent advances in patch-clamp and single-channel recording techniques give excellent promise of understanding the molecular basis of the activity of such agents on a variety of CNS cell types.

The tissue culture methodology has been useful in analyzing the presynaptic transmitter release mechanism. In particular, the relationship between the morphology and physiology of excitatory synaptic connections has been studied (32,33). The statistical properties of individual synaptic connections have been measured in conjunction with pre- and postsynaptic injection of fluorescent dyes and horseradish peroxidase to identify the synaptic structure involved in the synaptic activity. The physiological studies defined the number of functional release elements subserving a given connection. Each release element can release no more than one quantum of transmitter, and the probability that release of a quantum would occur following a presynaptic action potential has a value somewhere between 0 and 1. The number of release elements and their probability of release essentially define the *physiological* transmitter release apparatus. It was found that in some cases the number of anatomical synaptic boutons corresponded quite closely to the number of functional release elements. In a substantial proportion of cases, however, the number of boutons was much larger than the number of release elements, suggesting that up to one-half or two-thirds of boutons were not functional. This implies that a substantial reserve of functionally inactive synapses may be available for recruitment under appropriate circumstances.

Optical techniques, in conjunction with voltage or ion-sensitive dyes, provide a direct, relatively noninvasive and sensitive method for following different neuronal activities. A dye designed by Tsien and colleagues (34), Fura-2, has provided excellent quantitative measurement of cytosolic Ca^{2+} in single rat cerebellar granule cells in the outgrowth zone of explant cultures (35). The output of a CCD camera is recorded on a 320×512 pixel array, with exposure times of 0.25–0.5 sec being adequate to obtain each image. Emission at 500 nM with excitation at 340 versus 380 nM are compared to obtain Ca^{2+}-dependent emission. A formula exists for relating the 340/380 emission ratio to the free Ca^{2+} in the area corresponding to a given period, so that the processed data give a picture with $[Ca^{2+}]$ coded in color. High-potassium depolarization of the granule cells was accompanied by an increase in cytosolic Ca^{2+}; this effect was more pronounced in cells that had been maintained *in vitro* for longer periods. Furthermore, a pronounced accentuation of the rise in cytosolic calcium under depolarization was observed with repeated application of the high-K^+ solution. In intermediate stage cells (longer than 12 days *in vitro*), application of 25 mM K^+ raised cytosolic calcium from 100 mM to approximately 2 mM. Spike inactivation by TTX diminished by about one-half the calcium response to high-K^+ solutions, implying that spike activity was partly responsible for the Ca^{2+} rise. Nifedipine, an organic blocker of some types of voltage-sensitive calcium, also blocked about 50% of the calcium response to high-K^+ solutions. Applications of 10 μM GABA produced a consistent increase in cytosolic calcium, although this increase (a doubling or so) is much less than that produced by high K^+. Small, inconsistent calcium responses were produced by glutamate in younger cultures, but rarely in older cultures; more consistent responses were seen with kainate application.

This technology has been used in a number of studies of intracellular calcium in relation to neuronal structure (3).

TISSUE CULTURE METHODOLOGY

Quite recently, several presentations of neural tissue culture methodologies have appeared with both general discussion and detailed procedures (see ref. 24). We will make some comments on some preparations with which we are familiar, emphasizing those features that we feel are relevant to the design and utilization of an *in vitro* neurotoxicologic screen.

The overriding imperatives for toxicological testing using *in vitro* model systems are the three R's: relevance, reliability, and reproducibility. In addressing these imperatives for dissociated neural cultures, the ideal has been best achieved for reproducibility and reliability. Our experience with primary dissociated systems have indicated that the following variables are important in optimizing these systems for both analytical purposes and reproducibility: plating density, culture age, monitoring of electrical activity, cellular diversity, nutrient media, duration of test period, schedule of medium changes, and gestational age of tissue. Among the most important culture variables is plating density, requiring both a sufficient number of cells to allow survival yet few enough to retain cellular resolution. There exists a threshold of neuronal cell number that must be achieved to permit the survival of neurons, which probably is contingent on having enough background support cells and sufficient synaptic contact with other neurons. In the case of the dissociated spinal cord and hippocampal systems, low-density neuronal cultures can be achieved with a confluent layer of background cells with a high degree of reliability and reproducibility.

The number and type of support glial cells that are present in a test system are of major importance in several respects: The glia may themselves be the target of the test substance, thus producing neuronal damage indirectly by interfering with glial-derived support; in addition, the glia provide a cellular matrix upon which neurons can grow. These background cells can be manipulated in several ways to optimize a neuronal test system for toxicological screening. Of practical importance, by "seeding" neurons onto a confluent layer of astrocytes (typically from cerebral cortex), one can obtain an excellent dispersion of nonaggregated neurons at very high plating efficiency. Indeed, our experience with neuronal cultures from hippocampus and cerebral cortex has been that this seeding strategy provides cultures with greater reproducibility, increased longevity, and an impressive cellular resolution that is so important for many of the neuronal surface- and image-based assays. Another important aspect of the background cells is control of their cellular division to prevent astrocyte overgrowth and the proliferation of microglia. Typically, a 1- to 4-day treatment (depending on the culture) with uridine plus fluorodeoxyuridine provides adequate inhibition of the nonneuronal cells. In all systems we have worked with, this antimitotic treatment increased the longevity of the preparation and substantially improved the reliability of the test system.

Included in our list of important considerations for optimizing primary neuronal test systems is the *age* of the cultures when the test compound is added. The type and number of cellular processes which will be vulnerable to a test compound will vary depending on what age is chosen for the treatment period. For example, if the test compound is added at the time of plating or seeding, neuronal survival could be affected by substance that interferes with the attachment of the neurons to their background matrix. Because of this complication, we generally allow cultures to develop for a week before adding test compounds. This period allows for the neurons to migrate and establish a network of interacting, synaptically connected cells. Depending on the goals of the testing, one can limit the period to one in which the neurons are developing instead of one in which the neurons have matured. In general, this maturation requires 3–4 weeks *in vitro*. In screening compounds for their potential effects on developing systems, the concept of a "critical period" comes into consideration. A critical period is a finite stage of development during which the cultured cells are vulnerable to toxic effects of the test substance. Most often, this period occurs during a time when the system is undergoing rapid growth and differentiation. Indeed, this period varies with the type of preparation and brain area chosen, and thus this interval needs to be empirically determined for each test system. In the dissociated spinal cord/dorsal root ganglion preparation, this period exists for approximately 2 weeks, from day 7 to day 21 *in vitro*.

Another important variable in obtaining reproducible and reliable test cultures is the manipulation and control of the nutrient medium in which the cells grow. As mentioned previously, the cellular composition of the primary cultures can be manipulated by altering the growth medium and varying the number of complete changes of medium. In general, to obtain test cultures that are highly enriched in neurons versus nonneuronal cells, a serum-free, defined medium should be used. After plating the cells in a medium containing 10% fetal calf serum, we typically place the cultures into serum-free medium within 24 hr. Such cultures should be plated on poly-L-lysine or other suitable matrix protein such as collagen. Often a "sandwich" of matrix proteins is of value in optimizing cell adherence and stability in these preparations. Since there are very few nonneuronal cells in such preparations, the matrix protein becomes an important variable in maintaining cellular adherence and stability during the assay procedures. As previously discussed, such "pure" neuronal cultures probably are not the best initial screen for toxicity. Rather, a preparation which is comprised of a mixed population of cells including neurons and glia is more appropriate, so that indirect- as well as direct-acting agents will be detected. Other important medium-related variables include the number of complete medium changes and the age of the culture when these changes are made. The reason for this emphasis is the potential influence of conditioning substances that are released by cells over time in culture. The vulnerability of neurons can be dramatically affected by the absence or presence of conditioning factors. For instance, tetrodotoxin, a neurotoxin that blocks voltage-dependent sodium channels, produces a 30–50% loss of neurons when added to cultures after a complete exchange of medium, whereas the same treatment in cultures that have not received a complete change of medium actually prevents neuronal death that normally occurs in control cultures. Thus, an opposite pharmacological effect can be obtained depending on the manipulation of conditioning substances during medium exchanges. Thus, changes of medium should be made purposefully and under tight control to avoid inconsistencies during the screening process.

Many of the primary neuronal culture systems exhibit spontaneous electrical activity that can vary from an occasional postsynaptic potential to complex patterns of electrical bursting activity. In the case of *developing* neuronal cultures, the ability of a test compound to decrease this activity can itself result in neuronal cell death. Thus, the tested substance may not have an intrinsic toxic interaction with cellular metabolism yet still produce deleterious action through its alteration of the ionic milieu secondary to activity changes.

The most basic experiment for screening potentially toxic substances is the dose–response. Typically we screen substances at log concentration intervals over five orders of magnitude. The number of replications can be kept to a minimum (two to three) at this stage of screening. Although the broad range of concentrations chosen for the screen may appear excessive, we have found that by using this approach we have discovered atypical toxic effects that a more limited range would have missed. For example, our experiments with the envelope protein from the human immunodeficiency virus have shown that toxicity is observed primarily at very low concentrations (≤ 1 pM) of the purified protein, with higher amounts producing significantly less or no toxicity (51). The envelope protein studies serve to illustrate that in the case of peptide/protein test substances, higher concentrations don't necessarily produce greater toxicity. Whereas for most substances the dose–effect curve will be proportional, one should be aware of response properties that may be unique to a given class of substances.

ASSAYS OF TOXICITY

The intuitive strategy for screening compounds for their neurotoxic potential might be to devise a series of tests that proceed from a sensitive, albeit nonspecific measure of global cellular structure and function to assays that are directed at specific neuronal phenotypes or pointed at a specific biochemical pathway, which may explicate a neurochemical mechanism. Within this strategy proceeding from the general to specific, one has the option of employing either morphological or biochemically oriented measures to assess the level of toxicity in cultured cells. While primary neuronal cultures do provide for a degree of complexity that may increase the relevancy to effects *in vivo*, the morphological and neurochemical heterogeneity of the neurons that comprise the primary systems pose a problem in finding assays which are effective in assessing representative amounts of neurotoxic damage. However, it is our opinion that the advantage of having the interacting cell types present in the test system far outweigh any difficulty in estimating damage in such heterogeneous test systems. Indeed, large-scale studies conducted to determine the utility of assays using established cell lines have shown that they are not highly predictive of teratogenic potential (36). Hence, the need for relevant interacting cell types in the test system.

The prima facie approach in neurotoxic assessment is gross morphological evaluation for any abnormal appearance of neurons, including vacuolization, degeneration of axons or dendrites, lysis of cell bodies, and arborization shrinkage. In some types of preparations (e.g., dissociated spinal cord/dorsal root ganglion cultures), there is also a need to immunocytochemically identify neurons from glia because of their similar appearance. For this purpose, antisera to neuron-specific enolase is a good choice for immunocytochemical verification of neurons (37). Antisera to neurofilament proteins is also used to identify neurons, but this often results in a heavily stained neuropile, making somal body identification difficult in high-density cultures. We have used neuronal cell counts as the most direct assessment of neuronal survival in chronic (3–5 days) test paradigms (38). Counts are conducted from coded dishes on predetermined coordinate locations and, of course, without knowledge of the treatment group. With this method, one can evaluate neurotoxic effects on the number of morphologically distinct neurons (e.g., bipolar versus multipolar) or immunocytochemically identified neuronal phenotypes. Because these direct counting assays are time-consuming and laborious, we usually restrict their use to a confirmatory role of the more indirect screening assays enumerated below. With the advent of sophisticated computerized image analysis, it is now possible to count neurons and estimate neurite length by automated techniques (39,40). Although such systems can provide a rapid, quantitative method for obtaining morphometric parameters, the major disadvantages are cost and the specialized technical knowledge required for accurate image analysis.

For quantitative screening purposes employing biochemically oriented assays, there are several alternates that should be considered. In the most general category, the direct measurement of cellular protein or nucleic acid is commonly used. These, in general, are not very sensitive, and in complex systems of dissociated neural tissue the amount of protein associated with neurons may be an insignificant amount of the total culture protein. In preparations that are enriched for neurons in comparison to nonneuronal cells, the protein assay could be used with greater sensitivity and utility (41). Another general cytotoxic measure often employed is the release of the soluble enzyme lactate dehydrogenase (LDH) (42). Whereas this assay has no cellular specificity, it can be used advantageously in screening compounds for general cytotoxicity. The LDH assay can be automated and scaled down to achieve a rapid and quantitative measure of cytotoxicity (43). In addition, quantification of neurotoxic and neurotrophic effects has been reported using fluorescein diacetate, a dye taken up by living cells. For this assay, the total amount of fluorescein produced from the dye is measured in cell lysates (44). This method was found to be proportional to the number of cells counted under fluorescence microscopy.

In some cases, an assay more specifically directed at neurons is required. Options we have utilized for this purpose include iodinated tetanus toxin fixation, tritiated ouabain binding, and assay of neurotransmitter-related enzymes such as choline acetyltransferase (cholinergic neurons), glutamic acid decarboxylase (GABAergic neurons), or tyrosine hydroxylase (catecholiminergic neurons) (45,46). All of the above assays have interpretive disadvantages but possess the obvious benefit of speed and precise quantitation. In this brief discussion of these neuron-directed, biochemical methodologies, we should point out interpretive caveats inherent in the assay as well as indicate some of their potential applications. Radiolabeled tetanus toxin binds to neurons with very high affinity and can be used to estimate neuronal surface area (47). This method is rapid and easy to perform but has several limitations. Tetanus toxin does not bind well to newly dissociated neurons for as long as 4 days after plating. Thus, the utility of this assay is confined to neuronal cultures that have developed in cultures for about a week. In addition, tetanus toxin can bind to type II astrocytes, thereby limiting the conclusions that can be drawn. Tetanus toxin also can bind to dead neurons, and thus sufficient time must be allowed for cell lysis to occur to observe neuronal deficits by this method. More recently, ouabain binding has been employed to estimate neuronal damage (48). Ouabain binds with high affinity to the Na^+,K^+-ATPase which is enriched on neurons in comparison to nonneuronal cells. In addition, the binding of cardiac glycosides to various areas of rat brain have suggested that the high-affinity binding of ouabain selectively labels the neuronal form of the Na^+,K^+-ATPase (49). Membrane or whole-cell preparations may be used in the ouabain assay. Good correlations have been found between neuronal cell number and ouabain binding. Excitotoxin-mediated decrements have also been detected with high precision and reproducibility (49).

NEUROTOXICOLOGY

A basic distinction that should be kept in mind in neurotoxicology (as with other areas of toxicology) has to do with the design of a *screening* system for agents of unknown effect as compared to *analytic* systems for studying mechanisms that might be responsible for known toxic effects or related to structures having a high index of toxicological suspicion. In the latter case, experimental approaches analogous to those involved in mechanistic neurobiologic studies generally seem appropriate; that is, appropriate target neuronal or glial cell populations must be identified. These may be highly selective (i.e., only oligodendrocytes or cholinergic neurons) in some cases, whereas any neuronal, glial, or indeed any cell type may be usable in others. Possible involvement of specific molecular or cell biologic processes can then be investigated regarding their direct or secondary vulnerability to the toxic agent in question.

The design of an adequate screening system is perhaps conceptually more difficult. An extreme position that only the behaving human is an adequate test object is strictly correct, but not helpful. We will explore the characteristics of *in vitro* systems that may be useful in identifying compounds with neurotoxic potential, keeping in mind the necessity of avoiding both errors of omission (false-negative) and errors of commission (false-positive). For a *screening* system, the former sin would appear to be most serious in that, logically, an initial screen has utility if it removes from further consideration those compounds deemed *not* to be toxic. Therefore, a negative result on the screen needs to be quite well validated as strongly indicating that a compound will not have adverse effects on the intact nervous system. In general, studies that would justify using *in vitro* models in this strong, screening fashion are not available. It is beyond the scope of this review to provide a strategy for establishing such a role for *in vitro* systems; we believe it is possible to develop such a strategy, and if this is not done, the systems will be far less useful than would be desirable. Positive indications of toxicity require further investigation; if this reveals no significant effects, the initial false indicators will have resulted in "unnecessary" study of the compound, but no injury to the potential human population of exposed individuals. An excessively high proportion of false-positives, however, renders the initial screen of little utility.

As has been noted previously, the nervous system *in vitro* comes in three or four different general versions varying in complexity and the degree to which they retain structural and functional properties of the parent tissue. Detailed descriptions of these different types of cultures are available (24): (a) Continuously dividing tumor or transformed cell lines form the simplest preparation. These lines can be induced to stop dividing and exhibit a variety of neuronal or glial phenotypes including the formation of synapses with target cells. (b) Primary dissociated cell cultures are formed by growing a single-cell suspension from some central or peripheral neural structure on the surface of a culture dish. The single-cell suspension or the cultures themselves can be processed in various ways to produce pure neuronal or glial populations or even (with various marking and sorting methods) relatively pure populations of a given cell type, such as spinal motoneurons or a particular type of glia. (c) These cell suspensions can be manipulated to produce reaggregated cultures which may reconstitute various aspects of the parent tissue. (d) Small pieces or slices of neural tissue can be cultured, giving preparation preserving a considerable degree of homology with the parent brain structure. Different pieces of the brain can be positioned in the culture dish so that they establish appropriate synaptic connections with one another (spinal cord with muscle, retina with thalamus, etc.).

We will argue as have others (50) that (a) for an initial screening instrument, the more complex multicomponent systems are appropriate and (b) for the assay of toxic effect, more general indices of development and integrity are to be preferred.

A large number of assays are now available for evaluating the development and function of these preparations. These assays range in specificity from those reporting the activity of single molecules peculiar to an individual cell type (enzymes, receptors, specific antigens) to global indicators such as cell number, total proteins or RNA, general surface membrane markers, and so on. Intermediate markers are available for classes of cells (neurons versus glia; oligoglia versus astroglia).

The Use of More Highly Organized, Multicomponent Systems as a Screening Instrument

Since the utility of a screen depends on its being responsive to as broad a range of toxicological agents and mechanisms as possible, obviously for a preparation to signal an agent with a given target molecule (i.e., mechanism of action), that molecule must be present in the test system. The mixed or complex systems incorporate a wider range of cell types and hence should be responsive to a broader range of agents. Furthermore, some agents may act on mechanisms involved in the *interaction* between different types of cells. In such a case, *no* single-cell-type preparation would reveal a potentially significant toxic effect. An example may be useful in illustrating this situation. One of the distressing aspects of infection with the human immunodeficiency virus (HIV) experienced by many patients with acquired immunodeficiency syndrome (AIDS) is dementia. Histopathology has revealed that there is a loss of neurons in the cerebral cortex of some people infected with HIV, and experiments in cell cultures have demonstrated that gp120, an HIV coat protein shed from the virus and present in the blood of the infected individual, is capable of producing neuronal death (51). However, this is true in hippocampal cultures only if both neurons and glia cells are present, and neuronal killing is not produced by the gp120 protein when the glia population has been reduced or eliminated by appropriate culture conditions. One parsimonious interpretation is that the gp120 acts primarily on the astrocyte and that the neuronal death is a secondary effect of this primary action. Of course, this may not be the only action of the gp120, and indeed the death of retinal ganglion cells produced by gp120 may well be due to a direct effect of the peptide on those neurons (52).

The "excitotoxic" action of the amino acid alpha-amino-beta-methylamine propionic acid (BMAA) are thought to be indirect (50) because of the structural features of the BMAA, its relatively low potency, and the rather slow onset of excitant action following its administration.

THE USE OF GLOBAL MEASURES AS ASSAYS
FOR TOXICOLOGIC DAMAGE

Even extremely specific agents may have striking effects on general indicators of neuronal or glial well-being while leaving some more specific measures unaffected. An example is the voltage-sensitive sodium channel blocker, tetrodotoxin, as noted above. Incubation of fetal CNS cultures with 0.5 μM tetrodotoxin for a period of a few days results in a 30–50% decrease in neuronal number and of neuronal surface membrane as measured by tetanus toxin binding (15). The activity of GAD (glutamic acid decarboxylase) is, however, unchanged. Thus, while some neuronal populations are vulnerable to the effects of sodium channel blockade, others are not. If only selected subpopulations are affected, of course, this results in the signal indicative of toxic effect, which will be less than that of the culture as a whole. *The culture system must be extremely reliable and well characterized so that relatively small quantitative changes can be interpreted with confidence.* This requires that the large number of variables determining the development and maintenance of the culture will be controlled.

Of course, if structure–activity data or other information concerning a potential neurotoxicant are available and suggest a specific target or neuropathogenetic mechanism, a more targeted test system and assays would be appropriate.

SPECIFIC NEUROTOXICOLOGIC STUDIES

We will make no attempt to review the very large literature on *in vitro* neurotoxicologic testing (see refs. 53 and 54). Rather, we will take three examples which illustrate some of the problems and the promise of the field and discuss them in some detail. These are: (i) studies of the possible pathogenetic potential of various anticonvulsant medications; (ii) the excitotoxic responses exemplified by motor system damage produced in lathyrism, by nonprotein amino acids from the pathogenetic plant *Lathyrus sativus* and by domoic acid from some species of mussels; and (iii) issues related to heavy metal intoxication and neurotoxicology.

Phenobarbital, Phenytoin, and Other Anticonvulsant Agents

For many years and up until the 1970s, children with a febrile convulsion were treated for up to 5 years with phenobarbital. Dosage levels were such that blood levels were above 65 μmol (15 μg/ml) and up to 130 μmol (30 μg/ml). There was concern as to both the therapeutic need for treatment and effects on brain development in children, and in the 1970s and early 1980s a number of experimental studies in rats and mice suggested that phenobarbital administered pre- or postnatally did indeed impair brain growth (see, e.g., ref. 55). Several studies using *in vitro* methods have now been done to assess the neurotoxicity of phenobarbital and a number of other anticonvulsant medications.

In 1981, Bergey et al. (56) examined the effect of phenobarbital on developing dissociated cultures of mouse spinal cord. In 1983, Swaiman et al. (57) described similar experiments using phenytoin and mouse cortical cultures. A number of morphological and neurochemical markers were used to quantify the effects of various concentrations of the anticonvulsant agents on both neurons and glial cells. A more comprehensive pair of studies in 1985 (58,59) examined phenytoin, phenobarbital, carbamazepine, valproic acid, diazepam, and ethosuximide for their effect on mouse cerebral cortical culture, with the aim of determining the *relative* neurotoxicity of these different anticonvulsant agents. Parameters measured included the number of surviving neurons, total protein, tetanus toxin fixation (an indication of total neuronal surface membrane), high-affinity uptake of γ-aminobutyric acid and β-alanine, choline acetyltransferase activity, and specific and clonazepam-displaceable benzodiazepam binding. Ethosuximide and carbamazepine had minimal toxic effects, valproate and diazepam had modest effects, and phenobarbital and phenytoin were definitely detrimental to neuronal survival and development. Serrano et al. (60) performed a detailed morphological study of phenobarbital effects on neuronal development and concluded that phenobarbital produced a reduction in neuronal survival and that in surviving neurons, dendritic branching pattern and length were reduced in a dose-dependent manner.

The question of appropriate dosage is discussed in some detail in these papers and constitute a substantial problem of interpretation. Since the anticonvulsants are lipophilic molecules, much of the agents in serum is bound in some form or another. The question of whether to use total concentration or only the free form of the drug must be considered. Serrano et al. pointed out that in an equilibrium situation, brain levels may be closer to the total concentration in the serum than to the free concentration and that this may be particularly true in neonatal or young animals in which immaturity of the blood–brain barrier and reduced binding by plasma proteins may be important considerations.

Similar studies in 1990 by Regan et al. (61) used a shorter exposure period and also incorporated (in addition to primary mouse cerebral cortical culture) the use of neural (neuro-2A) and glial (C6) cell lines to test for anticonvulsant effects on cell proliferation. The cytotoxic effect of phenytoin was confirmed in these studies, and a specific effect on the mitotic rate in the cell lines by valproate and the benzodiazepines was noted.

One of the interesting features of the Serrano et al. study was that the effects of phenobarbital on cell number and process length and complexity was more pronounced for neurons treated from day 14 to week 6 of culture than for neurons treated from day 2 to week 6 despite the fact that the latter cultures were treated for a longer total time.

Do these *in vitro* studies have a parallel in *in vivo* or clinical situations? A number of experimental studies in rodents had demonstrated both structural and behavioral effects of phenobarbital given to neonates or to pregnant animals (effects on offspring). A randomized clinical study published by Farwell et al. (62) in 1990 compared the IQ of 217 children who had experienced at least one febrile seizure and who were randomly assigned to a treatment group or to a placebo control group. The children in the treatment group received 4–5 mg/kg body weight of phenobarbital. This group had blood levels of phenobarbital between 15 and 30 μg/ml during the course of the study. The treatment group had an average IQ score 8.4 points below that of the control group after 2 years of treatment, and at 6 months after cessation of treatment the IQ of the treated children was 5.2 points lower than that of the control placebo group. Thus it appears that phenobarbital treatment may well be accompanied by some decrement in tested intellectual function. In addition, this study showed a lack of clinical efficacy in that there was no difference between treatment group and placebo control in the number of seizures that were experienced.

Excitotoxins

Since the early descriptions by Olney and Sharpe (63) of neurotoxic damage to neural tissue by excitatory amino acids (EAAs), particularly glutamate, a fairly complete scheme has emerged for understanding this pathogenetic process. Receptors for EAAs exist in neurons and glia, and, in fact, these receptors are responsible for the normal excitatory synaptic interactions which occur between neurons and which are an essential feature of brain function. At least three or four pharmacologically and physiologically distinguishable species of these receptors exist, and molecular biological techniques have demonstrated several subspecies of receptor subunit polypeptides. Importantly, a number of agonists and specific competitive and noncompetitive blockers of these receptors have been developed which are extremely useful in testing whether a given neurotoxic result may be due to or involve a component of EAA excitotoxicity (see ref. 1 for review).

It seems likely excitotoxicity may contribute to the actions of a broad range of neurotoxins, and consideration of the cellular mechanisms involved in excitotoxic damage to the nervous system may be useful. Work from a number of laboratories have contributed to the scheme summarized by Choi (64).

Glutamate is present in very high (mM) concentrations in neural tissue, particularly in nerve terminals. It is released from excitatory terminals during normal physiological activity to mediate synaptic transmission between these terminals and postsynaptic receptor cells. The EAA receptors on these neurons are of at least two broad varieties termed N-methyl-D-aspartate (NMDA) and non-NMDA or kainate/quisqualate (K/Q) receptor. The NMDA receptor is characterized by its voltage-dependence, its permeability to both calcium and sodium, its blockability by Mg^{2+} ions, and its requirement for low levels of glycine for activation. The non-NMDA receptors exhibit none of these characteristics. The conductance change (channel openings) associated with synaptic activation of NMDA receptors is of considerably longer duration than that associated with non-NMDA receptor activation. The excitotoxicity hypothesis states that excessive uncontrolled activation of these EAA receptors produces a cascade of events resulting in brain damage.

A number of observations strongly suggest that an increase in intracellular calcium ion concentration is a key step in the excitotoxic process.

Cell biological investigations over the past two decades have revealed the central role that intracellular $[Ca^{2+}]_i$ plays in the regulation of cellular processes. Protein kinase, proteases, phospholipases, and xanthine oxidase are all affected, and in various ways these may contribute to cell damage. Proteases such as calpain I degrade cellular structural proteins, the phospholipases can break down cell membrane constituents, and xanthine oxidase and lipid breakdown products generate potentially destructive superoxide radicals.

Depolarization of neurons by the EAAs may initiate a cycle in which depolarization-induced release of EAAs produces further depolarization, EAA buildup, and pathological consequences.

It should be noted that these cell biologic effectors are extremely general and are impinged upon by a number of factors. Lebel and Bondy (65) have emphasized the potential importance of oxygen radicals as mediators of neurotoxicity and point out that six of eight common neurotoxic agents (including such diverse components as methyl mercury, toluene, and methamphetamines) increase cerebral oxygen radical formation. Such a "final common pathway," as these authors term it, would provide a basis for synergistic interactions between different types of neurotoxicants.

The neurotoxic effect of glutamate (and other EAAs) has been demonstrated by direct injection *in vivo* and by a number of *in vivo* experiments involving anoxia, ischemia, or physical trauma. The importance of EAAs in producing brain damage in these various models has been shown by the sparing effect that specific EAA receptor blockers produce. That is, NMDA receptor blockers are "neuroprotective in a variety of hypoxia paradigms" (59).

Two examples have been investigated in which ingestion of excitatory amino acids may be causal for neurodegenerative diseases. The most clear cut is that of lathyrism, caused by the toxin β-*N*-oxaly-lamino-L-alanine (BOAA) from the chick pea (50,66). The onset of symptoms occurs after prolonged periods of consumption of the agent—in contrast to the acute symptomatology seen with contaminated mussels (67,68), in which domoic acid is the EAA responsible for the neurotoxicity. A potentially important link has been suggested between ingestion of flour made from seeds of the cycad plant and development of amyotrophic lateral sclerosis–parkinsonism–dementia among people in the Western Pacific islands, particularly Guam (69). The suspect agent, β-methylaminoalanine (BMAA), is a weak and atypical EAA, and its mechanism of action is unclear; indeed its involvement in the Guam syndrome is challenged (70). The possibility, however, that such environmental agents may contribute through an excitotoxic mechanism to chronic neurodegenerative diseases is being considered most seriously. It is clear that while *in vitro* systems cannot be complete models for clinical conditions of such long time course, they provide excellent material for evaluating the excitotoxic potential of any suspect compounds.

Heavy Metals

Mercury, tin, and lead exemplify environmentally pervasive compounds that have a clear neurotoxic effect. Catastrophic acute effects have been conclusively shown at levels that occur in real-life situations as exemplified by the widespread mercury poisoning that occurred as a result of pollution of Minamata Bay in Japan (54,71). Acute lead poisoning is also an all-too-common clinical picture, and *in vitro* models have been useful in establishing possible molecular and cellular mechanisms underlying such toxicity (72). In those experiments, cells of the glial cell line C_6 were treated with various concentrations of lead, and the effect on two enzymes and on the induction of those enzymes by cortisol was noted. The two enzymes were glucose phosphate dehydrogenase (GPDH) and lactate dehydrogenase (LDH). Basal levels of the two enzymes were unaffected by lead doses up to the 1 mM range. The induction of GPDH, however, was inhibited in a dose-dependent manner by lead, and at 10^{-4} M the block of induction was 40–50%. The experiments showed that the failure of GPDH induction by cortisol under lead treatment was due to its block of synthesis of the enzyme; GPDH degradation was unaffected by lead treatment. The effect of lead seems to be quite specific with respect to GPDH induction; no effect is seen on basal enzyme levels, on norepinephrine induction of cAMP, on cell viability, or on protein synthesis generally. The authors conclude that lead acts at some point between cortical binding in the nucleus of the C_6 cells and translation of GPDH mRNA.

GPDH is a specific marker for oligodendrocytes and myelin-forming cells generally, and GPDH is thought to be involved in myelination. One of the symptoms of lead intoxication is a deficit in peripheral and central myelination. The demonstrated effects of lead on GPDH may well provide a molecular basis for some of the symptomatology of lead intoxication.

The discussion of lead as an environmental neurotoxicant has shifted considerably in recent years, because the possibility has been raised by epidemiological studies that very low levels of lead ingestion and blood concentration 10–100 times lower, for instance, than those explored in the study described above, over prolonged periods, may have a deleterious effect on intellectual performance (73). Intense controversy surrounds this issue (*Science*, August 23, 1991), and it poses one version of the neurotoxicology problem. For a compound known to be neurotoxic at high doses and for which total elimination may be difficult, or at least very expensive, can "acceptable" levels be satisfactorily established? This problem, of course, is a common and difficult one in other areas of toxicology, notably with respect to carcinogenic agents. How might *in vitro* methods contribute in this regard. Two possible strategies might be considered: (i) It is possible to maintain cultured preparations for relatively prolonged periods. Both dissociated cell culture preparations and organotypic slice preparations can be maintained for several months. While not approximating the lifetime exposure that might be involved with human populations, this may nevertheless allow longer-time-course pathogenetic processes to reveal themselves with very-low-dose exposures to neurotoxic agents.

(ii) Quantitative and precise indicators of toxic actions are provided by the many assays that are available for evaluating the *in vitro* system. Particularly if these assays are directed at the cell biologic and molecular entities directly affected by the neurotoxic agents, great sensitivity may be attained. Thus even quantitatively minor effects produced by very low levels of the agents may be unequivocally demonstrated in these systems at relatively short (days to weeks) periods. Although each situation would have to be evaluated carefully, such modest but reliable indications of damage might be useful in the context of evaluating the levels at which thresholds should be set. The epidemiological data provide the definitive basis for such threshold setting, but this sort of data is extremely difficult to obtain and evaluate and is costly. Exploring the degree to which data from *in vitro* test systems might be helpful in this regard would be well worthwhile.

PROBLEMS

1. A prominent difficulty or limitation of the *in vitro* system is that they do not deal at all with the process of biotransformation. Many environmental agents may not themselves be neurotoxic, but when metabolized in the liver or elsewhere, the products generated may be so. This may be offset in part by testing independently the known metabolites of potential neurotoxicants. Hybrid culture schemes have also been proposed combining potential biotransforming cellular components (such as liver or kidney cells) in some sort of co-culture with the test neural tissue. The presumption would be that such co-cultures might provide an efficient combination of high-resolution *in vitro* test systems with some component, at least, of whole-animal biotransformations of potential neurotoxicants.

2. Most primary neural cultures of either dissociated cells or organotypic explants are composed of nondividing neurons with, in many cases, a largely static population of glial cells. The effect of some neurotoxic agents may be on neuroblast division and differentiation, so that teratological, developmental abnormalities are dominant. As noted earlier, dividing cell lines with potential for neural expression may be useful in evaluating such agents. Such cell lines are useful in probing for molecular and cellular sites of action as well (see above for discussion of lead oligodendrocyte toxicity). A large number of cell lines are available which can be differentiated in various ways by different culture manipulation. Extremely interesting studies on viral transformation of neural and glial cells are creating material with rich potential for neurotoxicological evaluation.

PROSPECTS FOR *IN VITRO–IN VIVO* APPROACHES

There has been considerable recognition of the potential importance of *in vitro* approaches to neurotoxic evaluation of the very large number of essential untested chemicals in use (60,000–70,000) and being added to the inventory (1000–1500 per year) (74). After considering pros and cons of *in vitro* testing, a report by the OTA in 1990 (54) concluded the following: "Nevertheless all test systems have limitations, and there is general agreement that the many advantages of *in vitro* testing present a strong incentive for continued development and increased utilization." Reservations about the role of *in vitro* testing are summarized, however, by Tilson (74): "Clearly before *in vitro* techniques are adopted to problems of hazard detection in neurotoxicology, research will be needed to devise a strategy to develop, refine *and validate* these procedures" (emphasis added).

REFERENCES

1. Mayer ML, Westbrook GL. The physiology of excitatory amino acids in the vertebrate central nervous system. *Prog Neurobiol* 1987;28:197–276.
2. Mayer ML, Vyklicky L Jr, Patneau DK. Glutamate receptors in cultures of mouse hippocampus studied with fast application of agonists, modulators and drugs. In: Ben-Ari Y, ed. *Excitatory amino acids and neuronal plasticity*. New York, Plenum Press, 1990;3–11.
3. Kater SB, Mattson MP, Cohan CS, Connor JA. Calcium regulation of the neuronal growth cone. *Trends Neurosci* 1988;11:315–321.
4. Barde Y-A. Trophic factors and neuronal survival. *Neuron* 1989;2:1525–1534.
5. Patterson PH. Environmental determination of autonomic neurotransmitter function. *Annu Rev Neurosci* 1987;1:1–17.
5a. Yamamori T, Fukada K, Aebersold R, Korsching S, Fann M-J, Patterson PH. The cholinergic neuronal differentiation factor from heart cells is identical to leukemia inhibitory factor. *Science* 1989; 246:1412–1416.
6. McCarthy KD, De Vellis J. Preparation of separate astroglial and oligodendroglial cell cultures from rat cerebral tissue. *J Cell Biol* 1980;85:890.
7. Trimmer PA, Evans T, Smith MM, Harden TK, McCarthy KD. Combination of immunocytochemistry and radioligand receptor assay to identify β-adrenergic receptor subtypes on astroglia *in vitro. J Neurosci* 1984;4:1598.
8. Evans T, McCarthy KD, Harden TK. Regulation of cyclic AMP accumulation by peptide hormone receptors in immunocytochemically defined astroglial cells. *J Neurochem* 1984;43:131.
9. McCarthy KD, Prime J, Harmon T, Pollenz R. Receptor-mediated phosphorylation of astroglial intermediate filament proteins in cultured astroglia. *J Neurochem* 1985;44:723.
10. Cornell-Bell AH, Finkbeiner SM, Cooper MS, Smith SJ. Glutamate induces calcium waves in cultured astrocytes: long range glial signalling. *Science* 1990;247:470–473.
11. Fatatis A, Russell JT. Spontaneous changes in intracellular calcium concentration in Type I astrocytes from rat cerebral cortex in primary culture. *Glia* 1991.
12. Dodd J, Jessell TM. Lactoseries carbohydrates specify subsets of dorsal root ganglion neurons projecting to the superficial dorsal horn of rat spinal cord. *J Neurosci* 1985;5:3278.
13. Neale EA, Oertel WG, Bowers LM, Weise VK. Glutamate decarboxylase immunoreactivity and γ-[^{3}H]aminobutyric acid accumulation within the same neurons in dissociated cell cultures of cerebral cortex. *J Neurosci* 1983;2:376–382.
14. Neale EA, Matthew E, Zimmerman EA, Nelson PG. Substance P-like immunoreactivity in neurons in dissociated cell cultures of mammalian spinal cord and dorsal root ganglia. *J Neurosci* 1982;2: 169–177.
15. Brenneman DE, Nelson PG. Neuronal development in culture. Role of electrical activity. In: Bottenstein JE, Sato G, eds. *Cell culture in the neurosciences*. New York: Plenum Press, 1985;299–316.
16. Brenneman DE, Neale EA, Foster GA, d'Autremont SW, Westbrook GL. Nonneuronal cells mediate neurotropic action of vasoactive intestinal peptide. *J Cell Biol* 1987;104:1603–1610.
17. Brenneman DE, Foster GE. Structural specificity of peptides influencing neuronal survival during development. *Peptides* 1987;8:687–694.
18. Hill JM, Gozes I, Hill JL, Fridkin M, Brenneman DE. Vasoactive intestinal peptide antagonist retards the development of neonatal behavior in the rat. *Peptides* 1991;12:187–192.

19. Landis SC, Keefe D. Evidence for neurotransmitter plasticity *in vivo*: developmental changes in properties of cholinergic sympathetic neurons. *Dev Biol* 1983;98:349–372.
20. Schotzinger RS, Landis SC. Cholinergic phenotype developed by noradrenergic sympathetic neurons after innervation of a noval cholinergic target *in vivo*. *Nature* 1988;335:637–639.
21. Giller EL Jr, Neale JH, Bullock PN, Schrier BK, Nelson PG. Choline acetyltransferase activity of spinal cord cultures increased by co-culture with muscle and by muscle conditioned medium. *J Cell Biol* 1977;74:16–29.
22. McManaman JL, Crawford FG, Steward SS, Appel SH. Purification of a skeletal muscle polypeptide which stimulates choline acetyltransferase activity in cultured spinal cord neurons. *J Biol Chem* 1988;263:5890–5897.
23. Houenou LJ, McManaman JL, Prevette D, Oppenheim RW. Regulation of putative muscle-derived neurotrophic factors by muscle activity and innervation: *in vivo* and *in vitro* studies. *J Neurosci* 1991;11:2839–2837.
24. Banker G, Goslin K. *Culturing nerve cells.* Cambridge, MA: MIT Press, 1991.
25. Schaffner AE, St. John PA, Barker JL. Fluorescence-activated cell sorting of embryonic mouse and rat motoneurons and their long-term survival *in vitro*. *J Neurosci* 1987;7:3088–3104.
26. O'Brien RJ, Fischbach GD. Isolation of embryonic chick motoneurons and their survival *in vitro*. *J Neurosci* 1986;6:3265.
27. Huettner JE, Baughman RW. Primary culture of identified neurons from the visual cortex of postnatal rats. *J Neurosci* 1986;6:3044.
28. MacDermott AB, Mayer ML, Westbrook GL, Smith SJ, Barker JL. NMDA-receptor activation increases cytoplasmic calcium concentration in cultured spinal cord neurones. *Nature* 1986;321:519–522.
29. Mayer ML, MacDermott AB, Westbrook GL, Smith SJ, Barker JL. Agonist and voltage-gated calcium entry in cultured mouse spinal cord neurons under voltage clamp measured with arsenazo III. *J Neurosci* 1987;7:3230–3244.
30. Forsythe ID, Westbrook GL. Slow excitatory postsynaptic currents mediated by *N*-methyl-D-aspartate receptors on cultured mouse central neurones. *J Physiol* 1988;396:505–533.
31. Barker JL, Ransom BR. Pentobarbitone pharmacology of mammalian central neurones grown in tissue culture. *J Physiol (Lond)* 1987;280:355–372.
32. Neale EA, Nelson PG, Macdonald RL, Christian CN, Bowers LM. Synaptic interactions between mammalian central neurons in cell culture. III. Morphophysiological correlates of quantal synaptic transmission. *J Neurophysiol* 1983;49:1459–1468.
33. Pun RYK, Neale EA, Guthrie PB, Nelson PG. Active and inactive central synapses in cell culture. *J Neurophysiol* 1986;1242–1256.
34. Grybkiewicz G, Poenie M, Tsien RY. A new generation of Ca^{2+} indicators with greatly improved fluorescence properties. *J Biol Chem* 1985;260:3440–3450.
35. Hockberger PE, Tseng H-Y, Connor JA. Immunocytochemical and electrophysiological differentiation of rat cerebellar granule cells in explant cultures. *J Neurosci* 1987;7:1370.
36. Steele VE, Morrissey RE, Elmore EL, Gurganus-Rocha D, Wilkinson BP, Curren RD, Schmetter BS, Louie AT, Lamb JC, Yang LL. Evaluation of two *in vitro* assays to screen for potential developmental toxicants. *Fundam Appl Toxicol* 1988;11:673–684.
37. Schmechel D, Marangos PJ, Zis AP, Brightman M, Goodwin FK. Brain enolases as specific markers of neuronal and glial cells. *Science* 1978;199:313–315.
38. Brenneman DE, Buzy JM, Ruff MR, Pert CB. Peptide T sequences prevent neuronal cell death produced by the envelope protein (gp120) of the human immunodeficiency virus. *Drug Dev Res* 1988;15:361–369.
39. Clements JD, Buzy JM. Automated image analysis for counting unstained cultured neurones. *J Neurosci Methods* 1991;36:1–8.
40. Matsumoto T, Oshima K, Miyamoto A, Sakurai M, Goto M, Hayashi S. Image analysis of CNS neurotrophic factor effects on neuronal survival and neurite outgrowth. *J Neurosci Methods* 1990;31:153–162.
41. Hayashi M, Tanii H, Horiguchi M, Hashimoto K. Cytotoxic effects of acrylamide and its related compounds assessed by protein content, LDH activity and cumulative glucose consumption of neuron-rich cultures in a chemically defined medium. *Arch Toxicol* 1989;63:308–313.
42. Koh J, Choi DW. Quantitative determination of glutamate mediated cortical neuronal injury in cell culture by lactate dehydrogenase efflux assay. *J Neurosci Methods* 1990;20:83–90.
43. Klingman JG, Hartley DM, Choi DW. Automated determination of excitatory amino acid neurotoxicity in cortical culture. *J Neurosci Methods* 1990;31:47–51.

44. Didier M, Heaulme M, Soutrie P, Bockaert J, Pin JP. Rapid, sensitive and simple method for quantification of both neurotoxic and neurotrophic effects of NMDA on cultured cerebellar granule cells. *J Neurosci Res* 1990;27:25–35.
45. Brenneman DE. Role of electrical activity and trophic factors during cholinergic development in dissociated cultures. *Can J Physiol Pharmacol* 1986;64:356–362.
46. Brenneman DE, Neale EA, Habig WH, Bowers LM, Nelson PG. Developmental and neurochemical specificity of neuronal deficits produced by electrical impulse blockade in dissociated spinal cord cultures. *Dev Brain Res* 1983;9:13–27.
47. Dimpfel W, Huang RTC, Habermann E. Gangliosides in nervous tissue cultures and binding of ^{125}I-labeled tetanus toxin, a neuronal marker. *J Neurochem* 1977;29:329–334.
48. Markwell MAK, Sheng HZ, Brenneman DE, Paul SM. A rapid method to quantify neurons in mixed cultures based on the specific binding of [^{3}H]ouabain to neuronal Na$^+$,K$^+$-ATPase. *Brain Res* 1991;538:1–8.
49. Hauger R, Luu MD, Goodwin FK, Paul SM. Characterization of [^{3}H]ouabain binding in the rat central nervous system. *J Neurochem* 1985;33:1709–1715.
50. Spencer PS, Ross SM, Nunn PB, Roy DN, Seelig M. Detection and characterization of plant-derived amino acid motorsystem toxin in mouse CNS cultures. In: Shahar A, Goldstein AM, eds. *Model systems in neurotoxicologic alternative approaches to animal-testing.* New York: Alan R Liss, 1987;349–361.
51. Brenneman DE, Westbrook GL, Fitzgerald SC, Ennist DL, Elkins KL, Ruff MR, Pert CB. Neuronal cell killing by the envelope protein of HIV and its prevention by vasoactive intestinal peptide. *Nature* 1988;335:639–642.
52. Lipton SA. HIV-related neurotoxicity. *Brain Pathology* 1991;1:193–199.
53. Shahar A, Goldstein AM, eds. *Model systems in neurotoxicologic alternative approaches to animal-testing.* New York: Alan R Liss, 1987.
54. *Neurotoxicity. Identifying and controlling poisons of the nervous system. New developments in neuroscience.* Congress of the United States, Office of Technology Assessment, OTA-BA-436, Washington, DC: US Government Printing Office, 1990.
55. Yanai J, Bergman A. Neuronal deficits after neonatal exposure to phenobarbital. *Exp Neurol* 1981; 73:199–208.
56. Bergey GK, Swaiman KF, Schrier BK, Fitzgerald S, Nelson PG. Adverse effects of phenobarbital on morphological and biochemical development of fetal mouse spinal cord neurons in culture. *Annu Neurol* 1981;9:584–589.
57. Swaiman KF, Neale EA, Schrier BK, Nelson PG. Toxic effect of phenytoin on developing cortical neurons in culture. *Annu Neurol* 1983;13:48–52.
58. Neale EA, Sher PK, Graubard BI, Habig WH, Fitzgerald SC, Nelson PG. Differential toxicity of chronic exposure to phenytoin, phenobarbital, or carbamazepine in cerebral cortical cell cultures. *Pediatric Neurology* 1985;1:143–150.
59. Sher PK, Neale EA, Graubard BI, Habig WH, Fitzgerald SC, Nelson PG. Differnetial neurochemical effects of chronic exposure of cerebral cortical cell culture to valproic acid, diazepam, or ethosuximide. *Pediatric Neurology* 1985;1:232–237.
60. Serrano EF, Kunis DM, Ransom BR. Effects of chronic phenobarbital exposure on cultured mouse spinal cord neurons. *Annu Neurol* 1988;24:429–438.
61. Regan CM, Gorman AMC, Larsson OM, Maguire C, Martin ML, Schousboe A, Williams DC. *In vitro* screening for anticonvulsant-induced teratogenesis in neural primary cultures and cell lines. *Int J Dev Neurosci* 1990;8:143–150.
62. Farwell JR, Lee YS, Hirtz DG, Sulzbacher SI, Ellenberg JH, Nelson KB. Phenobarbital for fibril seizures—effects on intelligence and on seizure recurrence. *N Eng J Med* 1990;322:364–369.
63. Olney JW, Sharpe LG. Brain lesions in an infant rhesus monkey treated with monosodium glutamate. *Science* 1969;166:386–388.
64. Choi DW. Glutamate neurotoxicity and diseases of the nervous system. *Neuron* 1988;1:623–639.
65. Lebel CP, Bondy SC. Oxygen radicals' common mediators of neurotoxicity. *Neurotoxicol Teratol* 1991;13:341–346.
66. Spencer PS, Allen RG, Kisby GE, Ludolph AC. Excitotoxic disorders. *Science* 1990;245:144.
67. Perl TN, Bedard L, Kosatsky T, Hockin JC, Todd ECD, Remis RS. An outbreak of toxic encephalopathy caused by eating mussels contaminated with domoic acid. *N Engl J Med* 1990;322:1775–1780.
68. Teitelbaum JS, Zatorre RJ, Carpenter S, Gendron D, Evans AC, Gjedde A, Cashman NR. Neuro-

logic sequel of domoic acid intoxication due to the ingestion of contaminated mussels. *N Engl J Med* 1990;322:1781–1787.

69. Spencer PS, Nunn PB, Hugon J, Ludolph AC, Ross SM, Roy DN, Robertson RC. Guam amyotrophic lateral sclerosis Parkinsonian dementia linked to a plant excitant neurotoxin. *Science* 1987;237:517–522.

70. Duncan MW, Steele JC, Kopin IJ, Markey SP. 2-amino-3(methylamino)-propanoic acid (BMAA) in cycad flour: an unlikely cause of amyotrophic lateral sclerosis and Parkinsonism-dementia of Guam. *Neurology* 1990;40:767–772.

71. Chang LW. Mercury. In: Spencer PS, Schaumberg HH, eds. *Clinical and experimental neurotoxicology*. Baltimore: Williams & Wilkins, 1980;508–509.

72. DeVellis J, McGinn JF, Cole R. Selective effects of lead on the hormonal regulation of glial cell proliferation in cell culture. In: Shahar A, Goldstein AM, eds. *Model systems in neurotoxicologic alternative approaches to animal-testing*. New York: Alan R Liss, 1987;217–227.

73. Bellinger D, Leviton A, Waternaux C, Needleman H, Rabinowitz M. Longitudinal analyses of prenatal and postnatal lead exposure and early cognitive development. *N Engl J Med* 1987;316:1037–1043.

74. Tilson HA. Neurotoxicology in the 1990s. *Neurotoxicol Teratol* 1990;12:293–300.

In Vitro Toxicology,
edited by Shayne C. Gad.
Raven Press, Ltd., New York, © 1994.

9

In Vitro Assessment of Nephrotoxicity

Joan B. Tarloff* and Robin S. Goldstein†

*Department of Pharmacology and Toxicology, Philadelphia College of Pharmacy and
Science, Philadelphia, Pennsylvania 19104; and †Department of Investigative Toxicology,
SmithKline Beecham Pharmaceuticals, King of Prussia, Pennsylvania 19406*

The kidney is a complex and heterogeneous organ, composed of vascular as well as tubular components, and is frequently a site of injury following exposure to chemicals or during drug treatment. Susceptibility of the kidney to toxicity may be related to any one or more of a combination of factors. First, the kidneys receive a disproportionately high percentage of cardiac output (20% of total cardiac output distributed to organs accounting for less than 1% of body weight), thereby exposing renal tissue to high concentrations of toxicant. Second, potential toxicants may become highly concentrated within the tubular lumen following reabsorption of electrolytes, nutrients, and water by the nephron. Thus, tubular epithelial cells may be exposed to higher concentrations of toxicants than may be found in other tissues. Third, the proximal tubule actively reabsorbs solutes such as glucose and amino acids, while actively secreting metabolic products such as organic acids (e.g., urate, mercapturates) and organic bases (e.g., dopamine, creatinine). If a toxicant is reabsorbed or secreted, during active transport that toxicant may be concentrated within proximal tubular cells, causing site-specific injury. Fourth, proximal and distal tubular cells, as well as renomedullary interstitial cells, contain enzymes (e.g., cytochromes P450, cysteine conjugate β-lyase, prostaglandin H synthase) capable of bioactivating xenobiotics. Any one or a combination of these factors may contribute to the development of nephrotoxicity, and each is difficult to evaluate *in vivo* due to the complexity of the kidney. Therefore, investigators have developed *in vitro* methods in order to delineate more clearly the mechanisms involved in nephrotoxicity.

Preclinical toxicity studies of novel therapeutics or industrial chemicals in laboratory animals may reveal chemically induced nephrotoxicity. Since *in vivo* studies are time-consuming and expensive and may require that numerous animals be used, it would be desirable to rapidly and efficiently screen a series of compounds for nephrotoxic potential. Consequently, *in vitro* methods that can assess relative nephrotoxic potential have been developed and have been proven useful in the development of new drugs and chemicals.

Numerous *in vitro* methods which range from whole-organ perfusion to isolated cell systems are used by renal physiologists, pharmacologists, and toxicologists. The focus of this chapter is to review several of these *in vitro* methods by outlining the techniques and the specific advantages and limitations and by discussing several examples of studies utilizing each technique.

ISOLATED PERFUSED KIDNEY

Evaluation of the nephrotoxic potential of xenobiotics involves determining the effects of a toxicant on specific renal functions, such as urinary concentrating and diluting mechanisms, electrolyte reabsorption, and solute (e.g., glucose, amino acids) reabsorption. Traditionally, these renal functions have been assessed using *in vivo* clearance techniques or urinalysis. The isolated perfused kidney (IPK) may be used to assess renal function either following pretreatment of animals with toxicant (*ex vivo*) or during perfusion with a toxicant (*in vitro*). In addition, the IPK is used with increasing frequency to assess the role of the kidney in xenobiotic metabolism.

Methodology

An animal, usually a rat or rabbit, is anesthetized and the ureter is cannulated to enable collection of urine. The renal artery is cannulated, usually via the mesenteric artery, and arterial perfusion is established *in situ*. The kidney is removed from the animal, trimmed of fat, and placed in a perfusion chamber (Fig. 1). The kidney is perfused with a blood-free medium (e.g., Krebs–Ringer or Krebs–Henseleit buffers) containing glucose, amino acids, and albumin as an oncotic agent. A recirculating perfusion system is used and the perfusate is supplemented with metabolic substrates to prevent depletion (1). Perfusion may be set at constant speed or constant pressure (1,2). Inulin is generally present in the perfusate in order to determine glomerular filtration rate (GFR) (1). Recently, however, investigators have incorporated in-line features for instantaneous determination of GFR. For example, Cox et al. (3) included cyanocobalamin in the perfusate and incorporated a flow-through microcuvette in which urinary cyanocobalamin was determined colorimetrically. In this manner, GFR can be monitored continuously throughout an experiment, allowing an IPK to be discarded if functional capacity is not at the desired value.

During development of the IPK, investigators noted that GFR and sodium reabsorption were low compared to *in vivo* observations. In addition, in the IPK, high perfusion flow rates and pressures were required to maintain oxygenation, leading to impaired urinary concentrating ability that was not corrected by exogenous antidiuretic hormone (ADH) (4–6). These observations led investigators to question the stability and viability of the IPK. Subsequent studies indicated that early in the course of perfusion the IPK developed an irreversible lesion affecting the thick ascending limb of the loop of Henle (TALH) (6) and, in some instances, affecting the medullary portion of the proximal straight tubule (7). Morphologic damage,

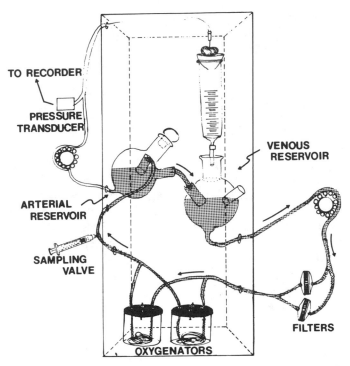

FIG. 1. Schematic diagram of apparatus used for isolated rat kidney perfusion. Shaded areas indicate perfusate that is undergoing rapid recirculation. Arrows indicate the direction of flow through the rapidly recirculating system. [Reproduced from Newton and Hook (1) and Academic Press, with permission.]

consisting of cytoplasmic flocculation and vacuolization, was apparent in the TALH as early as 15 min after initiating perfusion. Damage progressed to cytoplasmic disruption and nuclear pyknosis and extended to the distal tubule within 60–90 min of perfusion (6). Similar cytoplasmic and nuclear degeneration was observed in medullary proximal straight tubules after 100 or 200 min of perfusion (7). The lesion was exacerbated with low oxygen tension in the perfusate, but it was attenuated when erythrocytes or fluorinated hydrocarbons were used (8,9). When oxygen consumption by the IPK was reduced, by inhibiting sodium transport with ouabain or furosemide, morphologic damage to the TALH was minimized (10). These observations suggest that relative hypoxia/anoxia contributes importantly to the development of damage in the medullary proximal tubule and TALH. Furthermore, the IPK may be an unsuitable preparation to investigate toxic responses of the more distal portions of the nephron, such as the thick ascending limb, distal tubule, collecting tubule, and collecting duct. However, function and morphology in glomerular and early proximal tubular structures are well-maintained in the IPK (6,7), making this preparation useful in assessment of glomerular and proximal tubular integrity.

Advantages

For certain studies, the IPK presents distinct advantages that cannot be duplicated *in vivo* or by other *in vitro* techniques. Most importantly, the structural and morphological integrity of vascular and tubular components of the kidney is maintained in the IPK, unlike other *in vitro* techniques in which tubules are dissociated from glomeruli and capillaries. Structural integrity is a particular advantage in examining glomerular function in response to toxicants. Glomerular functional responses cannot be directly assessed with other currently available *in vitro* techniques, and evaluation of direct glomerular damage *in vivo* may be complicated by toxicant-induced changes in renal blood flow and/or cardiovascular function.

Another advantage of the IPK is that this technique utilizes an artificial perfusate, and the contents and composition of the perfusate may be rigorously defined and controlled. The ability to alter perfusate content is valuable in determining the roles of filtration and tubular transport in xenobiotic accumulation by tubular epithelial cells (see below). The ability to control perfusate composition allows the investigator to manipulate variables such as degree of protein binding of a xenobiotic, urinary pH, and urinary flow rate (2).

An important advantage of the IPK is that kidneys may be obtained from animals pretreated with toxicant as well as from naive animals, allowing for detailed *in vivo–in vitro* comparisons. In this manner, intrinsic responses of the kidneys may be differentiated from responses due to alterations in renal hemodynamics, cardiovascular function, or extrarenal factors such as hepatic metabolism and/or bioactivation.

The IPK offers substantial utility in the study of xenobiotic metabolism and disposition, and has been used in elucidating mechanisms by which the kidney handles drugs and toxicants. In the IPK, xenobiotics will undergo filtration, reabsorption, and/or secretion to the extent that those processes occur *in vivo*. Nonrenal factors that may influence xenobiotic disposition *in vivo*, such as extrarenal metabolism and binding to extrarenal tissue, may be circumvented by use of the IPK (2). For many xenobiotics, metabolism is catalyzed by cytochromes P450, enzymes present in both liver and kidney. It is difficult to quantitate the contribution of renal cytochromes P450 to overall xenobiotic metabolism, since renal P450 content is only about 10% of hepatic P450 content (11,12). However, renal concentrating mechanisms, active transport systems, and high intrinsic permeability of certain nephron segments may lead to intracellular concentrations of xenobiotics that are much higher in kidney than in other tissues (11,12). Isolated tissue preparations, such as tubules, cells, or microsomes, may allow xenobiotics to gain access to enzymes catalyzing metabolism whereas such access may be restricted *in vivo*. Metabolism of a xenobiotic by the IPK is convincing evidence that the xenobiotic can be metabolized by the kidney *in vivo* (13).

The IPK allows evaluation of the relative contribution of filtration (a glomerular function), tubular transport (largely a function of tubular basolateral and/or luminal membranes), and tubular reabsorption (largely a function of tubular luminal membranes) in xenobiotic accumulation and metabolism by tubular epithelial cells. Glomerular filtration *in vivo* can be reduced or abolished by maneuvers such as ligating the ureter or clamping the renal artery. Both of these procedures will eliminate glomerular filtration, but clamping the renal artery will also eliminate peritubular blood flow, making it impossible to assess the role of basolateral membrane transport in intrarenal accumulation of drugs. Ureteral ligation is a nonphysiological technique that relies on elevation of intraluminal pressure to eventually stop glomerular filtration. In contrast, glomerular filtration can be reduced in the IPK by raising perfusate albumin concentration so that perfusate colloid osmotic pressure approaches glomerular capillary hydrostatic pressure. In this manner, perfusate flow through the IPK is preserved, including flow through peritubular capillaries, while glomerular filtration is abolished. This maneuver allows clear dissociation of glomerular filtration from tubular transport and enables investigators to determine if xenobiotic accumulation in tubular epithelial cells is a consequence of basolateral or luminal transport (13).

Limitations

The IPK has several distinct weaknesses that limit its utility in toxicological studies. Considerable equipment is required to support the IPK. For example, custom-designed perfusion chambers, oxygenators, pumps, and filters are among a few of the items included in the perfusion circuit (Fig. 1). In addition, as with many *in vitro* techniques, the IPK is not a technically simple procedure. Great care must be taken in cannulating the renal artery so as not to produce ischemia (1). A significant limitation of the IPK is that renal function tends to decline over time: GFR and sodium reabsorption are stable for only 2 hr or so (1). If nephrotoxicity requires a period of several hours or longer to develop, the IPK may be unsuitable for *in vitro* monitoring of the progression of toxicity.

The morphologic lesion in the TALH as well as the inability to concentrate urine in the IPK, despite the presence of ADH, are significant limitations and make the IPK unsuitable for investigations of toxicants that injure distal nephron structures (e.g., TALH, distal tubule, collecting tubule, and collecting duct). Erythrocytes or fluorinated hydrocarbons cannot be included routinely in the perfusate of an IPK because of technical problems such as clumping and clotting with erythrocytes and uncertainty about inherent toxicity of fluorinated hydrocarbons. In particular, the concentrating defect may dilute luminal concentrations of some toxicants so that these compounds may not achieve sufficiently high concentrations in tubular epithelial cells to produce toxic responses (13).

Finally, functional assessments in the IPK do not allow identification of the site of nephrotoxic injury. For example, declines in GFR or increases in urine output are integrated responses of the whole kidney and cannot be ascribed to a single mechanism. Thus, the IPK continues the clearance "black-box" approach of comparing input with output except that extrarenal mechanisms, such as changes in renal hemodynamics or cardiovascular function, may be excluded from consideration.

Use of the IPK in Renal Toxicology

Acetaminophen Nephrotoxicity and Metabolism in the IPK

Acetaminophen overdosage is characterized primarily by hepatic necrosis. In addition, some patients may develop acute proximal tubular necrosis in the presence or absence of hepatotoxicity following acetaminophen overdosage. In rats, acetaminophen-induced hepatotoxicity occurs following cytochrome-P450-dependent formation of a reactive quinoneimine intermediate (14,15). In contrast, the precise pathways responsible for acute nephrotoxicity following acetaminophen overdosage in rats are unclear (16–18). The liver is the primary site of acetaminophen metabolism (14). The role of the kidney, if any, in the metabolism of acetaminophen is uncertain. Therefore, investigators have used the IPK to evaluate the ability of the kidney to metabolize acetaminophen and, in addition, to correlate acetaminophen metabolism with nephrotoxicity.

In the IPK, at toxicologically relevant concentrations of acetaminophen (1–3 mM), fractional excretion of acetaminophen was about 25%, indicating that approximately 75% of filtered acetaminophen was reabsorbed by the tubular epithelium (13,19). Acetaminophen metabolism by the kidney was suggested by the identification of glucuronide, sulfate, cysteine conjugates, and mercapturic acid metabolites of acetaminophen in urine, but not in the perfusate, of the IPK (13,19). All of these metabolic pathways were saturable with differing characteristic maxima (13), analogous to saturation of hepatic metabolism of acetaminophen (15). Thus, all major metabolites of acetaminophen formed in the liver are also formed in the kidney, although at considerably lower rates and in lower amounts than in the liver. Renal metabolism is unlikely to contribute importantly to overall acetaminophen elimination. However, intrarenal bioactivation of acetaminophen by cytochrome-P450-dependent pathways, such as occurs in the liver to produce hepatotoxicity, cannot be excluded as a possible factor in acetaminophen nephrotoxicity.

In examining acetaminophen metabolism in the IPK, investigators have tried to identify renal functions that are impaired by acetaminophen. Acetaminophen-induced nephrotoxicity requires about 24 hr to develop *in vivo*, and the IPK has not been particularly useful in investigating acetaminophen toxicity *in vitro*. For example, concentrations of acetaminophen in excess of 10 mM were required to produce diuresis and natriuresis in the IPK (13). In contrast, other investigators have observed no effects of 3×10^{-8} to 3×10^{-5} M acetaminophen on GFR, urine output, or sodium excretion (19). The only effect in IPKs perfused with acetaminophen was a 50% reduction of intracellular reduced glutathione (GSH) following 2 hr of drug treatment *in vitro* (19). Acetaminophen-induced GSH depletion was potentiated in kidneys from rats pretreated with polybrominated biphenyls, inducers of cyto-chromes P450, and was attenuated in kidneys from rats pretreated with piperonyl butoxide, an inhibitor of cytochromes P450 (19), suggesting a correlation between oxidative metabolism of acetaminophen and GSH depletion. However, recovery of sulfur-containing metabolites of acetaminophen could not quantitatively account for GSH depletion observed in these IPKs, leading to the suggestion that a portion of the GSH depletion seen with acetaminophen may be due to interaction of a reactive acetaminophen intermediate with enzymes responsible for GSH synthesis (19). Al-ternatively, oxidative stress may be a component of acetaminophen-induced neph-rotoxicity, similar to a mechanism proposed in acetaminophen-induced hepatotox-icity (20,21).

Thus, the IPK has been useful in defining the renal metabolism of acetaminophen (13,19). In addition, acetaminophen induced GSH depletion in the IPK; the magni-tude and time course of GSH depletion *in vitro* was similar to that observed *in vivo* (16,19). However, the time limitations of the IPK does not allow full expression of acetaminophen-induced nephrotoxicity, and the role of intrarenal metabolism in acetaminophen nephrotoxicity remains uncertain.

Cisplatin Nephrotoxicity in the IPK

A significant limitation in cisplatin therapy is the development of nephrotoxicity, characterized by reductions of renal plasma flow and GFR as well as tubular dys-function (22–24). It is not clear from *in vivo* clearance studies whether the effects of cisplatin on GFR are secondary to drug-induced changes in renal hemodynamics or tubular integrity or are due to direct glomerular injury. The IPK is an excellent technique to allow differentiation among effects on renal hemodynamics, glomeru-lar filtration, and tubular function, and it has been used to investigate cisplatin nephrotoxicity.

When rats were pretreated with cisplatin and kidneys perfused 48 hr later, GFR and sodium and glucose reabsorption were significantly reduced (25). Renal perfu-sion flow was similar in kidneys from naive or cisplatin-pretreated rats (25). Thus, cisplatin produced alterations in glomerular and tubular functional without apparent alterations of renal hemodynamics *ex vivo*. When 0.5 mM cisplatin was included in the perfusate, IPKs from naive rats showed a time-dependent decline in GFR and sodium and potassium reabsorption in the absence of changes in renal perfusate flow (Fig. 2) (25). The earliest manifestations of functional damage were reductions in GFR and sodium reabsorption within 30–40 min of perfusion (Fig. 2). Potassium reabsorption was not significantly reduced until 90–100 min of perfusion, whereas glucose reabsorption was unaltered during perfusion with cisplatin (25). In addition, clearances of *p*-aminohippurate (PAH) and tetraethylammonium (TEA) were mark-edly reduced during perfusion with cisplatin, when compared to those of controls (25).

In nonfiltering kidneys, inclusion of 0.5 mM cisplatin in the perfusate reduced

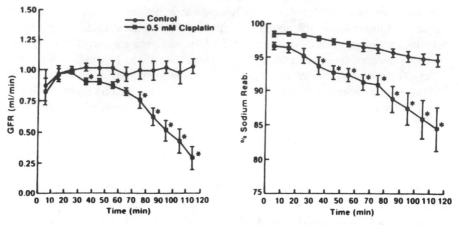

FIG. 2. Effects of cisplatin on glomerular filtration rate (GFR) **(left panel)** and sodium reabsorption (as percent of filtered load) **(right panel)** in the isolated perfused kidney. Asterisks indicate significant differences from control ($p < 0.05$). [Reproduced from Miura et al. (25) and Elsevier Scientific Publishers, with permission.]

renal perfusion pressure in a time-dependent manner (25). PAH and TEA clearances were also markedly reduced in the nonfiltering kidney perfused with cisplatin (25). Furthermore, reductions in PAH and TEA clearances were not due to reductions in perfusion pressure, since control kidneys perfused at flow rates comparable to those of the cisplatin-perfused kidneys maintained nearly normal cortical accumulation of PAH and TEA (25).

Thus, cisplatin treatment *in vivo* or *in vitro* markedly decreased GFR and tubular function. These effects were not mediated by changes in renal hemodynamics (25). However, since both glomerular and tubular functions were reduced by cisplatin, the primary site of cisplatin nephrotoxicity cannot be identified by these studies. The cisplatin-induced reduction in GFR may be related to changes in the ultrafiltration coefficient of the glomerulus and/or events subsequent to tubular damage—for example, tubular back-leak. Data from the nonfiltering IPK indicate that filtration is not a prerequisite for cisplatin nephrotoxicity and that transport and/or diffusion across the tubular basolateral membrane are sufficient for cisplatin to induce a tubular injury (25).

RENAL SLICES

Renal cortical slices were developed initially to investigate proximal tubular transport of organic anions (such as PAH) and organic cations [such as TEA or N-methyl-nicotinamide (NMN)]. These early studies indicated a reasonably good correlation between *in vivo* secretion and *in vitro* renal cortical slice accumulation of PAH and NMN or TEA (26). For example, substances that stimulated organic anion secretion *in vivo* (e.g., acetate or lactate) also stimulated renal cortical slice accumulation of these ions *in vitro*. Similarly, substances that decreased renal tubular secretion of organic ions *in vivo* (e.g., 2,4-dinitrophenol) also decreased renal cortical slice accumulation *in vitro*. In addition, xenobiotics such as the non-nutritive sweetener, saccharin, or drugs such as sulotroban and cimetidine have been shown to be actively secreted via organic ion transport *in vivo* and are accumulated by renal cortical slices *in vitro* via similar organic ion transporters (27–29). Thus, renal cortical slices have been established as a valuable technique to evaluate tubular transport of xenobiotics. More recently, the renal cortical slice technique has been used to evaluate the biochemical and functional responses to toxicants following either *in vivo* treatment or exposure to a nephrotoxicant *in vitro*.

Methodology

Several procedures are available for the preparation of renal slices. The oldest technique for the preparation of renal slices is a free-hand method in which slices of 0.2–0.5 mm in thickness can be prepared routinely. A Stadie–Riggs microtome also can be used, resulting in greater uniformity in thickness of tissue slices. Once prepared, 50–100 mg of tissue is transferred to flasks containing oxygenated buffer and then the flasks are placed in a metabolic shaker. Frequently, the Cross–Taggart medium (30) is used, although a Krebs–Ringer bicarbonate buffer also can be used. To maximize the renal cortical slice accumulation of organic anions, incubation medium is often supplemented with 10 mM lactate or acetate. Usually, tissue slices are shaken at either 25°C or 37°C in the presence of 100% oxygen or 95% O_2/5% CO_2, depending on the choice of buffered medium. Unless the flasks are stoppered, a continual flow of gas is needed. After an appropriate amount of time, slices are removed from the incubation flask, blotted, and weighed. Slices are then processed for determination of the biochemical end points of interest. For example, to assess the effects of a xenobiotic on PAH and TEA transport in renal cortical slices, renal cortical slices are incubated in a medium supplemented with PAH and TEA. Subsequently, slices are homogenized and assayed for PAH and TEA content; an aliquot of the incubation media is similarly processed. Data obtained from such an experiment are expressed in terms of the slice/medium (S/M) concentration ratio of PAH and TEA. In general, S/M ratios exceeding unity are indicative of active transport. Renal cortical slices also have been used either *ex vivo* or *in vitro* to monitor the effects of a toxicant on gluconeogenesis, formation of peroxidative products such as malondialdehyde (MDA), enzyme (i.e., lactate dehydrogenase (LDH), alkaline phosphatase, maltase) leakage, oxygen consumption, covalent binding, and intracellular content of ATP and GSH (31,32). In addition, metabolism of a xenobiotic by renal cortical slices can be assessed (33).

One limitation of the renal cortical slice method is that although cell–cell contact is maintained, site-selective injury cannot be assessed morphologically due to difficulties in identifying cell types in this particular preparation. To circumvent this problem, positional renal slices have been developed, allowing identification of renal cell types by their anatomical location within the slice (34). Briefly, kidneys from rabbits are removed and decapsulated, and then cylindrical cores (6 mm in diameter) are made through the kidney along its cortical–papillary axis. Cores are obtained from the kidney by gently pushing the kidney against a cork borer mounted to a variable-speed drill motor rotating at approximately 300 rpm. Cores are then sliced perpendicular to this axis using a mechanical slicer. Up to 100 cortical slices (300 μm) from a single rabbit can be collected. Incubations are carried out in vessels designed to support several slices on a porous surface submerged beneath a constantly circulating aerated medium. Slices are incubated in a buffered medium gassed with 95% O_2/5% CO_2 at room temperature. Similar to renal cortical slices, positional slices may be used either *ex vivo* or *in vitro* to monitor the effects of a toxicant on biochemical (intracellular potassium, DNA and ATP content, oxygen consumption) and functional (organic ion transport) indices. In addition, positional slices may be evaluated by light and/or electron microscopy to identify the exact site of damage. Thus, positional renal slices can be used to evaluate and compare effects of xenobiotics on renal tubular biochemistry and function versus morphology. Ruegg et al. (34) have demonstrated that viability (intracellular potassium/DNA) and structural integrity of positional slices can be maintained for at least 30 hr.

Advantages

Renal slices offer several advantages over other techniques. The use of renal slices is relatively straightforward and inexpensive. Slices prepared from animals challenged with a toxicant can be used to provide more sensitive indices of chemically induced damage than standard estimates such as blood urea nitrogen (BUN) or serum creatinine concentrations. Indeed, studies from several laboratories have demonstrated that the *in vitro* renal cortical slice accumulation of PAH and TEA are among the most sensitive and versatile indicators of proximal tubular injury when compared to other renal functional tests such as uninalyses or serum biochemistry (BUN, creatinine) (35–37). It is possible to assess a variety of biochemical and functional end points in a single sample. For example, organic ion transport, oxygen consumption, enzyme leakage, and lipid peroxidation can be measured in slices from a single incubation vessel, thus providing an economical means of assessing nephrotoxic potential. Positional renal slices offer the added advantage of assessing site-selective morphologic injury. In addition to *ex vivo* evaluation, slices can be prepared from naive animals and exposed to toxicants *in vitro*. Thus, the *in vivo* and *in vitro* effects of a toxicant can be compared in similar tissue preparations, and such a comparison allows assessment of direct (intrarenal) versus indirect (extrarenal) effects. Evaluation of the temporal sequence of biochemical and functional changes produced by nephrotoxicants *in vitro* can provide valuable information on mechanisms of nephrotoxicity.

Renal slices can be prepared from a number of mammalian species, including mouse, rat, rabbit, hamster, guinea pig, dog, monkey, and human; within any given species, strain-, sex-, and age-related differences can be assessed. This wide range of populations from which renal slices can be prepared, coupled with the ease of preparation, facilitates species-, strain-, sex-, and age-related comparisons of toxicant-induced renal damage both *ex vivo* and *in vitro* and ultimately may provide information on more appropriate animal models for toxicologic evaluation.

Limitations

Renal cortical slices contain a heterogeneous population of tubules, and it is difficult to identify the site of injury. In addition, the lumens of the tubules in a slice are collapsed; hence the basolateral membrane may be preferentially exposed to toxicants in slice preparations. Thus, renal slices may not be appropriate in evaluating the nephrotoxic potential of drugs or chemicals which normally enter the proximal tubular cell via the luminal membrane. Using standard incubation conditions, renal cortical slice preparations have a limited viability of approximately 3 hr, although viability may be extended from 8 to 30 hr using specialized incubation methods (34,38). Limited viability may pose some problems when determining the relevance of data gathered from short-term incubations, particularly when toxicity *in vivo* may take days to become manifest.

An additional limitation of renal cortical slices is the potential for generating false-positives in assessing nephrotoxicity *in vitro*. Smith (32) investigated the *in vitro* nephrotoxic effects of a wide variety of chemicals, including mercuric chloride, cephaloridine, gentamicin, carbon tetrachloride, hexachlorobutadiene, potassium dichromate, and 4-ipomeanol. Although the nephrotoxic potential of most of these chemicals and drugs *in vitro* correlated well with their known nephrotoxic potential *in vivo*, 4-ipomeanol, which is not nephrotoxic *in vivo*, also produced nephrotoxic effects *in vitro*, albeit at relatively high concentrations. Thus, the use of renal cortical slices to screen unknown chemicals and drugs for nephrotoxicity may not be appropriate. Rather, the greatest utility of this technique relates to screening of a known nephrotoxic class of compounds and/or investigating biochemical mechanisms of a nephrotoxicant.

Use of Slices in Renal Toxicology

Biochemical Mechanisms of Nephrotoxicity: Cephalosporin Antibiotics

Cephaloridine is a broad-spectrum cephalosporin antibiotic which produces dose-related nephrotoxicity when administered in large doses to laboratory animals (39). Cephaloridine nephrotoxicity *in vivo* has been fairly well characterized, and several studies have indicated that renal cortical slice function *ex vivo* is an exquisitely sensitive indicator of nephrotoxicity. For example, cephaloridine-induced elevations in BUN concentrations occurred in rabbits receiving dosages of 150 mg/kg or greater, whereas decreased renal cortical slice accumulation of PAH and TEA and gluconeogenesis were observed at dosages as low as 50–100 mg/kg (40). Similarly, in cephaloridine-treated F344 rats, renal cortical slice accumulation of PAH and TEA and gluconeogenic capacity were decreased as early as 1 hr following administration of 2000 mg/kg of cephaloridine, a time preceding any detectable change in BUN or serum creatinine concentrations (41). Importantly, the early biochemical effects of cephaloridine observed following *in vivo* treatment (i.e., organic ion transport, gluconeogenesis, intracellular GSH depletion, lipid peroxidation) have been reproduced in renal cortical slices harvested from naive animals and exposed to cephaloridine *in vitro* (31). Thus, the similar nephrotoxic effects of cephaloridine observed in renal cortical slices following either *ex vivo* or *in vitro* treatment provided the basis to investigate the mechanisms of cephaloridine nephrotoxicity using renal cortical slices *in vitro*.

In vivo studies have indicated that the incidence and severity of cephaloridine nephrotoxicity were related to the renal cortical concentrations of this drug. For example, both renal cortical concentrations and nephrotoxicity of cephaloridine were greatest in rabbits, intermediate in guinea pigs, and least in rats (42), suggesting a relationship between cortical accumulation and toxicity of this antibiotic. The exact mechanisms mediating the renal cortical accumulation of cephaloridine have been studied in detail in the rabbit. Pretreatment of rabbits with inhibitors of organic anion transport such as probenecid decreased the cortex/serum concentration ratio of cephaloridine (42), suggesting that cephaloridine is actively transported into proximal tubular cells by an organic anion transporter. That organic anion transport plays an important role in cephaloridine accumulation and nephrotoxicity has been suggested by the observation that pretreatment of rabbits with probenecid or other competitive inhibitors of organic anion transport, such as PAH or benzylpenicillin, decreased both renal accumulation and nephrotoxicity of cephaloridine (43). Unlike other cephalosporins, however, cephaloridine is a zwitterion containing a positive charge at the 3 position of the cephem ring, and organic cation transport also seems to be important to the renal tubular handling of cephaloridine. Wold and Turnipseed (44) demonstrated that the renal cortical concentrations and nephrotoxicity of cephaloridine were significantly greater following *in vivo* treatment with an inhibitor of organic cation transport, cyanine. To investigate the mechanisms mediating the effects of cyanine on renal cortical concentrations of cephaloridine, Wold and Turnipseed (44) studied the effects of cyanine on the *in vitro* uptake and efflux of cephaloridine in renal cortical slices from naive rabbits. Indeed, cyanine did not affect the uptake of cephaloridine, but did significantly decrease its efflux by renal cortical slices, suggesting that cephaloridine transport from the proximal tubular cell into the tubular fluid was dependent on an organic cation transporter. Thus, the increased severity of cephaloridine nephrotoxicity following cyanine pretreatment was attributed to the ability of cyanine to decrease efflux (excretion) and, hence, increase net renal cortical concentrations of this antibiotic. These studies further demonstrate (a) the utility of renal cortical slices in dissecting the mechanisms of tubular transport of xenobiotics and (b) the potential relationship of tubular transport processes to drug-induced nephrotoxicity.

Although the role of renal tubular transport in cephaloridine nephrotoxicity has been fairly well defined, the exact biochemical mechanisms mediating cephaloridine cytotoxicity are less well understood. Several lines of evidence suggest that lipid peroxidation may play an important role. Most notably, Kuo et al. (45) have reported that conjugated dienes, products of lipid peroxidation, were increased in renal cortical tissue shortly following cephaloridine administration, prior to the detection of other biochemical or functional evidence of tubular injury. Furthermore, cephaloridine also depleted renal cortical GSH concentrations and increased GSSG concentrations, consistent with cephaloridine-induced oxidative stress. However, these *in vivo* observations do not provide direct evidence of a causal link between cephaloridine-induced oxidative stress and nephrotoxicity. To more precisely determine whether cephaloridine-induced oxidative stress is an initiating event mediating cephaloridine nephrotoxicity, the time course of biochemical effects were monitored in renal cortical slices exposed to cephaloridine *in vitro*. These studies revealed that incubation of renal cortical slices with cephaloridine resulted in a time- and concentration-related increase in lipid peroxidation, reflected by MDA production (31). Furthermore, the onset of cephaloridine-induced peroxidation preceded cephaloridine-induced inhibition of organic ion transport. More definitive evidence supporting a role for lipid peroxidation in cephaloridine nephrotoxicity was obtained from studies evaluating the effects of antioxidants on cephaloridine-induced alterations in organic ion transport. Incubation of renal cortical slices with antioxidants such as promethazine or N,N'-diphenyl-p-phenylenediamine (DPPD) blocked the effects of cephaloridine on both lipid peroxidation and organic ion transport (31,46), suggesting a cause–effect relationship between cephaloridine-induced lipid peroxidation and inhibition of organic ion transport. Thus, these *in vitro* studies using renal cortical slices have defined more precisely the role of lipid peroxidation in cephaloridine nephrotoxicity.

In addition, *in vitro* biochemical studies of cephaloridine nephrotoxicity indicated that cephaloridine impaired certain metabolic functions of the proximal tubule by mechanisms other than lipid peroxidation. For example, cephaloridine profoundly inhibited pyruvate-supported gluconeogenesis in renal cortical slices *in vitro*, an effect which occurred prior to the onset of lipid peroxidation (31). Furthermore, antioxidants such as promethazine or DPPD did not block cephaloridine inhibition of gluconeogenesis, suggesting that the effects of cephaloridine on gluconeogenesis were independent of peroxidation. Further *in vitro* studies were designed to test the hypothesis that cephaloridine-induced inhibition of renal cortical slice gluconeogenesis was related to inhibition of any one or more of the rate-limiting enzymes of gluconeogenesis, specifically, pyruvate carboxylase, phosphoenolpyruvate carboxykinase, fructose diphosphatase, and/or glucose-6-phosphatase. To test this hypothesis, gluconeogenesis was evaluated using substrates supporting each of the rate-limiting reactions, namely, pyruvate (pyruvate carboxykinase), oxaloacetate (phosphoenolpyruvate carboxykinase), fructose-1,6-diphosphate (fructose diphosphatase), and glucose-6-phosphate (glucose-6-phosphatase) (47). These studies indicated that cephaloridine inhibited gluconeogenesis supported by each of these substrates, suggesting either that cephaloridine inhibited each of the rate-limiting enzymes in a nonspecific manner or, alternatively, that cephaloridine inhibited the final step in glucose synthesis, namely, the conversion of glucose-6-phosphate to glucose. Further assessment of the effects of cephaloridine on enzymatic activity in subcellular fractions indicated that cephaloridine specifically inhibited glucose-6-phosphatase activity, suggesting that cephaloridine inhibition of gluconeogenesis was due to inhibition of the final step in glucose synthesis (47).

In summary, studies using renal cortical slices have yielded valuable information concerning cephaloridine-induced nephrotoxicity. First, *ex vivo* renal cortical slice functions are exquisitely sensitive indicators of cephaloridine nephrotoxicity. Second, the effects of cephaloridine on renal cortical slice functions and biochemistry *in vitro* are consistent with the effects observed following cephaloridine administration *in vivo*. Third, *in vitro* evaluation of the temporal sequence of biochemical effects as well as the effects of antioxidants on cephaloridine nephrotoxicity have more precisely defined the role of lipid peroxidation in cephaloridine nephrotoxicity. Finally, there are multiple mechanisms of cephaloridine nephrotoxicity which are characterized by both peroxidative-dependent and peroxidative-independent effects.

Site-Selective Nephrotoxic Injury

Most nephrotoxicants appear to have their primary effects on discrete segments or regions of the nephron. The proximal tubule, for example, is the primary target for many nephrotoxic antibiotics, antineoplastics, halogenated hydrocarbons, and heavy metals, whereas the glomerulus is the primary target for immune complexes, the loop of Henle/collecting duct is the primary target for fluoride ions, and the medulla/papilla is the primary target for chronically consumed analgesic mixtures. Although the reasons underlying this site-selective injury are complex, segmental differences in morphology, physiology, and biochemistry appear to play important roles. For example, blood flow to the cortex is disproportionately high compared to other regions of the kidney; thus, blood-borne toxicants likely will be delivered preferentially to the cortical region, rendering cortical structures (predominantly proximal tubules) more vulnerable to chemically induced injury. However, in certain instances, site-selective injury does persist *in vitro* under conditions in which all cell types are exposed to identical extracellular concentrations of a given nephrotoxicant. Thus, under these conditions, site-selective injury cannot be attributed solely to systemic delivery of toxicants but rather may be due to the biochemical properties of the cell type(s) in question.

Using positional renal slices, work from Gandolfi's laboratory has indicated that nephrotoxicants as diverse as mercuric chloride, potassium dichromate, cisplatin, hexachlorobutadiene, and *S*-(1,2-dichlorovinyl)-L-cysteine (DCVC) produce the same pattern of selective cellular injury *in vitro* as reported by others following *in vivo* exposure (48–51). More specifically, both *in vivo* and *in vitro* exposure to mercuric chloride resulted in nephrotoxic lesions to the straight segment (pars recta), whereas *in vivo* and *in vitro* exposure to potassium dichromate produced selective injury to the convoluted segment (pars convoluta) of the proximal tubule (48). More recently, Wolfgang et al. (51) have used positional renal cortical slices to delineate the temporal sequence of biochemical and histopathological changes leading to the site-specific injury to the pars recta following exposure to DCVC. In these studies, ^{35}S-DCVC uptake by renal cortical slices was shown to be time- and concentration-dependent. Autoradiography indicated that ^{35}S-DCVC was distributed fairly equally among all proximal tubular segments within the slice, suggesting that the site-selective injury to the pars recta could not be attributed solely to a preferential uptake and/or accumulation of DCVC by the pars recta. Following DCVC uptake, the initial events related to DCVC toxicity were characterized by covalent binding followed by alterations in intracellular ATP content, changes in oxygen consumption, and leakage of brush-border enzymes. These temporal data further suggested that covalent binding preceded ultrastructural damage to both mitochondria and brush border, both of which appear to be early targets of DCVC toxicity. Light microscopy revealed a sequence of histopathologic changes beginning with a selective lesion to the pars recta followed by lesions to all other proximal tubular segments. Thus, these studies demonstrated that the site-selective injury to the pars recta by DCVC was preceded by covalent binding, followed by effects on mitochondria and brush border.

Although these studies indicated that the nature of chemically induced site-selective injury observed *in vitro* is comparable to that observed *in vivo*, Ruegg et al. (48) have reported that the site of nephrotoxic injury following hypoxia is different *in vitro* from that observed *in vivo*. Renal cortical slices rendered hypoxic *in vitro* sustained a selective injury to the convoluted portion of the proximal tubule (48), a finding which contrasts with *in vivo* observations indicating that the pars recta is the primary site of injury following renal ischemia. Ruegg and Mandel (52) have suggested that under reduced oxygen delivery conditions *in vivo*, a nonuniform oxygen gradient renders the pars recta (perfused by distal capillary beds) anoxic because other nephron segments, perfused by the proximal capillary beds, maximally extract the available oxygen when oxygen delivery is reduced. Thus, transient or sustained hypotension *in vivo* results in poor perfusion of the outer medullary stripe, leaving the pars recta anoxic. In contrast, uniform oxygen deprivation (i.e., *in vitro* hypoxia/anoxia) results in selective injury to the proximal convoluted tubule, suggesting that in the absence of regional differences in oxygen delivery and regional blood flow, these cells are intrinsically more susceptible to the effects of oxygen deprivation. Taken together, these *in vivo/in vitro* comparisons demonstrate how *in vitro* slice studies can be used to enhance our understanding of the intrinsic biochemical properties which render certain cell types susceptible to nephrotoxic injury.

TUBULE SUSPENSIONS

Several methods have been utilized to investigate biochemical responses of renal epithelial cells to potential toxicants. In large part, these methodologies have been adapted from physiological studies examining renal metabolism and transport properties. In general, *in vitro* preparations used for biochemical studies include semi-purified portions of tubular epithelium (tubule suspensions) or individual tubular epithelial cells (cell suspensions, cell cultures).

Methodology

Usually, tubules are harvested from rabbits, although tubule suspensions have been prepared from rats and mice (53–58). Several methods have been published describing preparation of tubule suspensions (59–62).

Many investigators use *in situ* and/or *ex vivo* perfusion with collagenase in order to isolate tubules from supporting tissue. Following anesthesia, the renal artery is cannulated either directly (62) or through the aorta (54,63). Kidneys are perfused initially with a collagenase-free solution to remove blood. The perfusate is then switched to a solution containing collagenase, and perfusion is continued for several minutes. Following perfusion, the kidneys are removed from the animal and tubules are obtained by manual dispersion of kidney tissue. The tubules are separated from cellular debris by a variety of methods, including filtering through gauze or centrifugation through discontinuous gradients of Percoll or Ficoll. Alternatively, kidneys may be perfused with a collagenase solution containing magnetic iron oxide. Following perfusion and manual dispersion of the tissue, the tubule suspension is strained through a series of wire sieves and glomeruli are removed magnetically (62).

Other investigators use *in vitro* incubation of kidney tissue with collagenase in order to disperse tubules. In this method, kidneys may be perfused initially with collagenase-free buffer in order to remove blood cells. Kidneys are then removed from the animal, placed on ice, and minced into small pieces. The kidney pieces are incubated in collagenase-containing buffer for 30–60 min at 37°C. The resulting tubule suspension is washed and centrifuged several times to remove cellular debris, then further purified by centrifugation through a Percoll or Ficoll gradient (54, 64–66).

Advantages

Tubule suspensions have several distinct advantages over other *in vitro* methods, such as kidney slices, cell suspensions, or cultured cells. A significant advantage of tubule suspensions is that the nephron segments maintain morphologic integrity and display metabolic characteristics and transport properties similar to those observed *in vivo*. For example, proximal tubules in suspension actively accumulated α-methylglucose approximately 20-fold, and this active accumulation was reduced by phloretin or phloridzin, inhibitors of sugar transport (65). Tubule suspensions responded appropriately to addition of hormones: Proximal tubules produced cAMP in response to parathyroid hormone (PTH) but not ADH, whereas distal tubules produced cAMP in response to ADH but not PTH (64,67).

Another advantage of this technique is that relatively pure suspensions containing the nephron segment of interest may be prepared by careful choice of starting material and/or purification method. For example, by limiting the starting tissue to the outer cortex, investigators have prepared suspensions containing greater than 90% proximal tubules (61,64). By limiting dispersion to medullary tissue, other investigators have prepared suspensions containing greater than 90% medullary TALH (68). Responses of specific nephron segments to potential toxicants may be examined *in vitro* using these purified tubule suspensions.

Tubule suspensions maintain viability for at least several hours (57,58) or longer (65), a longer lifespan than observed for the IPK. Thus, toxicants may be tested in tubule suspensions over a period of several hours or more. As with any *in vitro* technique, use of tubule suspensions allows the investigator to precisely control the incubation medium and substrate concentrations. Toxicants may be included for the duration of the incubation period or removed after some specified time. In evaluation of proximal tubular function, transport substrates such as PAH, TEA, or α-methylglucose may be included to assess tubular integrity following exposure to a potential toxicant.

An additional advantage of this technique is that tubule suspensions yield a relatively large amount of tissue, particularly if a large animal such as a rabbit is used or if kidneys from several rats or mice are pooled. Thus, characterization of concentration—and time—response curves and/or structure—activity relationships may be evaluated in a relatively homogeneous preparation.

Tubule suspensions offer the ability to directly or indirectly probe intracellular sites of toxicity. For example, oxygen consumption, cAMP production, hormone responsiveness, transport capabilities, substrate-supported gluconeogenesis, and leakage of intracellular enzymes are among the numerous responses to toxicants that may be measured in tubule suspensions. Since the starting material (i.e., the nephron segment contained in the suspension) is relatively well defined, the responses elicited by toxicant exposure *in vitro* should resemble the characteristic responses of that nephron segment following toxicant exposure *in vivo*. Lack of correlation between responses obtained with tubule suspensions *in vitro* and nephrotoxic responses observed *in vivo* would suggest that extrarenal factors are involved in the nephrotoxicity of a compound.

Limitations

Tubule suspensions have several limitations that must be borne in mind when using this technique. When kidneys are perfused *in situ* or *ex vivo*, there is a risk of producing anoxia and/or ischemia. When magnetic iron is used to separate glomeruli from tubules, clumping and inadequate perfusion may occur with these iron-containing perfusates (61). By whatever method tubules are prepared, initial steps involve limited collagenase digestion in order to free tubules from the supporting extracellular matrix. Collagenase digestion may compromise the integrity of tubule membranes, making these membranes leakier and allowing diffusion to occur more readily than in intact tubules. Although tubule suspensions are purified, purification is not complete and trace contamination by other tubular segments and/or vascular tissue will probably occur to some degree. Therefore, the preparation needs to be carefully evaluated, preferably by microscopic methods, to assess purity. In most cases, suspensions will be enriched greater than 90% in the nephron segment of interest, so that contamination by other nephron segments does not confound interpretation of data.

Compared to the IPK or renal slices, considerably more time is required to make a tubule suspension. Equipment required to support tubule suspensions is not as extensive as with the IPK, but somewhat more equipment is needed than with kidney slices. In addition, cost of collagenase and other chemicals required to prepare tubule suspensions makes the technique more costly than renal slices or the IPK.

Other disadvantages include (a) the finite lifespan of any preparation, which must be rigorously defined by the investigator prior to toxicity testing or biochemical studies, and (b) the small amount of tissue contained in tubule incubations, compared to the IPK or renal slices. Typically, renal slices use 50–100 mg of tissue per incubation, whereas tubule suspensions use 10–50 μg of tissue for each incubation. Thus, assays need to be down-sized or modified to detect small amounts of compounds. Often, investigators will use radiolabeled compounds or custom-made equipment to measure experimental end points, further driving up the cost of an experiment.

Finally, limited information is available concerning *in vivo* and *in vitro* correlations for tubule suspensions. As with the IPK and renal slices, since some toxicities are slow to develop, the relatively short lifespan of tubule preparations may make them unsuitable for some studies.

With renal slices and the IPK, tissue may be obtained from animals pretreated with toxicants. The ability to obtain tubule suspensions from animals pretreated with toxicants has not been rigorously investigated or reported, although one group has obtained tubules from rats at various times after renal arterial occlusion and reflow (69). These investigators obtained viable proximal tubule suspensions from rats that were subjected to 45 min of renal arterial occlusion followed by 15 min, 2 hr, or 24 hr of reflow. Tubules were prepared according to a method that yielded primarily proximal convoluted tubules. Viability was monitored by ouabain-sensitive and nystatin-stimulated oxygen consumption, and these indices were reduced compared to those of control rats only after 15 min or 2 hr of reflow (69). Viability returned to control values within 24 hr of reflow (69). In addition, the authors provided morphologic evidence of tubular damage following ischemic insult and 15 min of reflow; however, they failed to comment on the progression or lack of progression of tubular injury at longer reflow times (69). In contrast, *in vivo* renal arterial occlusion (25 min) and 24 hr of reflow in rats produced marked proximal tubular injury, primarily affecting proximal straight tubules (70). Longer periods of ischemia (45–60 min) with 24 hr of reflow produced extensive damage to both proximal convoluted and proximal straight tubules (71). Based on these *in vivo* studies, one would expect some degree of damage to be detectable in proximal convoluted tubules harvested from rats subjected to 45 min of ischemia and 24 hr of reflow, as used by Gaudio et al. Alternately, if 45 min of ischemia and reflow produced damage only in proximal straight tubules, then Gaudio et al. isolated tubules that were undamaged by ischemia and reflow, since their procedure harvested primarily proximal convoluted tubules. It is difficult to reconcile the discrepancies between these *in vivo* and *in vitro* studies (69–71). One possible explanation may be that severely damaged tubules may be difficult or impossible to obtain by conventional procedures, and that the tubule suspension prepared from rats subjected to *in vivo* ischemia represents uninjured or minimally injured tubules. Thus, it is unclear whether damaged tubules may be obtained following toxicant exposure *in vivo*. Certainly, more work is required to validate this technique for use following pretreatment regimens.

Use of Tubule Suspensions in Renal Toxicology

Comparison of Tubular Segments: Proximal versus Distal Tubules

The kidney is a heterogeneous organ, comprised of discrete and unique portions. Nowhere is this complexity more evident than in the tubule itself. Each renal tubule contains at least eight segments, differentiated by morphology, localization, and function. In the past, it has been difficult to purify different tubule segments, with the exception of proximal tubules, in quantities necessary to determine intracellular contents, enzymatic components, and other biochemical characteristics. Tubule suspensions have helped overcome some of these difficulties by allowing differential preparation of fractions enriched in particular nephron segments—for example, proximal versus distal segments.

By centrifugation of partially digested kidney cortex through a Percoll gradient, several groups have prepared suspensions enriched in proximal or distal tubules (54,67). These suspensions, containing greater than 90% proximal or distal tubules, allowed comparison of biochemical characteristics of these tubular segments. Oxygen consumption and ATP content were similar in proximal and distal tubule suspensions (67). Alkaline phosphatase, γ-glutamyl-transpeptidase, fructose-1,6-diphosphatase, and glucose-6-phosphatase activities were significantly higher in proximal tubules, whereas hexokinase and kallikrein activities were significantly greater in distal tubules (67). Gluconeogenesis in the distal tubule suspensions was less than 10% of that in proximal tubule suspensions. Cytochrome P450 content and PAH uptake in proximal tubules were significantly greater than in distal tubules. Nonprotein sulfhydryl content (primarily GSH) was similar in proximal and distal tubules. Although xenobiotic metabolism is most commonly associated with proximal rather than distal tubules, distal tubular enzymes catalyzed glucuronidation of 4-methylumbelliferone (Fig. 3), although activity in distal tubules was only about 50% of that in proximal tubules (54).

Thus, by use of suspensions containing proximal or distal tubules, direct compar-

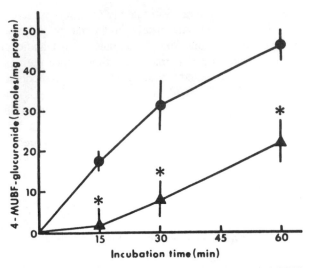

FIG. 3. Time course of glucuronidation of 4-methylumbelliferone (4-MUBF) to 4-MUBF-glucuronide by proximal (●) and distal (▲) tubule fractions. Asterisks indicate significant differences between proximal and distal tubular suspensions ($p < 0.05$). [Reproduced from Cojocel et al. (54) and Pergamon Press, with permission.]

ison of these segments was possible and biochemical similarities and differences were identified. As expected, proximal tubule suspensions had greatest activity in those functions previously associated with the proximal tubule, such as PAH uptake, gluconeogenesis, and cytochrome-P450-dependent metabolism. These activities were minimal or not detectable in distal tubule suspensions. In contrast, distal tubules had significant glucuronidation capacity, as evidenced by glucuronidation of 4-methylumbelliferone (Fig. 3). Previously, glucuronidation in the kidney was thought to occur only in the proximal tubule. The significance of distal tubule glucuronidation capacity remains unclear, and further investigations to more fully characterize glucuronidation, as well as other biochemical functions, of the distal tubule would help clarify the role of this nephron segment in xenobiotic metabolism.

Biochemical Mechanisms of Toxicity: Bromobenzene and Bromoquinones

Bromobenzene is a hepatotoxicant requiring cytochrome-P450-dependent metabolic bioactivation to produce cellular injury (72). Bromobenzene and *o*-bromophenol, a major metabolite of bromobenzene, both produce acute proximal tubular necrosis in rats (73). Evidence suggests that bromobenzene is metabolized via cytochrome P450 to 2-bromohydroquinone (2-BrHQ) and that 2-BrHQ is a more potent nephrotoxicant than either bromobenzene or *o*-bromophenol (74,75). In contrast to bromobenzene, 2-BrHQ produces negligible hepatotoxicity (73). GSH conjugates of 2-BrHQ are produced in liver, released into blood, and transported into proximal tubular cells to exert cytotoxic activity (74,75). However, the precise mechanism(s) involved in activation of 2-BrHQ to the ultimate nephrotoxicant and the subsequent mechanism(s) leading to lethal cell injury were unknown and proved difficult to investigate using *in vivo* methodology. Schnellmann and associates have used proximal tubule suspensions to investigate 2-BrHQ metabolism and cytotoxicity.

Proximal tubule suspensions prepared from rabbit kidneys were evaluated for their susceptibility to toxicity induced by bromobenzene and bromobenzene metabolites (59). Bromobenzene was the least potent compound, producing cytotoxicity at 5 mM bromobenzene. In contrast, 2-BrHQ was the most potent compound, with cytotoxicity elicited by 0.1 mM 2-BrHQ (59). Other metabolites (2-, 3-, and 4-bromophenol) were of intermediate potency with respect to cytotoxicity. The rank order of potency observed *in vitro* (59) was in excellent agreement with that observed *in vivo* (74–76), suggesting that rabbit proximal tubule suspensions would be a suitable system to explore mechanisms of bioactivation and cytotoxicity of bromobenzene and metabolites.

Further studies focused on 2-BrHQ, since this was the most cytotoxic bromobenzene metabolite, and initially addressed mechanism(s) of bioactivation of 2-BrHQ. When added to proximal tubule suspensions, 2-BrHQ was metabolized to glucuronide and mono- and di-GSH conjugates (77). Also, a significant amount of 2-BrHQ became covalently bound to renal tubular proteins (77). Cytochrome P450 was not involved in 2-BrHQ bioactivation, since inhibitors of cytochrome P450 (e.g., piperonyl butoxide and SKF 525A) failed to attenuate 2-BrHQ cytotoxicity (59). Furthermore, prostaglandin H synthase (PHS) was not involved in 2-BrHQ bioactivation, since inhibitors of PHS activities (e.g., indomethacin, methimazole) did not prevent 2-BrHQ-induced cytotoxicity (59). GSH conjugates of 2-BrHQ were potent nephrotoxicants *in vivo* (78). However, GSH conjugates of 2-BrHQ were not primarily responsible for cytotoxicity *in vitro*, since depletion of GSH in proximal tubule suspensions potentiated 2-BrHQ toxicity and AT-125, an inhibitor of γ-glutamyl transpeptidase, failed to attenuate 2-BrHQ-induced cytotoxicity (77). Thus, the mechanism of 2-BrHQ bioactivation remains unresolved.

Proximal tubule suspensions yielded considerable information concerning the mechanism(s) of cytotoxicity of 2-BrHQ. The earliest change induced by 2-BrHQ in proximal tubules was a decrease in GSH content, followed by decreases in basal and nystatin-stimulated oxygen consumption (59,79). These alterations occurred without detectable loss of LDH activity (79). Cellular ATP content was reduced by 2-BrHQ, as was mitochondrial state 3 respiration and electron transport through cytochrome c–cytochrome oxidase (79). Covalent binding occurred within 15 min of exposure of proximal tubules to 2-BrHQ, prior to overt signs of toxicity (77). In addition, depletion of GSH from proximal tubules increased covalent binding of 2-BrHQ and potentiated mitochondrial toxicity, whereas supraphysiological concentrations of GSH (achieved by incubating tubules with GSH) reduced covalent binding and attenuated mitochondrial toxicity (77). Redox cycling and/or oxidative stress did not appear to be involved in 2-BrHQ-induced cytotoxicity (80). Currently, the precise mechanisms of 2-BrHQ cytotoxicity are not entirely clear, but may involve covalent binding of 2-BrHQ or a metabolite to cellular proteins, consequently resulting in mitochondrial dysfunction and cell death.

CELL SUSPENSIONS

The utility of hepatocyte preparations led investigators to try similar techniques with kidneys, with varying degrees of success. Whereas the liver contains only a few cell types, the kidney is a complex organ containing numerous cell types. Therefore, methodology had to be developed to obtain fairly homogeneous preparations of the desired cell population. Essentially, two different approaches may be employed. One approach is to prepare tubule fragments, as described above, and further dissociate those fragments into single cells. This method is complicated by inherent heterogeneity of several nephron segments. For example, collecting tubules are composed of two cell types, principal and intercalated cells. Therefore, dissociation of collecting tubule fragments into single cells will yield a heterogeneous population. However, for other nephron segments that are more homogeneous in nature, such as the thick ascending limb of the loop of Henle, dissociation of fragments into single cells works fairly well. The second approach is to dissociate renal tissue directly into single cells, then isolate a homogeneous population of cells using a variety of methods, including those based on buoyant density (isopycnic density gradient centrifugation, sedimentation), different rate of migration in a density gradient (isokinetic gradients) or electric field (free-flow electrophoresis), or differences in fluorescence (cell sorter) (81).

Methodology

Most investigators who use renal cell suspensions start with *in situ* and/or *ex vivo* collagenase perfusion of donor kidneys, similar to the process described for preparation of renal tubule suspensions (see above). Perfusion is initiated *in vivo* and continued *in vitro* in a recirculating perfusion apparatus similar to that described for the IPK (Fig. 4) (82). A major difference is that, to prepare cell suspensions, perfusion is continued for a longer period of time (usually 15–30 min) than the time required to prepare tubule suspensions (usually 5–10 min). Following perfusion, further procedures are necessary to isolate individual cells. Generally, separation of proximal and distal tubule cells from loop of Henle and collecting duct cells is achieved by selecting cortical tissue for processing, while discarding medullary tissue (83). Alternately, medullary tissue is retained for processing and cortical tissue discarded when suspensions of medullary cells are desired (84).

When cortical tissue is processed, glomeruli may be removed by taking advantage of size differences. For example, the diameter of a rat glomerulus is approximately 100 μm whereas the diameter of a tubular epithelial cell is considerably less (83). Thus, sieving tissue digest through a series of screens serves to remove larger

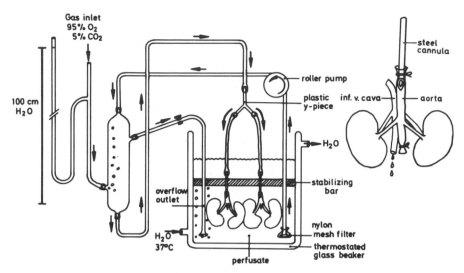

FIG. 4. Left: Schematic drawing of apparatus for isolating kidney cells. Arrows indicate direction of perfusate flow through recirculating system. The apparatus allows for simultaneous perfusion of two pairs of kidneys. **Right:** Illustration of placement of steel cannula into aorta for *in situ/ex vivo* perfusion. [Reproduced from Ormstad et al. (82) and Academic Press, with permission.]

tissue fragments, glomeruli, blood vessels, and connective tissue. However, the resulting preparation contains cells of proximal as well as distal tubule origin, and further purification is necessary to obtain a more homogeneous cell suspension. Numerous purification procedures have been described, most involving centrifugation through discontinuous gradients of Ficoll, Percoll, or other polymers (83). The final preparation is highly enriched in proximal tubule cells, although heterogeneity still exists in that cells are derived from S_1 and S_2 subtypes (83).

For whatever perfusion and purification method employed, cells must be characterized as to nephron segment of origin and extent of contamination by other cell types in the suspension. A variety of methods have been employed to characterize cell suspensions, including morphologic examination of cells in suspension (Table 1), distribution of marker enzymes (e.g., hexokinase for distal tubule cells, alkaline phosphatase and γ-glutamyl transpeptidase for proximal tubule cells), and oxygen consumption (inhibited by furosemide in TALH cells, inhibited by amiloride in distal tubule cells) (83–85).

Advantages

In general, cell suspensions share the same advantages as do tubule suspensions. A fairly homogeneous population of the desired cell type may be prepared and cell population may be exposed to a toxicant over a short period of time. Viability parameters, such as oxygen uptake, LDH content, dye exclusion, and calcium con-

TABLE 1. *Structural markers for identification of single isolated cells from rabbit renal medulla*[a]

Cells	Plasma membrane	Nucleus	Mitochondria	Cytoplasmic inclusions
Proximal tubule (pars recta)	Long microvilli, thick baso-lateral mem-brane infoldings	Round, elon-gated, often indented	Small, ovoid, dark	Numerous vesi-cles (mean diameter ~ 0.7 μm), electron-dense mate-rial[b]
TALH	Few short microvillus projections, basolateral membrane is highly folded	Elongated with indentations	Numerous, large, dark, densely packed, filling up most of cell, mostly round, larger than in proxi-mal and col-lecting tubule cells, visible	Vesicles mostly smaller than mitochondria[b]
Collecting duct (principal cells)	A few short mi-crovilli, infold-ings	Large, round	Dark, small, less nu-merous than in proximal tubule	Small, light ves-icles (mean diameter ~ 0.3 μm)
Thin loop, inter-stitial, and endothelial cells	Irregular sur-face with mi-crovillous-like extrusions	Irregular shape	Very few	Some vesicles, cytoplasm is only a small ring around the nucleus

[a]Reproduced from Eveloff et al. (84), with permission from the Rockefeller University Press.
[b]Vesicles may include naturally occurring vesicle structures and cross sections of basolateral membranes.

tent, may be measured in cell suspensions. Intracellular contents of metabolic sub-strates, such as adenine nucleotides and GSH, may be monitored, as well as intra-cellular ion concentrations (e.g., sodium and potassium). All of these parameters may provide valuable information concerning cell viability.

Cell suspensions offer additional advantages over previously discussed *in vitro* methods. In cell suspensions, unstirred layers and anoxic and/or ischemic damage are minimized since cells are individually and uniformly exposed to medium on all sides. In tubule suspensions, the lumen is open and accessible during separation and purification procedures, but it is not certain that the lumen remains open during subsequent incubations (83). Thus, during incubation with tubule suspensions, compounds that gain access to tubular epithelial cells by luminal transport or diffu-sion may not accumulate if tubular lumens do indeed collapse. In contrast, cell suspensions are continually exposed to toxicant throughout an incubation, and ac-cess of toxicant to intracellular compartments is not a problem. In addition, cell suspensions may be "pulsed" with toxicant. For example, cells may be incubated with toxicant for a short period of time, then washed and resuspended in incubation medium free of toxicant. In this manner, sequential responses to short toxicant exposures may be studied.

Limitations

As with other *in vitro* techniques, cell suspensions have a limited lifespan of 2–4 hr, similar to tubule suspensions. In addition, a significant amount of time is required to prepare cell suspensions, negating an advantage of renal slices in terms of ease and rapidity of preparation. As mentioned, enzymatic digestion is required to loosen cells from underlying extracellular matrix. Since the incubation and/or perfusion time required to prepare cells is longer than the time required to prepare tubules, it is possible that membrane integrity may be compromised during digestion and that epithelial cells may lose some specific membrane functions (83).

Another disadvantage of cell suspensions is loss of *in situ* polarity. In suspension, cells are evenly exposed to medium on all sides. Luminal and basolateral attachments are lost, as is luminal and basolateral polarity. Consequently, in renal cell suspensions, more membrane surface area is exposed to toxicants than in renal slices or tubule suspensions, creating a potential for enhanced diffusion of toxicant into tubular cells.

Another limitation of cell suspensions is the relatively low yield of tissue. Typically, only $25–50 \times 10^6$ cells are recovered from rat kidneys following digestion and purification (85,86). Cell yield is usually sufficient to allow experimental maneuvers with appropriate controls. However, analytical techniques may need to be adapted to detect small quantities of substances, and specialized equipment may be necessary to monitor desired parameters.

Use of Cell Suspensions in Renal Toxicology

Comparison of Renal Tubular Cells: Proximal versus Distal Tubular Cells

Most nephrotoxicants injure renal proximal tubules, although several compounds that injure distal tubules have been identified (amphotericin B, lithium). However, the identification of the proximal tubules as the more common site of chemical-induced injury may reflect a greater ability to detect proximal tubular damage. For example, the proximal tubule has well-defined, unique functions, such as organic anion and cation transport, that make detection of injury relatively easy. The distal tubule has fewer unique functions than does the proximal tubule, making it difficult to identify toxicity in the distal tubule. As noted above, Cojocel et al. (54) used suspensions enriched in proximal or distal tubules to quantitate differences in between these tubular segments. Lash and co-workers have taken advantage of different densities of proximal and distal tubular cells to prepare purified proximal or distal tubular cell suspensions (85,87,88).

In a series of studies, Lash and co-workers tested cytotoxic responses of proximal or distal tubular cells to three different classes of compounds: cephalosporin antibiotics, specifically cephaloridine (85); oxidizing agents, specifically *tert*-butylhydroperoxide (tBH), menadione, and hydrogen peroxide (87); and alkylating agents, specifically methyl vinyl ketone (MVK), allyl alcohol, and *N*-dimethylnitrosamine (NDMA) (88). Cephaloridine produces proximal tubular necrosis *in vivo* (89), and produces cytotoxicity only in proximal tubular cells (85). Cell viability, measured as trypan blue exclusion, was reduced in a time- and concentration-dependent manner in proximal tubular cells, whereas distal tubular cells incubated with cephaloridine showed no loss of viability over 2 hr (85). Thus, *in vitro* cell suspensions were in excellent agreement with *in vivo* studies and showed that proximal tubular cells were susceptible to cephaloridine-induced cytotoxicity whereas distal tubular cells were not.

In contrast to selective susceptibility of proximal tubular cells to cephaloridine, distal tubular cells were much more susceptible than proximal tubular cells to cytotoxicity induced by oxidizing agents (87). All three oxidizing agents produced cytotoxicity, measured as LDH leakage, in both proximal and distal tubular cells. However, LDH leakage was significantly greater in distal than in proximal tubular cells (Fig. 5) (87). Oxidative stress is known to alter GSH redox status in cells (90,91). To elucidate the mechanism(s) underlying greater susceptibility of distal versus proximal tubular cells to oxidative stress, GSH and oxidized glutathione (GSSG) were measured in cell suspensions following exposure to tBH. As expected, incubation of either proximal or distal tubular cells with tBH produced loss of GSH and accumulation of GSSG (87). In addition, incubation of proximal tubular cells in GSH-containing buffer failed to protect against tBH cytotoxicity, whereas incubation with GSH exerted a protective effect in distal tubular cells (87). However, exogenous dithiothreitol protected distal tubular cells from tBH-induced cytotoxicity to the same extent as did exogenous GSH, suggesting that protection was due to nonspecific thiol reductant properties rather than GSH-dependent enzyme-catalyzed reactions (87). Further studies indicated that GSH status could be dissociated from oxidative injury. For example, preincubation with buthionine sulfoximine, an inhibitor of GSH synthesis, plus acivicin, an inhibitor of GSH degradation, reduced GSH concentration to a similar extent in both proximal and distal tubular cells. However, cytotoxicity of tBH was more pronounced in distal than in proximal tubular cells, despite comparable concentrations of GSH (87). In addition, increases in cellular GSSG were not uniformly accompanied by increases in LDH leakage. Examination of enzymes involved in GSH status indicated that distal tubular cells had lower activities of GSH peroxidase, GSSG reductase, catalase, and DT-diaphorase than did proximal tubular cells (87). Thus, distal tubular cells may be more susceptible to oxidative stress than proximal tubular cells due to a reduced ability of distal tubular cells to detoxify reactive species generated by oxidizing agents.

Both proximal and distal tubular cells were susceptible to cytotoxicity induced by

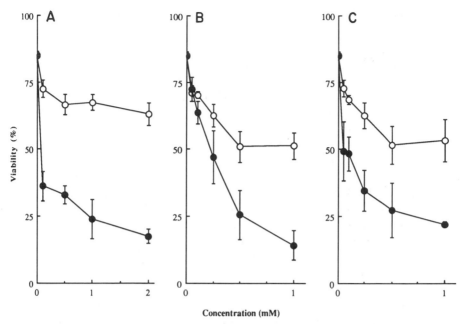

FIG. 5. Concentration dependence of cytotoxicity in isolated rat kidney proximal tubule (PT) and distal tubular (DT) cells. Isolated renal PT (○) and DT (●) cells were incubated for 1 hr with indicated concentrations of *tert*-butyl hydroperoxide **(A)**, menadione **(B)**, or hydrogen peroxide **(C)**. Viability was measured as fraction of cells that did not leak LDH. [Reproduced from Lash and Tokarz (87) and the American Physiological Society, with permission.]

alkylating agents (88). Distal tubular cells were significantly more susceptible than proximal tubular cells to MVK-induced LDH leakage and moderately more susceptible to cytotoxicity induced by allyl alcohol. Both MVK and allyl alcohol react with soft nucleophiles such as GSH and protein sulfhydryl groups. Thus, agents that react directly with GSH are more cytotoxic to distal tubular cells than to proximal tubular cells, consistent with decreased ability of distal tubular cells to detoxify reactive intermediates through GSH metabolism (see above). In contrast, NDMA was equally cytotoxic to proximal and distal tubular cells (88). NDMA undergoes cytochrome-P450-dependent metabolism to generate formaldehyde and a methylating intermediate, or undergoes denitrosation to form formaldehyde and mono-methylamine, a metabolically inert species (92). Similar susceptibility of proximal and distal tubular cells to NDMA cytotoxicity suggests that both cell populations are able to bioactivate NDMA. This observation is somewhat at odds with previous work suggesting that cytochromes P450 are present in the proximal tubule and virtually absent from the distal tubule (11,54). It is possible that cytochrome P450 content is higher or a specific cytochrome P450 isozyme is higher in distal tubules than previously thought. Cytochrome P450 content of proximal versus distal tubular cells could be reexamined, perhaps using cell suspensions, to resolve this discrepancy.

Biochemical Mechanisms of Cytotoxicity: Halogenated Hydrocarbons

GSH and cysteine-S-conjugates of halogenated hydrocarbons, such as S-(1,2-dichlorovinyl)GSH (DCVG) and DCVC, are potent nephrotoxicants, causing necrosis of renal proximal tubules, elevations of BUN concentration, and glucosuria (93–96). Nephrotoxicity of these compounds depends on metabolic bioactivation: DCVG is metabolized to DCVC via γ-glutamyl transferase and cysteinylglycine dipeptidase (or aminopeptidase M), and DCVC is further metabolized to pyruvate, ammonia, and a reactive thiovinyl intermediate via cysteine conjugate β-lyase (95–99). However, the mechanism whereby the reactive intermediate produces cytotoxicity was not entirely clear. Previous studies suggested that mitochondria are a primary target of DCVC cytotoxicity (100,101), and cell suspensions were employed to more precisely define the events involved in DCVC-induced cytotoxicity.

Incubation of proximal tubular cell suspensions with either DCVG or DCVC caused time- and concentration-dependent loss of viability (measured as trypan blue exclusion and LDH leakage) (102). DCVG cytotoxicity was attenuated when AT-125, an inhibitor of γ-glutamyl transpeptidase, was included in the incubation medium, and cytotoxicity due to either DCVG or DCVC was attenuated when aminooxyacetic acid (AOAA), an inhibitor of cysteine conjugate (β-lyase, was included in the incubation medium (102). Thus, cytotoxicity of both agents in cell suspensions required the same metabolic steps as did nephrotoxicity *in vivo*, supporting the utility of cell suspensions in investigating DCVG and DCVC cytotoxicity.

Incubation of cells with DCVC for 30 min caused marked declines in cellular GSH and glutamate concentrations without significantly changing GSSG concentrations (102). The lack of change in GSSG concentration, as well as absence of thiobarbituric acid (TBA)-reactive material (indicative of lipid peroxidation), suggested that DCVC cytotoxicity did not involve oxidative stress. The decline in glutamate concentration was interpreted to suggest that DCVC induced alterations in cellular energy metabolism.

Subsequent studies monitored the effects of DCVC on three parameters of mitochondrial function: adenine nucleotide status, oxygen consumption, and calcium sequestration. DCVC produced a rapid and pronounced decline in cellular ATP content, coupled with modest increases in cellular ADP and AMP content. The cellular ATP/ADP ratio and energy charge fell dramatically, suggesting that proximal tubule cells exposed to DCVC would have impaired ability to maintain ATP-dependent functions (102). DCVC decreased oxygen consumption with succinate as substrate; however, oxygen consumption with glutamate plus malate or ascorbate plus N,N,N', N'-tetramethyl-p-phenylenediamine as electron donors was unaltered by DCVC (102). Thus, DCVC specifically inhibited succinate oxidation. Both mitochondria and endoplasmic reticulum play major roles in regulation of intracellular calcium homeostasis (103,104). Incubation of proximal tubule cells with DCVC reduced mitochondrial calcium sequestration by 62% in 2 hr without altering microsomal calcium sequestration (102). A strong correlation existed between DCVC-

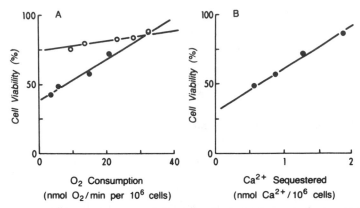

FIG. 6. Correlation between effects of DCVC on renal cell viability and mitochondrial function. **A:** Relationship between effects of 1 mM DCVC (●) or 1 mM DCVC + 0.1 mM AOAA (○) on cell viability and oxygen consumption. **B:** Relationship between effects of 1 mM DCVC on cell viability and mitochondrial calcium sequestration. [Reproduced from Lash and Anders (102) and the American Society of Biological Chemists, with permission.]

induced loss of cell viability and cellular oxygen consumption or mitochondrial calcium sequestration (Fig. 6) (102). Thus, the primary target of DCVC-induced cytotoxicity appears to be mitochondria, leading to alterations in energy charge and calcium sequestration. However, the precise steps leading to cell death remain uncertain.

CELL CULTURES

The major disadvantage of previously discussed *in vitro* techniques is the limited lifespan of each preparation. With renal slices, tubule suspensions, or cell suspensions, investigators routinely use high concentrations of toxicant to accelerate the onset of cytotoxic events. However, higher concentrations of toxicants may introduce complications in interpretation. Many toxicities depend on enzyme-catalyzed metabolism for bioactivation and/or detoxification. Since enzyme-catalyzed processes saturate at finite substrate concentrations, use of high toxicant concentrations may distort normal metabolic pathways—for example, by inappropriately saturating detoxification pathways. It would be more desirable to be able to produce toxicity using concentrations of toxicant similar to those found *in vivo*. Thus, some toxicologists have turned to cell culture systems to investigate mechanisms of cytotoxicity.

Cell culture systems may be divided into established cell lines and primary cell cultures. Established cell lines frequently used in renal toxicology include: MDCK cells, considered to be of distal tubular or cortical collecting duct origin and derived from cocker spaniel kidney (105–107); LLC-PK$_1$, considered to be of proximal tubular origin and derived from Hampshire pig (108,109); and OK cells, considered to be of proximal tubular origin and derived from opossum kidney (110,111). Primary cultures are established by isolating cells from donor kidneys (usually rat) and allowing these cells to grow and proliferate in defined culture conditions (83,112).

Methodology

Cell culture techniques are well established. Cells are grown on plastic dishes or on porous membranes under controlled conditions (CO_2 tension, humidity, temperature, oscillations) in medium containing metabolic substrates and growth factors, such as fetal calf serum. Cultures are allowed to grow to confluency (i.e., form a monolayer), then are replated at lower cell density (subculture). Established cell lines may be subcultured infinitely, whereas primary cell cultures may be subcultured a limited number of times before dedifferentiation and loss of specific functions occurs (83).

Primary cultures are initiated by obtaining cells from a donor kidney. In general, the procedure is the same as that used to obtain cell suspensions. Cells are harvested by collagenase digestion, purified as previously discussed, and placed in a Petri dish or other culture system in appropriate medium. Unfortunately, purification is never complete, and some contamination with cells other than those desired will invariably occur. An additional complication of trace contamination in the initial preparation is that all cells do not grow at the same rate. Therefore, it is possible that a contaminating cell type may grow faster than the desired cell type, eventually overgrowing and replacing the desired cells in the culture system. In particular, overgrowth of fibroblasts is a problem with proximal tubular cells in culture. Fibroblast contamination may be minimized by including D-valine and ornithine rather than L-valine and arginine in the culture medium, since proximal tubular cells, but not fibroblasts, can convert D-valine and ornithine into L-valine and arginine, respectively (113,114).

Traditionally, cells in culture are grown on plastic dishes or plates. Cells attach to the plastic surface, forming a basement-membrane-like structure. With polarized cells, such as kidney tubule cells, the basolateral surface of the cell is oriented against the plastic support, thereby making the basolateral membrane inaccessible to incubation medium. The luminal (apical) membrane of kidney cells develops normally in culture, exhibiting microvilli and other characteristic features, and is accessible to incubation medium (106–109,115). When grown on plastic supports, both established cell lines and primary cell cultures develop "domes," areas in which fluid accumulates under the epithelial sheet. Dome formation can be abolished by including an inhibitor of sodium transport, such as ouabain or amiloride, in the incubation medium (106,109), suggesting that dome formation is due to transepithelial "reabsorption" of solutes and water. Glucose reabsorption in the proximal tubule occurs via a luminal transporter that is inhibited by phloridzin, and kidney proximal tubular cells grown on plastic supports accumulated α-methylglucose via a phloridzin-sensitive pathway (112). In contrast, PAH accumulation by

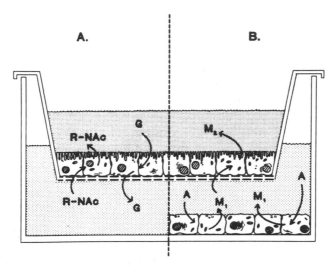

FIG. 7. Schematic drawing of proximal tubule cells cultured on a porous membrane, illustrating several possible pathways involved in nephrotoxicity. In panel **A**, mercapturic acids (R-NAc) applied to the basolateral membrane (lower compartment) may be transported into proximal tubular cells, then secreted across the luminal membrane into the upper compartment. Glucose (G) applied to the luminal membrane (upper compartment) may be taken up by proximal tubular cells and transported out of cells at the basolateral membrane into the medium (lower compartment). This system allows selective exposure of the luminal and basolateral membranes as well as separate analysis of unidirectional cellular fluxes. In panel **B**, the porous membrane support system allows the co-culture of different cell types on a rigid support system (bottom chamber). In this example, compound A is metabolized by co-cultured cells (bottom of the well) to a metabolite (M_1). M_1 is cytotoxic to proximal tubular cells after M_1 is accumulated by transport across the basolateral membrane. Alternately, M_1 may be further metabolized to M_2, which may be excreted into the medium. [Reproduced from Boogaard et al. (83) and Elsevier Scientific Publishers, with permission.]

proximal tubular cells occurs via a probenecid-sensitive basolateral transport pathway, and PAH was not accumulated by proximal tubular cells in primary culture grown on plastic supports (112), indicating that, with conventional cell culture systems, the basolateral membrane is not accessible to incubation medium. To overcome this difficulty, investigators have turned to growing cells on porous filters that may be suspended in incubation medium, as illustrated in Fig. 7 (83). When primary cultures of proximal tubular cells were grown on porous membranes, probenecid-sensitive PAH uptake was observed (112). In addition, primary cultures of proximal tubular cells grown on porous membranes acidified the medium bathing the apical surface, whereas cells grown on plastic dishes did not acidify the incubation medium (116). Therefore, the support system (plastic versus porous membrane) may be an important consideration when establishing cell cultures, since processes that rely on accessibility of the basolateral membrane, such as organic anion accumulation or acidification, may not occur when that membrane is in close contact with the support system.

Advantages

The primary advantage of cell culture over other *in vitro* techniques is that cells may be exposed to toxicant for long periods of time (several days to weeks for established cell lines) at concentrations that are relevant to those observed *in vivo*. No other *in vitro* technique retains viability for longer than 24–30 hr. The ability to use pharmacologically or toxicologically relevant concentrations of a compound cannot be overemphasized. Many compounds depend on enzymatic bioactivation and/or detoxification in order to exert cytotoxicity. By definition, enzyme-mediated processes may be saturated at sufficiently high concentrations of substrate. If a minor metabolic pathway for a compound involves bioactivation by an enzyme-mediated reaction, such as occurs with acetaminophen in the liver, then the traditional method of using high concentrations of substrate with renal slices, tubule suspensions, or cell suspensions will result in production of a greater amount of reactive metabolite than found *in vivo*. Furthermore, some toxicants may produce injury by multiple, concentration-dependent mechanisms. Exposure of tissue to high concentrations of toxicant for short-term incubations may alter the balance of mechanisms involved in cytotoxicity, such as increased bioactivation when detoxification is saturated. Thus, when investigators use short-term systems that rely on high concentrations of toxicants, they should be aware of the potential for differences between *in vitro* and *in vivo* metabolism. Cell culture systems, whether established cell lines or primary cultures, avoid problems with metabolic differences by allowing cells to be exposed to pharmacologically or toxicologically relevant concentrations of toxicant over an extended period of time. In addition, cell cultures may be used for "pulsed" experiments, when toxicant is introduced for a period of time and then removed, allowing cells to fully develop injury and/or recovery. While "pulsing" is possible with previously discussed *in vitro* techniques, the short lifespan of other preparations makes it more difficult to monitor expression of cytotoxicity and/or recovery (repair).

For established cell lines, a unique advantage is that these cells are theoretically immortal and can be reseeded and subcultured repeatedly without change in phenotype or function. In practice, however, established cell lines may undergo some changes over time, so that cell lines need to be characterized periodically by each investigator.

Primary cell cultures, on the other hand, do have a finite lifetime and undergo phenotypic and functional changes (see below). Thus, a primary culture established at a different point in time may differ somewhat from a previously established culture. However, if rigorous care is taken so that starting material and culture conditions are constant for each experiment, primary cell cultures should remain sufficiently homogeneous to allow comparison of data from different cultures.

Limitations

A major limitation of cell culture techniques is the inherent heterogeneity of any preparation. While heterogeneity may be overcome by using established cell lines, these cell lines have several other limitations. In particular, LLC-PK₁ cells, derived from proximal tubule, lack several specific proximal tubular functions such as organic anion and glucose transport (117). In addition, LLC-PK₁ cells display some characteristics of distal tubule and TALH cells, including (a) vasopressin- and calcitonin-sensitive adenylate cyclases (118,119) and (b) high transepithelial resistance similar to that of the collecting duct (120–122). Thus, the use of established cell lines may incorporate some difficulties in interpretation due to ambiguous origin of those cells.

Primary cultures theoretically avoid the problems of heterogeneity, but in practice it is nearly impossible to completely purify the starting preparation (83). However, if culture conditions are optimized as previously discussed, and cultures are carefully and thoroughly characterized as to purity of cells of interest, considerable information may be gained by using primary cultures.

When establishing primary cell cultures, proliferating cells go through a series of dedifferentiations, reverting to a more juvenile cell type, and redifferentiations, acquiring characteristics of the origin cell line (83). In an ultrastructural study, Koechlin et al. (123) described these processes for rabbit proximal tubular cells grown in culture. Through the first 6 days in culture, proximal tubular cells progressively dedifferentiated, losing brush border, basal interdigitations, and many intracellular organelles. From day 6 through day 20, cells underwent progressive redifferentiation, acquiring microvilli, forming basal interdigitations, and replacing intracellular organelles. However, redifferentiating cells also acquired glycogen granules not seen in proximal tubular cells *in situ*, which Koechlin et al. suggested might be due to overloading the culture medium with glucose. In addition, the apical microvilli of cells in culture were not as prevalent or well developed as microvilli of cells *in situ*, basal interdigitations remained poorly developed, and mitochondria were less numerous in cultured cells than in proximal tubular cells *in situ*. From day 20 through day 39, cells in culture became overloaded with glycogen granules and other cellular debris, suggesting that cells were undergoing degenerative processes (123). These data suggest that primary cell cultures do not retain uniform phenotypical characteristics throughout the life of the culture, and timing of experiments relative to days in culture may be a critical variable in studies using cell culture. In addition, cells in culture do not exactly duplicate the appearance of cells *in situ*. The extent to which cells in culture resemble cells *in situ* functionally must be defined by the investigator.

In cultured hepatocytes, investigators have observed a rapid and irreversible decline in cytochrome-P450- and glucuronyl-transferase-dependent metabolism (124–126). In a recent investigation, Bruggeman et al. (127) observed that cytochrome P450 was undetectable in microsomes prepared from 3- to 5-day-old cultured proximal tubular cells. Furthermore, GSH concentrations and glutathione S-transferase contents (determined by measuring glutathione S-transferase subunits by high-performance liquid chromatography) were lower in proximal tubular cells cultured from day 1 through day 5 than in freshly isolated proximal tubular cells (127). Thus, it may be that proximal tubular cells in culture undergo dedifferentiation with loss of enzymes catalyzing metabolism of xenobiotics, similar to the process observed in hepatocytes. To some extent, loss of enzyme activity in cultured proximal tubular cells may be circumvented by including renal S9 fraction (128). In addition, investigators are exploring culture systems designed to preserve enzyme activities in cultured hepatocytes (129), and these techniques could easily be extended to cultured renal tubular cells.

Cell culture is a difficult and expensive technique. Considerable equipment is needed to support cell cultures, including sterile facilities for isolating, seeding, and replating cells, incubators for maintaining cells during proliferation, and miscellaneous supplies, solutions, and chemicals, all of which make experiments rather costly. Unfortunately, it is easy to lose a culture to bacterial contamination or fibroblast overgrowth, so that rigorous control of sterility and culture conditions is essential. In addition, a relatively small amount of tissue is contained in a monolayer, so that sensitive methodology is required to detect cytotoxicity (83).

Use of Cell Cultures in Renal Toxicology

Biochemical Mechanisms of Lethal Cell Injury: Halogenated Hydrocarbons

Cysteine conjugates of halogenated hydrocarbons, such as DCVC and DCVG, have been extensively investigated in numerous *in vitro* systems, as previously discussed. However, the intracellular events leading to cell death have been difficult to identify. Studies in proximal tubular cell suspensions indicated that loss of mitochondrial integrity and/or impaired ability to sequester calcium contributed to DCVC-induced cytotoxicity.

The role of altered calcium distribution in DCVC cytotoxicity was further investigated using cultured LLC-PK$_1$ cells. Intracellular calcium concentration and localization were determined using fura-2, a calcium-sensitive fluorescent dye. In control cells, intracellular calcium was localized primarily in mitochondria, as shown by rhodamine-123 staining. In contrast, incubation of LLC-PK$_1$ cells for 24 hr with 10^{-4} M DCVC increased intracellular calcium concentration approximately fourfold while greatly reducing mitochondrial calcium concentration (130). Mitochondria remained viable despite calcium loss, as indicated by rhodamine-123 staining properties (130). Longer incubations with DCVC (up to 96 hr) caused further increases in intracellular calcium concentration, as well as plasma membrane blebbing. Membrane blebs contained high calcium concentrations, whereas calcium was virtually absent from mitochondria. In addition, with longer incubations, mitochondria became nonviable and could no longer be detected by rhodamine-123 staining (130). Thus, these studies demonstrated that DCVC produced major alterations in intracellular calcium concentration and distribution. Depletion of mitochondrial calcium preceded bleb formation and cell death. In addition, loss of mitochondrial calcium preceded collapse of mitochondrial membrane potential (130). Vamvakas et al. (130) suggested that calcium release from mitochondria prior to loss of mitochondrial membrane potential may be related to oxidation and hydrolysis of mitochondrial pyridine nucleotides and ADP-ribosylation of mito-chondrial membrane proteins.

Chen et al. (131) tested a variety of cytoprotective agents for their ability to prevent DCVC-induced cytotoxicity in LLC-PK$_1$ cells. Inhibitors of proteolysis (leupeptin, antipain, methylamine) or phospholipase (dibucaine, *p*-bromophenyl-acyl bromide), calcium channel blockers (nifedipine, verapamil) or a calmodulin antagonist (calmidazolium) were ineffective in preventing LDH leakage following incubation of LLC-PK$_1$ cells with DCVC (131). In contrast, both AOAA and DPPD were extremely effective in ameliorating DCVC-induced cytotoxicity (131). AOAA was included as a positive control, since AOAA competitively inhibits cysteine conjugate β-lyase, the enzyme responsible for bioactivation of DCVC (see above). Several other antioxidants were tested for protective effects against DCVC: hydro-philic antioxidants (uric acid, ascorbic acid) were ineffective, whereas lipophilic antioxidants (butylated hydroxyanisole, propyl galate, butylated hydroxytoluene, and butylated hydroxyquinone) were very effective inhibitors of DCVC toxicity (131). In contrast to AOAA, which inhibits both DCVC bioactivation and covalent binding, DPPD prevented DCVC-induced cytotoxicity without altering covalent binding of ^{35}S derived from DCVC. Thus, DCVC cytotoxicity may be dissociated from covalent binding of a reactive intermediate of DCVC.

The inability to demonstrate protection against DCVC cytotoxicity by calcium channel blockers (nifedipine, verapamil) observed by Chen et al. (131) appears to be in direct contrast to calcium-dependent DCVC cytotoxicity proposed by Vam-vakas et al. (130). However, Chen et al. noted a biphasic protective effect of DPPD that depended on the concentration of DCVC in the incubation medium. Specifi-cally, DPPD was effective in blocking toxicity at low concentrations of DCVC (25–50 μM) but ineffective at higher DCVC concentrations (250–500 μM) (131). Thus, the mechanisms of DCVC cytotoxicity are concentration-dependent. Specifically, lipid peroxidation and/or oxidative stress may be involved in DCVC cytotoxicity at low DCVC concentrations, whereas antioxidant-insensitive pathways may be in-volved at higher DCVC concentrations (131). Concentration-dependent toxicity in cultured or freshly prepared hepatocytes has been described for several compounds, including acetaminophen (132) and carbon tetrachloride (133). Thus, toxicant con-centration may be a critical determinant of the mechanism of cytotoxicity.

The ability of DPPD and other antioxidants to protect cells from DCVC cytotox-icity suggested that lipid peroxidation was a factor in DCVC-induced cell injury. Indeed, TBA-reactive products, indicative of lipid peroxidation, were detectable in LLC-PK$_1$ cells incubated with DCVC prior to the onset of LDH leakage, suggesting that lipid peroxidation was occurring prior to, rather than coincident with, cell death. Coincubation of cells with DCVC and DPPD prevented both formation of TBA-positive material and LDH leakage, indicating protection from DCVC cyto-toxicity (131). Deferoxamine, an iron chelator, prevented formation of TBA-posi-tive material and LDH leakage without altering covalent binding of radiolabel de-rived from DCVC (131), supporting a role for iron-dependent lipid peroxidation in DCVC-induced cell injury. Dithiothreitol, a thiol reducing agent, also protected against DCVC cytotoxicity without altering covalent material of radiolabel derived from DCVC (131). Thus, DCVC-induced cell death may be due to oxidative stress. The mechanism of initiation of DCVC-induced oxidative stress remains unclear.

Cellular Accumulation and Metabolism: Aminoglycoside Antibiotics

Aminoglycoside antibiotics, such as gentamicin, are used clinically to treat gram-negative bacterial infections. Nephrotoxicity is a major complication associated with aminoglycoside therapy and has been the subject of numerous investigations (134,135). However, gentamicin nephrotoxicity is relatively slow to develop. In rats, repeated administration of gentamicin is necessary to produce renal injury (136,137). Gentamicin nephrotoxicity *in vivo* is characterized by multiple and diffuse abnormalities, including accumulation of myeloid bodies in proximal tubular cells, enzymuria and proteinuria, and decreases in GFR (134,135). While some tubular epithelial cells may undergo necrosis and death during continuing administration of gentamicin, other cells may undergo regeneration. These regenerating cells are relatively undifferentiated and immature, and retain normal morphology despite the presence of gentamicin (138), suggesting that immature cells are not susceptible to gentamicin toxicity.

In vitro methods have been used to investigate the mechanisms leading to gentamicin nephrotoxicity. Alterations in plasma membrane function (e.g., disturbances of phospholipid metabolism, changes in intracellular calcium concentration, alterations in membrane transport properties), alterations in mitochondrial function (e.g., uncoupling of respiration, inhibition of calcium accumulation), and lysosomal membrane alterations (e.g., lysosomal destabilization, diminished phospholipase activity) have been implicated in the development of gentamicin nephrotoxicity (135). However, the precise mechanisms involved in gentamicin-induced cell injury remain unclear.

Cell culture is an excellent system in which to investigate slowly developing toxicities, such as that caused by gentamicin. However, it should be noted that gentamicin toxicity in cell culture systems generally requires exposure to concentrations higher than those seen *in vivo* (see below). Presumably, the higher gentamicin concentrations necessary to injure cultured cells may be due to the dedifferentiated and/or immature state of cultured cells, making them less susceptible to gentamicin-induced cytotoxicity than proximal tubular cells *in vivo*.

It is well established that gentamicin is accumulated within proximal tubular cells via endocytosis across the luminal membrane of proximal tubular cells (134,135). Cultured LLC-PK$_1$ cells accumulated gentamicin via energy-dependent pathways, inhibited by rotenone and dinitrophenol (139). Gentamicin accumulation occurred against a concentration gradient, and intracellular gentamicin concentration in LLC-PK$_1$ cells was approximately three times greater than the gentamicin concentration in the incubation medium (139). Furthermore, A23187, a calcium ionophore, stimulated gentamicin accumulation whereas EGTA, a calcium chelator, reduced gentamicin uptake (139). In addition, gentamicin uptake was sensitive to alterations in calcium concentration of the medium. A23187-stimulated gentamicin uptake was minimal at low external calcium concentrations, whereas gentamicin uptake was maximally stimulated by A23187 at high external calcium concentrations (139). These studies suggested that LLC-PK$_1$ cells might be a suitable *in vitro* system to investigate gentamicin nephrotoxicity because active gentamicin uptake occurred in these cells. Furthermore, these *in vitro* studies supported the hypothesis that gentamicin accumulation occurred via an endocytotic process by demonstrating that uptake required the presence of calcium ions.

Using LLC-PK$_1$ cells, Schwertz et al. (140) investigated morphological and functional alterations following incubation with gentamicin. Cells were incubated with concentrations of gentamicin ranging from 0.1 to 2 mM, considerably higher than the desired therapeutic range of 2–10 µg/ml (134,135), for up to 7 days. Within 4 days of incubation with gentamicin, LLC-PK$_1$ cells developed myeloid bodies characteristic of gentamicin accumulation (140). However, cell death, indicated by nigrosin permeability, required incubation for at least 7 days with gentamicin, and even then some cells remained viable despite continued exposure to gentamicin (140). Incubation of cells for 4 days with up to 2 mM gentamicin did not alter DNA, RNA, protein, or ATP content in LLC-PK$_1$ cells. In contrast, total phospholipid content increased in LLC-PK$_1$ cells incubated with gentamicin, with increased concentrations of phosphatidylinositol and phosphatidylcholine (140). Gentamicin also altered neutral lipid turnover in LLC-PK$_1$ cells, with increased incorporation of label from [^{3}H]arachidonic acid or [^{14}C]acetate into free fatty acids, monoglyceride, diglyceride, and nonesterified cholesterol, and reduced labeling of triglycerides in cells incubated with gentamicin (140). Whereas gentamicin might require calcium ions to enter proximal tubular cells, gentamicin-induced alterations in phospholipid metabolism were not dependent on calcium concentration in the incubation medium: Raising calcium concentration in the incubation medium from 0.2 through 0.6 mg/ml did not alter the gentamicin-induced stimulation of phosphatidylinositol and phosphatidylcholine in LLC-PK$_1$ cells (140). Thus, in LLC-PK$_1$ cells, gentamicin was accumulated and caused phospholipidosis similar to that observed *in vitro*. However, a correlation between phospholipidosis and lethal cell injury could not be established in these studies.

In primary cultures of rabbit proximal tubular cells, incubation with 10^{-3} M gentamicin for up to 6 days failed to alter cell viability, whereas by day 12 of incubation, cell viability was reduced by about 35% (141). In addition, gentamicin failed to consistently alter protein and DNA content, or protein and DNA synthesis (measured as [^{14}C]leucine or [^{3}H]thymidine incorporation) until day 12 of incubation (141). In contrast, gentamicin produced a marked phospholipidosis in cultured rabbit proximal tubular cells as early as day 2 of incubation (Fig. 8) (141). All phospholipids examined, including phosphatidylcholine, phosphatidylserine, and sphingomyelin, were significantly increased after exposure of cells to gentamicin for 6 days (Fig. 9) (141). These studies indicate that one of the earliest functional changes associated with gentamicin toxicity was phospholipidosis affecting all ma-

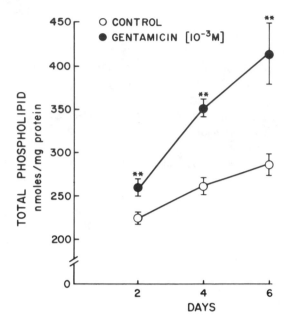

FIG. 8. Effect of 10^{-3} M gentamicin on total phospholipid of cultured rabbit proximal tubular cells as a function of drug exposure. Double asterisks indicate significant difference between control and gentamicin groups, $p < 0.01$. [Reproduced from Ramsammy et al. (141) and the American Physiological Society, with permission.]

jor phospholipids. Gentamicin-induced phospholipidosis was due, at least in part, to reduced degradation of phospholipids, as indicated by slower turnover of prelabeled phospholipids in cultured cells (141). In addition, at least a portion of the phospholipidosis is secondary to more rapid synthesis of selected phospholipids. In particular, incorporation of [³H]myoinositol and [³H]ethanolamine was markedly stimulated by incubating prelabeled cells with gentamicin, whereas incorporation of [³H]choline and [³H]serine was unaltered during gentamicin exposure (141). Cell culture techniques were essential in these studies characterizing degradation and synthesis of phospholipids because cells could be incubated with labeled precursors, allowing uniform labeling of intracellular precursor pools as well as labeling of synthesized phospholipids. These studies demonstrate that phospholipid metabolism is markedly altered during exposure to gentamicin. However, whether these alterations contribute to or are simply coincident with gentamicin cytotoxicity remains to be established.

CONCLUDING REMARKS

Considerable progress has been made over the last 10–20 years in developing and refining *in vitro* techniques for the assessment of nephrotoxicity. As in all areas, considerably more research is needed to expand and extend upon the fundamental information obtained thus far. In particular, more studies examining *in vivo–in vitro* or *in vivo–ex vivo* correlations in nephrotoxicity are needed. Furthermore, the implications of relying upon relatively high concentrations of a toxicant in *in vitro*

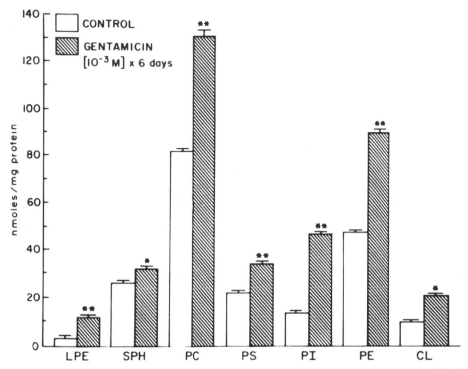

FIG. 9. Effect of 10^{-3} M gentamicin on phospholipid composition of cultured rabbit proximal tubular cells exposed to drug for 6 days. Asterisks indicate significant differences between control and gentamicin groups; $*p<0.05$, $**p<0.01$. LPE, lysophosphatidylethanolamine; SPH, sphingomyelin; PC, phosphatidylcholine; PS, phosphatidylserine; PI, phosphatidylinositol; PE, phosphatidylethanolamine; CL, cardiolipin. [Reproduced from Ramsammy et al. (141) and the American Physiological Society, with permission.]

systems need to be better understood. As previously discussed, some toxicities depend upon a balance between bioactivation and detoxification pathways. For example, when high concentrations of a toxicant are used, one or more pathways involved in either bioactivation or detoxification may become saturated, and the possibility exists that toxicity may be either exacerbated or attenuated in an *in vitro* system under saturation conditions. In addition, we have discussed several examples of concentration-dependent toxicity in which different mechanisms seem to contribute to cytotoxicity at low and high concentrations of toxicant, as with acetaminophen and DCVC. With concentration-dependent toxicities, mechanistic *in vitro* studies that use high concentrations of toxicant may give erroneous or irrelevant information concerning mechanisms of cytotoxicity occurring *in vivo*.

Recently, investigators have recognized the importance of preserving metabolic capabilities (such as cytochromes P450) in cell culture systems, and are devising methods and strategies that make cell culture systems resemble more closely the *in vivo* biochemical systems originally present in the cells. Such efforts will greatly extend the utility of cell culture systems in evaluation of nephrotoxicity, as well as in mechanistic studies.

REFERENCES

1. Newton JF, Hook JB. Isolated perfused rat kidney. In: Jakoby WB, ed. *Methods in enzymology*, vol 77. New York: Academic Press, 1981;94–105.
2. Bekersky I. Use of the isolated perfused kidney as a tool in drug disposition studies. *Drug Metab Rev* 1983;14:931–960.
3. Cox PGF, Moons MM, Slegers JFG, Russel FGM, van Ginneken CAM. Isolated perfused rat kidney as a tool in the investigation of renal handling and effects of nonsteroidal antiinflamatory drugs. *J Pharmacol Methods* 1990;24:89–103.
4. Ross BD, Epstein FH, Leaf A. Sodium reabsorption in the perfused rat kidney. *Am J Physiol* 1973;225:1165–1171.
5. Ross BD. The isolated perfused rat kidney. *Clin Sci Mol Med* 1978;55:513–521.
6. Alcorn D, Emslie KR, Ross BD, Ryan GB, Tange JD. Selective distal nephron damage during isolated kidney perfusion. *Kidney Int* 1981;19:638–647.
7. Schurek HJ, Kriz W. Morphologic and functional evidence for oxygen deficiency in the isolated perfused rat kidney. *Lab Invest* 1985;53:145–155.
8. Brezis M, Rosen S, Silva P, Epstein FH. Selective vulnerability of the medullary thick ascending limb to anoxia in the isolated perfused rat kidney. *J Clin Invest* 1984;73:182–190.
9. Lieberthal W, Stephens GW, Wolf EF, et al. Effect of erythrocytes on the function and morphology of the isolated perfused rat kidney. *Renal Physiol* 1987;10:14–24.
10. Brezis M, Rosen S, Spokes K, Silva P, Epstein FH. Transport-dependent anoxic cell injury in the isolated perfused rat kidney. *Am J Pathol* 1984;116:327–341.
11. Tarloff JB, Goldstein RS, Hook JB. Xenobiotic biotransformation by the kidney: pharmacological and toxicological aspects. *Prog Drug Metab* 1990;12:1–39.
12. Hewitt WR, Goldstein RS, Hook JB. Toxic responses of the kidney. In: Amdur MO, Doull J, Klaassen CD, eds. *Casarett and Doull's toxicology: the basic science of poisons*, 4th ed. New York: Pergamon Press, 1991;354–382.
13. Ross BD, Tange J, Emslie K, Hart S, Smail M, Calder I. Paracetamol metabolism by the isolated perfused rat kidney. *Kidney Int* 1980;18:562–570.
14. Mitchell JR, Jollow DJ, Potter WZ, David DC, Gillette JR, Brodie BB. Acetaminophen-induced hepatic necrosis. I. Role of drug metabolism. *J Pharmacol Exp Ther* 1973;187:185–194.
15. Hinson JA, Pohl LR, Monks TJ, Gillette JR. Acetaminophen-induced hepatotoxicity. *Life Sci* 1981;29:107–116.
16. McMurtry RJ, Snodgrass WR, Mitchell JR. Renal necrosis, glutathione depletion, and covalent binding after acetaminophen. *Toxicol Appl Pharmacol* 1978;46:87–100.
17. Newton JF, Yoshimoto M, Bernstein J, Rush GF, Hook JB. Acetaminophen nephrotoxicity in the rat. I. Strain differences in nephrotoxicity and metabolism. *Toxicol Appl Pharmacol* 1983;69:291–306.
18. Newton JF, Bailie MB, Hook JB. Acetaminophen nephrotoxicity in the rat. Renal metabolic activation *in vitro*. *Toxicol Appl Pharmacol* 1983;70:433–444.
19. Newton JF, Braselton WE, Kuo CH, et al. Metabolism of acetaminophen by the isolated perfused kidney. *J Pharmacol Exp Ther* 1982;221:76–79.
20. Gerson RJ, Casini A, Gilfor D, Serroni A, Farber JL. Oxygen-mediated cell injury in the killing of cultured hepatocytes by acetaminophen. *Biochem Biophys Res Commun* 1985;126:1129–1137.
21. Adamson GM, Harman AW. A role for the glutathione peroxidase/reductase enzyme system in the protection from paracetamol toxicity in isolated mouse hepatocytes. *Biochem Pharmacol* 1989; 38:3323–3330.
22. Madias NE, Harrington JT. Platinum nephrotoxicity. *Am J Med* 1978;65:307–314.
23. Blachley JD, Hill JB. Renal and electrolyte disturbances associated with cisplatin. *Ann Intern Med* 1981;95:628–632.
24. Meijer M, Sleijfer DT, Mulder NH, et al. Some effects of combination chemotherapy with cis-platinum on renal function in patients with nonseminomatous testicular carcinoma. *Cancer* 1983; 51:2035–2040.

25. Miura K, Goldstein RS, Pasino DA, Hook JB. Cisplatin nephrotoxicity: role of filtration and tubular transport of cisplatin in isolated perfused kidneys. *Toxicology* 1987;44:147–158.
26. Berndt WO, Davis ME. Renal methods for toxicology. In: Hayes AW, ed. *Principles and methods of toxicology*, 2nd ed. New York: Raven Press, 1989;629–648.
27. Goldstein RS, Hook JB, Bond JT. Renal tubular transport of saccharin. *J Pharmacol Exp Ther* 1978;204:690–695.
28. Mann WA, Welzel GE, Goldstein RS, et al. Characterization of the renal effects and renal elimination of sulotraban in the dog. *J Pharmacol Exp Ther* 1991;259:1231–1240.
29. Cacini W, Keller MB, Grund VR. Accumulation of cimetidine by kidney cortex slices. *J Pharmacol Exp Ther* 1982;221:342–346.
30. Cross RJ, Taggart VJ. Renal tubular transport: accumulation of *p*-aminohippurate by rabbit kidney slices. *Am J Physiol* 1950;161:181–190.
31. Goldstein RS, Pasino DA, Hewitt WR, Hook JB. Biochemical mechanisms of cephaloridine nephrotoxicity: time and concentration dependence of peroxidative injury. *Toxicol Appl Pharmacol* 1986;83:261–270.
32. Smith JH. The use of renal cortical slices from the Fischer 344 rat as an *in vitro* model to evaluate nephrotoxicity. *Fundam Appl Toxicol* 1988;11:132–142.
33. Smith JH, Hewitt WR, Hook JB. Role of intrarenal biotransformation in chloroform-induced nephrotoxicity in rats. *Toxicol Appl Pharmacol* 1985;79:166–174.
34. Ruegg CE, Gandolfi AJ, Nagle RB, Krumdieck CL, Brendel KP. Preparation of positional renal slices for study of cell-specific toxicity. *J Pharmacol Methods* 1987;17:111–123.
35. Kluwe WM. Renal function tests as indicators of kidney injury in subacute toxicity studies. *Toxicol Appl Pharmacol* 1981;57:414–424.
36. Kyle GM, Luthra R, Bruckner JV, MacKenzie WF, Acosta D. Assessment of functional, morphological, and enzymatic tests for acute nephrotoxicity induced by mercuric chloride. *J Toxicol Environ Health* 1983;12:99–117.
37. Miyajima H, Hewitt WR, Cote MG, Plaa GL. Relationships between histological and functional indices of acute chemically induced nephrotoxicity. *Fundam Appl Toxicol* 1983;3:543–551.
38. Tarloff JB, Goldstein RS, Silver AC, Hewitt WR, Hook JB. Intrinsic susceptibility of the kidney to acetaminophen toxicity in middle-aged rats. *Toxicol Lett* 1990;52:101–110.
39. Atkinson RM, Currie JP, Davis B, Pratt DAH, Sharpe HM, Tonich EG. Acute toxicity of cephaloridine, an antibiotic derived from cephalosporin C. *Toxicol Appl Pharmacol* 1966;8:398–406.
40. Wold JS. Antibiotic nephropathies. In: Hook JB, ed. *Toxicology of the kidney*. New York: Raven Press, 1981;251–266.
41. Kuo CH, Hook JB. Depletion of renal glutathione content and nephrotoxicity of cephaloridine in rabbits, rats and mice. *Toxicol Appl Pharmacol* 1982;63:292–302.
42. Tune BM. Relationship between the transport and toxicity of cephalosporins in the kidney. *J Infect Dis* 1975;122:33–44.
43. Tune BM. Effect of organic acid transport inhibitors on renal cortical uptake and proximal tubular toxicity of cephaloridine. *J Pharmacol Exp Ther* 1972;181:250–256.
44. Wold JS, Turnipseed SA. The effect of renal cation transport inhibitors on the *in vivo* and *in vitro* accumulation and efflux of cephaloridine. *Life Sci* 1980;27:2559–2564.
45. Kuo CH, Maita K, Sleight SD, Hook JB. Lipid peroxidation: a possible mechanism of cephaloridine-induced nephrotoxicity. *Toxicol Appl Pharmacol* 1983;67:78–88.
46. Cojocel C, Laeschke KH, Inselmann G, Baumann K. Inhibition of cephaloridine-induced lipid peroxidation. *Toxicology* 1985;35:295–305.
47. Goldstein RS, Contardi LR, Pasino DA, Hook JB. Mechanisms mediating cephaloridine inhibition of renal gluconeogenesis. *Toxicol Appl Pharmacol* 1987;87:297–305.
48. Ruegg CE, Gandolfi AJ, Brendel K. Differential patterns of injury to the proximal tubule of renal cortical slices following in vitro exposure to mercuric chloride, potassium dichromate or hypoxic conditions. *Toxicol Appl Pharmacol* 1987;90:261–273.
49. Phelps JS, Gandolfi AJ, Brendel K, Dorr RT. Cisplatin nephrotoxicity: *in vitro* studies with precision-cut rabbit renal cortical slices. *Toxicol Appl Pharmacol* 1987;90:501–512.
50. Wolfgang GHI, Gandolfi AJ, Brendel K. Evaluation of organic nephrotoxins in rabbit renal cortical slices. *Toxicol In Vitro* 1989;31:341–350.
51. Wolfgang GHI, Gandolfi AJ, Nagle RB, Brendel K, Stevens JL. Assessment of *S*-(1,2-dichlorovinyl)-L-cysteine induced toxic events in rabbit renal cortical slices. Biochemical and histological evaluation of uptake, covalent binding and toxicity. *Chem Biol Interact* 1990;75:153–170.

52. Ruegg CE, Mandel LJ. Bulk isolation of renal PCT and PST. II. Differential responses to anoxia and hypoxia. *Am J Physiol* 1990;259:F176–F185.
53. Porter KE, Dawson AG. Inhibition of respiration and gluconeogenesis by paracetamol in rat kidney preparations. *Biochem Pharmacol* 1979;28:3057–3062.
54. Cojocel C, Maita K, Pasino DA, Kuo C-H, Hook JB. Metabolic heterogeneity of the proximal and distal kidney tubules. *Life Sci* 1983;33:855–861.
55. Bastin J, Cambon N, Thompson M, Lowry OH, Burch HB. Change in energy reserves in different segments of the nephron during brief ischemia. *Kidney Int* 1987;31:1239–1247.
56. Uchida S, Endou H. Substrate specificity to maintain cellular ATP along the mouse nephron. *Am J Physiol* 1988;255:F977–F983.
57. Aleo MD, Rankin GO, Cross TJ, Schnellmann RG. Toxicity of N-(3,5-dichlorophenyl)succinimide and metabolites to rat renal proximal tubules and mitochondria. *Chem Biol Interact* 1991; 78:109–121.
58. Aleo MD, Wyatt RD, Schnellmann RG. The role of altered mitochondrial function in citrinin-induced toxicity to rat renal proximal tubule suspensions. *Toxicol Appl Pharmacol* 1991;109:455–463.
59. Schnellmann RG, Mandel LJ. Cellular toxicity of bromobenzene and bromobenzene metabolites to rabbit proximal tubules: the role and mechanism of 2-bromohydroquinone. *J Pharmacol Exp Ther* 1986;237:456–461.
60. Schnellmann RG, Mandel LJ. Multiple effects of presumed glutathione depletors on rabbit renal proximal tubules. *Kidney Int* 1986;29:858–862.
61. Sina JF, Noble C, Bean CL, Bradley MO. Renal tubules *in vitro* as a model for nephrotoxicity. In: McQueen C, ed. *In vitro toxicology: model systems and methods*. Caldwell, NJ: Telford Press, 1989;263–290.
62. Rush GF, Ponsler GD. Cephaloridine-induced biochemical changes and cytotoxicity in suspensions of rabbit isolated proximal tubules. *Toxicol Appl Pharmacol* 1991;109:314–326.
63. Balaban RS, Soltoff S, Storey JM, Mandel LJ. Improved renal cortical tubule suspension: spectrophotometric study of O_2 delivery. *Am J Physiol* 1980;238:F50–59.
64. Vinay P, Gougoux A, Lemieux G. Isolation of a pure suspension of rat proximal tubules. *Am J Physiol* 1981;241:F403–411.
65. Sina JF, Bean CL, Noble C, Bradley MO. Isolation and characterization of proximal tubule suspensions from rabbits for *in vitro* studies. *In Vitro Toxicol* 1986;1:5–12.
66. Sina JF, Bean CL, Bland JA, et al. An *in vitro* assay for cytotoxicity to proximal tubule suspensions from rabbit kidney. *In Vitro Toxicol* 1986;1:13–22.
67. Gesek FA, Wolff DW, Strandhoy JW. Improved separation method for rat proximal and distal renal tubules. *Am J Physiol* 1987;253:F358–F365.
68. Beach RE, Watts BA, Good DW, Benedict CR, DuBose TD. Effects of graded oxygen tension on adenosine release by renal medullary and thick ascending limb suspensions. *Kidney Int* 1991; 39:836–842.
69. Gaudio KM, Thulin G, Ardito T, Kashgarian M, Siegel NJ. Metabolic alterations in proximal tubule suspensions obtained from ischemic kidneys. *Am J Physiol* 1989;257:F383–F389.
70. Venkatachalam MA, Bernard DB, Donohoe JF, Levinsky NG. Ischemic damage and repair in the rat proximal tubule: differences among the S_1, S_2, and S_3 segments. *Kidney Int* 1978;14:31–49.
71. Shanley PF, Rosen MD, Brezis M, Silva P, Epstein FH, Rosen S. Topography of focal proximal tubular necrosis after ischemia with reflow in the rat kidney. *Am J Pathol* 1986;122:462–468.
72. Lau SS, Monks TJ. The contribution of bromobenzene to our current understanding of chemically-induced toxicities. *Life Sci* 1988;42:1259–1269.
73. Monks TJ, Highet RJ, Lau SS. 2-Bromo-(diglutathion-S-yl)hydroquinone nephrotoxicity: physical, biochemical, and electrochemical determinants. *Mol Pharmacol* 1988;34:492–500.
74. Lau SS, Monks TJ, Gillette JR. Identification of 2-bromohydroquinone as a metabolite of bromobenzene and o-bromophenol: implications for bromobenzene-induced nephrotoxicity. *J Pharmacol Exp Ther* 1984;230:360–366.
75. Lau SS, Monks TJ, Greene KE, Gillette JR. The role of *ortho*-bromophenol in the nephrotoxicity of bromobenzene in rats. *Toxicol Appl Pharmacol* 1984;72:539–549.
76. Reid WD. Mechanism of renal necrosis induced by bromobenzene or chlorobenzene. *Exp Mol Pathol* 1973;19:197–214.
77. Schnellmann RG, Monks TJ, Mandel LJ, Lau SS. 2-Bromohydroquinone-induced toxicity to rabbit renal proximal tubules: the role of biotransformation, glutathione, and covalent binding. *Toxicol Appl Pharmacol* 1989;99:19–27.

78. Monks TJ, Lau SS, Highet RL, Gillette JR. Glutathione conjugates of 2-bromohydroquinone are nephrotoxic. *Drug Metab Dispos* 1985;13:553–559.
79. Schnellmann RG, Ewell FPQ, Sgambati M, Mandel LJ. Mitochondrial toxicity of 2-bromohydroquinone in rabbit renal proximal tubules. *Toxicol Appl Pharmacol* 1987;90:420–426.
80. Schnellmann RG. 2-Bromohydroquinone-induced toxicity to rabbit renal proximal tubules: evidence against oxidative stress. *Toxicol Appl Pharmacol* 1989;99:11–18.
81. Kinne R. New approaches to study renal metabolism: isolated single cells. *Miner Electrolyte Metab* 1983;9:270–275.
82. Ormstad K, Orrenius S, Jones DP. Preparation and characteristics of isolated kidney cells. In: Jakoby WB, ed. *Methods in enzymology*, vol 77. New York: Academic Press, 1981:137–146.
83. Boogaard PJ, Nagelkerke JF, Mulder GJ. Renal proximal tubular cells in suspension or in primary culture as *in vitro* models to study nephrotoxicity. *Chem Biol Interact* 1990;76:251–292.
84. Eveloff J, Haase W, Kinne R. Separation of renal medullary cells: isolation of cells from the thick ascending limb of Henle's loop. *J Cell Biol* 1980;87:672–681.
85. Lash LH, Tokarz JJ. Isolation of two distinct populations of cells from rat kidney cortex and their use in the study of chemical-induced toxicity. *Anal Biochem* 1989;182:271–279.
86. Boogaard PJ, Mulder GJ, Nagelkerke JF. Isolated proximal tubular cells from rat kidney as an *in vitro* model for studies on nephrotoxicity. I. An improved method for preparation of proximal tubular cells and their functional characterization by α-methylglucose uptake. *Toxicol Appl Pharmacol* 1989;101:135–143.
87. Lash LH, Tokarz JJ. Oxidative stress in isolated rat renal proximal and distal tubular cells. *Am J Physiol* 1990;259:F338–F347.
88. Lash LH, Woods EB. Cytotoxicity of alkylating agents in isolated rat kidney proximal tubular and distal tubular cells. *Arch Biochem Biophys* 1991;286:46–56.
89. Tune BM, Fravert D. Mechanisms of cephalosporin nephrotoxicity: a comparison of cephaloridine and cephaloglycin. *Kidney Int* 1980;18:591–600.
90. Reed DJ. Regulation of reductive processes by glutathione. *Biochem Pharmacol* 1986;35:7–13.
91. Lash LH, Anders MW, Jones DP. Glutathione homeostasis and glutathione-*S*-conjugate toxicity in the kidney. *Rev Biochem Toxicol* 1988;9:29–67.
92. Streeter AJ, Nims RW, Sheffels PR, et al. Metabolic denitrosation of *N*-nitrosodimethylamine *in vivo* in the rat. *Cancer Res* 1990;50:1144–1150.
93. Terracini B, Parker VH. A pathological study on the toxicity of *S*-dichlorovinyl-L-cysteine. *Food Cosmet Toxicol* 1965;3:67–74.
94. Gandolfi AJ, Nagle RB, Soltis JJ, Plescia FH. Nephrotoxicity of halogenated vinyl cysteine compounds. *Res Commun Chem Pathol Pharmacol* 1981;33:249–261.
95. Elfarra AA, Anders MW. Renal processing of glutathione conjugates. Role in nephrotoxicity. *Biochem Pharmacol* 1984;33:3729–3732.
96. Elfarra AA, Lash LH, Anders MW. Metabolic activation and detoxication of nephrotoxic cysteine and homocysteine-*S*-conjugates. *Proc Natl Acad Sci USA* 1986;83:2667–2671.
97. Jones DP, Moldeus P, Stead AH, Ormstad K, Jornvall H, Orrenius S. Metabolism of glutathione and a glutathione conjugate by isolated kidney cells. *J Biol Chem* 1979;254:2787–2792.
98. Hassall CD, Gandolfi AJ, Duhamel RC, Brendel K. The formation and biotransformation of cysteine conjugates of halogenated ethylenes by rabbit renal tubules. *Chem Biol Interact* 1984;49:283–297.
99. Elfarra AA, Jakobson I, Anders MW. Mechanism of *S*-(1,2-dichlorovinyl)glutathione-induced nephrotoxicity. *Biochem Pharmacol* 1986;35:283–288.
100. Parker VH. A biochemical study of the toxicity of *S*-dichlorovinyl-L-cysteine. *Food Cosmet Toxicol* 1965;3:75–87.
101. Stonard MD, Parker VH. The metabolism of *S*-(1,2-dichlorovinyl)-L-cysteine by rat liver mitochondria. *Biochem Pharmacol* 1971;20:2429–2437.
102. Lash LH, Anders MW. Cytotoxicity of *S*-(1,2-dichlorovinyl)glutathione and *S*-(1,2-dichlorovinyl)-L-cysteine in isolated rat kidney cells. *J Biol Chem* 1986;261:13076–13081.
103. Mandel LJ, Murphy E. Regulation of cytosolic free calcium in rabbit proximal renal tubules. *J Biol Chem* 1984;259:11188–11196.
104. Murphy E, Mandel LJ. Cytosolic free calcium levels in rabbit proximal kidney tubules. *Am J Physiol* 1982;242:C124–C128.
105. Gaush CR, Hard WL, Smith TF. Characterization of an established line of canine kidney cells (MDCK). *Proc Soc Exp Biol Med* 1966;122:931–935.

106. Cereijido M, Robbins ES, Dolan WJ, Rotunno CA, Sabatini DD. Polarized monolayers formed by epithelial cells on a permeable and translucent support. *J Cell Biol* 1978;77:853–880.
107. Rindler MJ, Chuman LM, Shaffer L, Saier MH. Retention of differentiated properties in an established dog kidney epithelial cell line (MDCK). *J Cell Biol* 1979;81:635–648.
108. Hull RN, Cherry WR, Weaver GW. The origin and characteristics of a pig kidney cell strain, LLC-PK$_1$. *In Vitro* 1976;12:670–677.
109. Handler JS, Perkins FM, Johnson JP. Studies of renal cell function using cell culture techniques. *Am J Physiol* 1980;238:F1–F9.
110. Malstrom K, Stange G, Murer H. Identification of proximal tubular transport functions in the established kidney cell line, OK. *Biochem Biophys Acta* 1987;902:269–277.
111. Van den Bosh L, DeSmedt H, Borghgraef R. Characteristics of Na$^+$-dependent hexose transport in OK, an established renal epithelial cell line. *Biochem Biophys Acta* 1989;979:91–98.
112. Boogaard PJ, Zoeteweij JP, van Berkel TJC, van't Noordende JM, Mulder GJ, Nagelkerke JF. Primary culture of proximal tubular cells from normal rat kidney as an *in vitro* model to study mechanisms of nephrotoxicity. Toxicity of nephrotoxicants at low concentrations during prolonged exposure. *Biochem Pharmacol* 1990;39:1335–1345.
113. Leffert H, Paul D. Serum dependent growth of primary cultured differentiated fetal rat hepatocytes in arginine-deficient medium. *J Cell Physiol* 1973;81:113–124.
114. Gilbert SF, Migeon BR. D-Valine as a selective agent for normal human and rodent epithelial cells in culture. *Cell* 1975;5:11–17.
115. Elliget KA, Trump BF. Primary cultures of normal rat kidney proximal tubule epithelial cells for studies of renal cell injury. *In Vitro Cell Dev Biol* 1991;27A:739–748.
116. Ford SM, Williams PD, Grassl S, Holohan PD. Transepithelial acidification by cultures of rabbit proximal tubules grown on filters. *Am J Physiol* 1990;259:C103–C109.
117. Rabito CA. Occluding junctions in a renal cell line (LLC-PK$_1$) with characteristics of proximal tubular cells. *Am J Physiol* 1986;250:F734–F743.
118. Chabardes D, Imbert-Teboul M, Montegut M, Clique A, Morel F. Distribution of calcitonin-sensitive adenylate cyclase activity along the rabbit kidney tubule. *Proc Natl Acad Sci USA* 1976;73:3608–3612.
119. Morel F, Chabardes D, Imbert-Teboul M. Vasopressin action sites along the nephron. *J Physiol Paris* 1981;77:615–620.
120. Helman SI, Grantham JJ, Burg MB. Effect of vasopressin on electrical resistance of renal cortical collecting tubules. *Am J Physiol* 1971;220:1825–1832.
121. Ausiello DA, Hall DH, Dayer J-M. Modulation of cyclic AMP-dependent protein kinase by vasopressin and calcitonin in cultured porcine renal LLC-PK$_1$ cells. *Biochem J* 1980;186:773–780.
122. Gstraunthaler G, Handler JS. Isolation, growth, and characterization of a gluconeogenic strain of renal cells. *Am J Physiol* 1987;252:C232–C238.
123. Koechlin N, Pisam M, Poujeol P, Tauc M, Rambourg A. Conversion of a rabbit proximal convoluted tubule (PCT) into a cell monolayer: ultrastructural study of cell dedifferentiation and re-differentiation. *Eur J Cell Biol* 1991;54:224–236.
124. Bridges JW, Wiebkin P, Fry JR. Rate-limiting factors in xenobiotic metabolism by cytochrome P-450, sulphotransferase, and glucuronyl transferase. In: Coon MJ, Conney AH, Estabrook RW, Gelboin HV, Gillette JR, O'Brien PJ, eds. *Microsomes, drug oxidations, and chemical carcinogenesis*, vol 2. New York: Academic Press, 1980;619–627.
125. Holme JA, Soderlund E, Dybing E. Drug metabolism activities of isolated rat hepatocytes in monolayer culture. *Acta Pharmacol Toxicol* 1983;52:348–356.
126. Niemann C, Gauthier JC, Richert L, Ivanov MA, Melcion C, Cordier A. Rat adult hepatocytes in primary pure and mixed monolayer culture. Comparison of the maintenance of mixed function oxidase and conjugation pathways of drug metabolism. *Biochem Pharmacol* 1991;42:373–379.
127. Bruggeman IM, Mertens JJWM, Temmink JHM, Lans MC, Vos RME, van Bladeren PJ. Use of monolayers of primary rat kidney cortex cells for nephrotoxicity studies. *Toxicol In Vitro* 1989; 3:261–269.
128. Williams PD, Laska DA, Tay LK, Hottendorf GH. Comparative toxicities of cephalosporin antibiotics in a rabbit kidney cell line (LLC-RK$_1$). *Antimicrob Agents Chemother* 1988;32:314–318.
129. Schuetz EG, Li D, Omiecinski CJ, et al. Regulation of gene expression in adult rat hepatocytes cultured on a basement membrane matrix. *J Cell Physiol* 1988;134:309–323.
130. Vamvakas S, Sharma VK, Sheu SS, Anders MW. Pertubations of intracellular calcium distribution in kidney cells by nephrotoxic haloalkenyl cysteine S-conjugates. *Mol Pharmacol* 1990;38:455–461.

131. Chen Q, Jones TW, Brown PC, Stevens JL. The mechanism of cysteine conjugate cytotoxicity in renal epithelial cells. Covalent binding leads to thiol depletion and lipid peroxidation. *J Biol Chem* 1990;265:21603–21611.
132. Farber JL, Leonard TB, Kyle ME, Nakae D, Serroni A, Rogers SA. Peroxidation-dependent and peroxidation-independent mechanisms by which acetaminophen kills cultured hepatocytes. *Arch Biochem Biophys* 1988;267:640–650.
133. Albano E, Carini R, Parola M, et al. Effects of carbon tetrachloride on calcium homeostasis. A critical reconsideration. *Biochem Pharmacol* 1989;38:2719–2725.
134. Kaloyanides GJ, Pastoriza-Munoz E. Aminoglycoside nephrotoxicity. *Kidney Int* 1980;18:571–582.
135. Humes HD. Aminoglycoside nephrotoxicity. *Kidney Int* 1988;33:900–911.
136. Houghton DC, Plamp CE, DeFehr JM, Bennett WM, Porter G, Gilbert D. Gentamicin and tobramycin nephrotoxicity. *Am J Pathol* 1978;93:137–152.
137. Cohen L, Lapkin R, Kaloyanides GJ. Effect of gentamicin on renal function in the rat. *J Pharmacol Exp Ther* 1975;193:264–273.
138. Gilbert DN, Houghton DC, Bennett WM, Plamp CE, Reger K, Porter G. Reversibility of gentamicin nephrotoxicity in rats: recovery during continuous drug administration. *Proc Soc Exp Biol Med* 1979;160:99–103.
139. Saito H, Inui KI, Hori R. Mechanisms of gentamicin transport in kidney epithelial cell line (LLC-PK$_1$). *J Pharmacol Exp Ther* 1986;238:1071–1076.
140. Schwertz DW, Kreisberg JI, Venkatachalam MA. Gentamicin-induced alterations in pig kidney epithelial (LLC-PK$_1$) cells in culture. *J Pharmacol Exp Ther* 1986;236:254–262.
141. Ramsammy LS, Josepovitz C, Lane B, Kaloyanides GJ. Effect of gentamicin on phospholipid metabolism in cultured rabbit proximal tubular cells. *Am J Physiol* 1989;256:C204–C213.

In Vitro Toxicolog
edited by Shayne C
Raven Press, Ltd.,

10

Primary Hepatocyte Culture as an *In Vitro* Toxicological System of the Liver

A. P. Li

Surgical Research Institute, St. Louis University Medical School, St. Louis, Missouri 63110

As the body's second largest organ (next to the skin), the liver is no doubt one of the key organs in toxicology. A large variety of chemicals, including pharmaceuticals and environmental agents, are known to induce liver toxicity in the human population. Examples of liver toxicants include: (a) the widely used over-the-counter analgesic acetaminophen, which, when taken in large quantities, is responsible for a significant number of suicidal or accidental hepatotoxic events, sometimes resulting in death; (b) the key ingredient of alcoholic beverages, ethanol, prolonged exposure to which is known to lead to liver cirrhosis in both laboratory animals and man; and (c) the naturally occurring mushroom hepatotoxins, the thermal stable cyclic octapeptides α-, β-, and γ-amanitins, which are believed to be responsible for most of the clinically observed hepatotoxicity after ingestion of the poisonous mushroom *Amanita phalloides*.

Besides being one of the organs sensitive to toxic agents, the liver plays an important role in metabolic transformation, leading to detoxification or activation (metabolism of the relatively inert parent compound to highly reactive metabolites) of blood-borne xenobiotics. This metabolic transformation, commonly called *xenobiotic metabolism*, is performed by the parenchymal cells in the liver. The parenchymal cells, also commonly referred to as *hepatocytes*, which constitute over 80% of the liver by weight, have a high level of the inducible P450 mixed function oxygenases (MFOs). The MFOs are membrane-bound enzymes, mainly located on the endoplasmic reticulum, especially the smooth endoplasmic reticulum. The MFOs are responsible for the Phase I reactions such as oxidations, reductions, and hydrolyses, and are found to be isozymes which can be distinguished based on antigenicity and substrate specificity. Different animal species are known to have different isozyme patterns. This difference in MFO activity is believed to play a significant role in the species differences in toxicity of some toxicants. Oxidation of xenobiotics by the MFO is followed by phase II metabolism, in which the metabolites are made more polar by conjugation to highly polar small molecules such as glutathione, sulfate, and glucuronic acid. Phase II conjugation enzymes, including glutathione-S-transferases, sulfatases, and UDP-glucuronosyltransferases, are abundant in the liver, found both in the cytosol and on the endoplasmic reticulum. The conjugated metabolites are usually excreted directly from the liver as bile, or from the kidney as components of the urine. The importance of metabolism in chemical toxicity in the human population can be illustrated by the finding that alcoholics are more sensitive to chemical toxicity. Normal doses of acetaminophen, for instance, can induce hepatotoxicity—and, in some cases, liver failure—in the alcoholic population. One explanation for this observation is that alcohol consumption leads to the induction of P450 MFO activities, thereby increasing the rate of formation of the toxic metabolites from acetaminophen.

Because of the metabolic and toxicological importance of the liver, *in vitro* experimental systems have been developed. These include the use of subcellular fractions, isolated hepatocytes, liver slices, and isolated perfused livers. Of these systems, the most versatile and well-characterized is the cultured parenchymal cells or hepatocytes. In this chapter, the culturing of hepatocytes and their applications in toxicological studies are reviewed.

ISOLATION OF PRIMARY HEPATOCYTES

The liver contains multiple cell types. Based on stereological analysis, the parenchymal cells, commonly referred to as *hepatocytes*, are found to constitute 92.5% of the total volume of liver cells. The remainder of the cells are sinusoidal and perisinusoidal cells, including the fenestrated endothelial cells, the stationary macrophage Kupffer cells, and the vitamin-A-storing stellate cells or lipocytes (3).

Dispersion of liver cells is commonly performed using a two-step perfusion procedure, firstly perfusing the liver with a calcium removal agent, and followed by perfusing with a solution containing a digestive enzyme such as collagenase to achieve cell dissociation. In small experimental animals, the procedure can be performed *in situ* (2a,58,59). After achieving anesthesia, the animal's abdomen is cut open and the portal vein is cannulated with a cannula connected to a perfusion solution. The inferior vena cava is severed and perfusion is initiated. The initial perfusion solution usually consists of an isotonic calcium-free buffer, sometimes containing a chelating agent such as EGTA, serving to clear the blood in the liver as well as to prevent blood coagulation. The removal of calcium ions by EGTA has been reported to enhance the viability of the isolated hepatocytes. The perfusion solution is then changed to that containing collagenase, which serves to dissociate the liver cells. Upon completion of collagenase digestion, the liver is removed, placed in an isotonic buffer solution, and gently agitated to release the dissociated cells.

While the *in situ* procedure is appropriate for small animals such as rats and mice, the "biopsy" procedure is used for larger animals with which a dissected portion of the liver rather than the whole organ is perfused. The biopsy procedure, first described by Reese and Byard (54), involved the perfusion of the dissected lobe via one of the major blood vessels exposed at the cut surface (Fig. 1). This procedure is

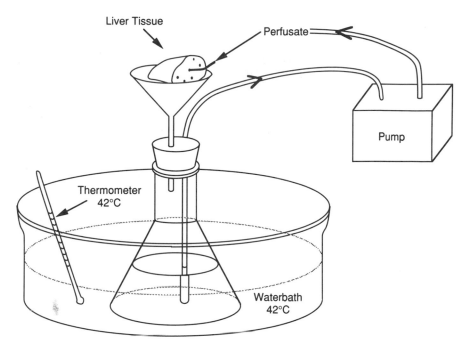

FIG. 1. Schematic drawing of the perfusion system for the isolation of hepatocytes. This is the procedure commonly referred to as "biopsy perfusion," developed by Reese and Byard (54). The procedure has been used successfully in our laboratory for the isolation of hepatocytes from multiple animal species, including human.

useful with livers from small animals as well as with liver portions from large animals, including human. The advantage of the "biopsy" procedure is that surgical specimens, which sometimes are the only specimens available from humans, can be used for hepatocyte isolation. Furthermore, while flow rate is extremely critical to hepatocyte viability for the *in situ* procedure, it is less critical for the biopsy procedure. This is probably due the numerous channels at the cut surface for the exudation of perfusate in the biopsy samples, resulting in a lower pressure buildup. In our laboratory, we recently modified the procedures of Reese and Byard (54) for the isolation of human hepatocytes from surgical specimen (42). Using our procedure, we have an extremely high success rate in the isolation of highly viable (over 80% viability) human hepatocytes (Table 1). The parameters we found critical to a successful isolation include the perfusion of a limited size (up to 50 g), the use of specimen with only one cut surface and intact capsule on the uncut surfaces, perfusion via one or sometimes two blood vessels rather than all visible vessels (to allow circulation), and the use of an appropriate concentration of collagenase. As will be discussed later, the ability to culture hepatocytes from multiple animal species, including human, allows one to perform experiments on species comparison of xenobiotic metabolism and toxicity.

TABLE 1. *Isolation of hepatocytes from human liver portions: results of 19 consecutive isolations*

Donor		Weight of liver portion (g)	Hepatocytes	
Sex	Age		Yield ($\times$ 10^6)	Viability(%)[a]
M	73	8.3	13.0	92.0
M	66	17.7	52.0	85.0
F	40	19.6	212.3	94.7
F	37	17.6	68.5	86.0
M	76	32.8	114.0	92.0
F	27	9.4	52.0	91.2
F	27	12.3	96.0	90.5
F	69	19.4	129.0	90.2
M	79	11.8	136.0	93.4
M	73	9.0	34.5	90.2
M	53	3.2	11.3	82.0
F	66	10.7	28.5	95.0
M	[b]	4.9	41.3	92.7
M	49	8.2	51.5	91.5
F	34	7.2	10.8	63.2
M	57	11.3	53.0	77.7
M	[b]	46.7	671.3	84.0
F	43	38.3	1010.3	83.0
M	58	19.2	195.0	91.0

[a]Determined by trypan blue exclusion.
[b]Not available.

After cell dissociation, the most common procedure is to partially purify the parenchymal cells by several low-speed (50g) centrifugation steps. The parenchymal cells will pellet while the nonparenchymal cells will stay in the supernatant. Further purification of each cell population can be performed via density centrifugation. Using Percoll, Smedsrod et al. (61a) developed a procedure for the purification of parenchymal cells and nonparenchymal cells. The Kupffer and endothelial cell populations can be further separated from each other via differential attachment: The Kupffer cells, like most macrophages, attach quickly onto a plastic substratum and are thereby separated from the less adherent endothelial cells.

For most toxicological studies, the parenchymal cells are used. Although the endothelial and Kupffer cells are known to play critical roles in liver toxicity, including parenchymal cell toxicity and regeneration, they have been generally ignored by toxicologists in their studies. In terms of xenobiotic metabolism, the nonparenchymal cells probably play a rather minor role when compared to the parenchymal cells. In our laboratory, we found that xenobiotic metabolism measured based on the activation of promutagens dimethyl nitrosamine and 3-methyl cholanthrene, and the measurement of 7-deoxycoumarin-O-deethylase activity, was near undetectable in the nonparenchymal cells isolated from rat livers (64). Our study therefore confirms that parenchymal cells, rather than the nonparenchymal cells, are the cells primarily responsible for xenobiotic metabolism in the liver.

CULTURING OF ISOLATED HEPATOCYTES

Freshly isolated hepatocytes are routinely cultured as monolayer cells on collagen-coated plastic, although extremely short-term experiments (hours) can be performed with hepatocytes in suspension. In suspension, the freshly isolated hepatocytes rapidly lose viability, with nearly 100% cell death after a 24-hr period. As monolayer culture on plastic or collagen-coated plastic surfaces, the hepatocytes assume an epithelial cell morphology (Fig. 2). The cells are polygonal, with distinct nuclei and cytoplasmic inclusions. Binucleated cells are often seen, reflecting the occurrence of both mononucleated and binucleated cells in the liver *in vivo*. The cells retain viability, but gradually (over a period of several days) they will lose their liver functions, including albumin synthesis and P450 MFO activities. The phase II conjugating enzymes, however, do not appear to decrease with culturing time, at least for the initial several days during which the phase I enzymes show a dramatic decrease (12).

Recently, hepatocytes have been found to retain more of their functional characteristics when cultured on a murine tumor cell [Engelbreth–Holm–Swarm sarcoma (EHS)]-derived reconstituted basement membrane matrix called *Matrigel*, as compared to culturing on collagen (56,60). Matrigel is a mixture of components extracted from the EHS tumor that spontaneously form a stable gel at 37°C. The components of matrigel are similar to that found in basement membrane, including laminin (60%), type IV collagen (30%), heparin sulfate proteoglycan (3%), nidogen (5%) and entactin (1%) (33). On Matrigel, the hepatocytes assume a rounded cell morphology (Fig. 2). Hepatocytes cultured on matrigel were found to secrete higher levels of liver-specific proteins, including albumin, transferrin, haptoglobin, and hemopexin. The interaction of the basement membrane matrix components with membrane receptors, as well as the rounded cell shape, may be involved in the prolonged maintenance of differentiated functions.

Another approach to maintaining the differentiated properties is to co-culture the hepatocytes with another cell type. Hepatocytes co-cultured with rat liver epithelial cells are found to express high levels of liver functions, including acute-phase protein synthesis and both phase I and phase II drug metabolism (1a,24), even after weeks of culturing. After co-culturing with a variety of transformed epithelial-like cell lines, Donato et al. (12) reported that in general the hepatocytes retained a higher level of xenobiotic metabolism activities than did pure cultures after several days in culture.

Recently, methods for the culturing of hepatocytes as cell aggregates (multicellular spheroids) have been developed (e.g., see refs. 40 and 66). Such a culturing system allows hepatocytes to retain the cuboidal cell shape and three-dimensional cell–cell contact, similar to the liver *in vivo*. Hepatocytes cultured as spheroids may maintain differentiated functions better than monolayer cultures. Detailed characterization of hepatocytes cultured as spheroids and their applications in toxicology studies have yet to be reported. Another development is the culturing of hepatocytes as entrapped aggregates in a packed bed bioreactor (42a). The hepatocytes in the

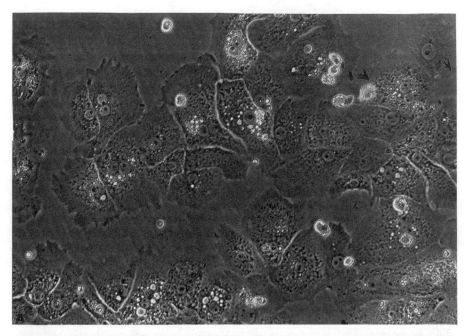

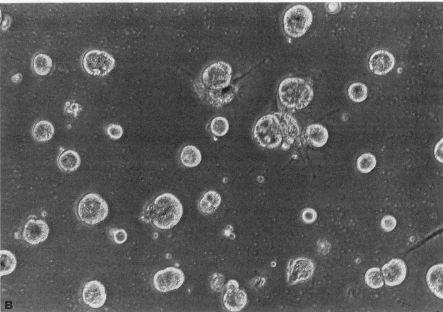

FIG. 2. Morphology of human hepatocytes cultured on collagen-coated plastic **(A)** and Matrigel **(B)**. The cells shown were cultured for 24 hr. The cells on collagen have an epithelial morphology, whereas on Matrigel they have a rounded cell shape. This difference in cell shape on the two attachment substrata may be one of the factors contributing to the differences in cell properties.

bioreactor resemble those of the liver *in vivo*, with the cuboidal cell shape, three-dimensional cell-cell contact, and nutrient perfusion. The hepatocyte bioreactor has the potential to be a more realistic model of the liver *in vivo* in drug metabolism and toxicology.

In spite of the above-mentioned advances in maintaining differentiation of hepatocytes in culture, in toxicology, hepatocytes and still mainly used as short-term suspension cultures and monolayer cultures on collagen-coated surfaces.

XENOBIOTIC METABOLISM

Phase I Oxidation: P450 Isozymes

A major problem with prolonged hepatocyte cultures is the decline of cytochrome P450 mixed function oxygenase (MFO) activities with time in culture (Fig. 3). Moreover, different P450 isozymes appear to decline at different rates (25), and, amidst the decline of most of the isozymes, induction of a few specific isozyme has been observed (15). Attempts to maintain P450 content as well as MFO isozymes include the supplementation of medium with multiple agents such as thyroid and pituitary hormones, sex steroids, glucocorticoid hormones, and DMSO (10,16,19, 50,52), the culturing of hepatocytes on reconstituted basement membrane (57), and co-culturing hepatocytes with other cell types (1a,12,23a). However, none of these approaches has been shown to maintain the multiple P450 isozymes. For instance, while co-culturing of hepatocytes with liver epithelial cells is believed to be the most effective, differential decline of P450 isozymes is still observed (51a). Short-term cultures of freshly isolated hepatocytes therefore remain preferable over prolonged cultures for metabolism studies.

While the P450 isozymes decline in culture, some are found to be inducible by the addition of specific inducers in the culture medium, usually after a 2- to 3-day incubation period. The inducibility of some of the isozymes appears to be a function of the culturing conditions. For instance, cytochrome P450IIE and IIB1/2 could only be induced when hepatocytes were cultured on reconstituted basement membrane. Phenobarbital, a known P450 inducer, was found to induce cytochrome P450IIB1/2 and P450IIIA1 (34) in rat hepatocytes cultured on Matrigel, a reconstituted basement membrane. Ethanol was found to induce cytochromes P450IIE, IIB1/2, and IIIA in cultured rat hepatocytes on Matrigel (61). Similar isozymes are induced in cultured hepatocytes and *in vivo*, illustrating that isolated hepatocytes are a relevant experimental system for cytochrome P450 induction studies. It is interesting to note that P450 induction performed *in vivo* is found to lead to induced activities in the isolated hepatocytes for at least 24 hr in culture. After administration of several cytochrome P450 inducers (phenobarbitone, β-naphthoflavone, dexamethasone, and isoniazid), the induced cytochrome P450 enzyme activities found *in vivo* were found to be maintained in the isolated hepatocytes for 24 hr in culture on a positively charged plastic surface, namely, a Primaria culture plate (26). This observation further confirms the appropriateness of using freshly isolated hepatocytes for xenobiotic metabolism studies.

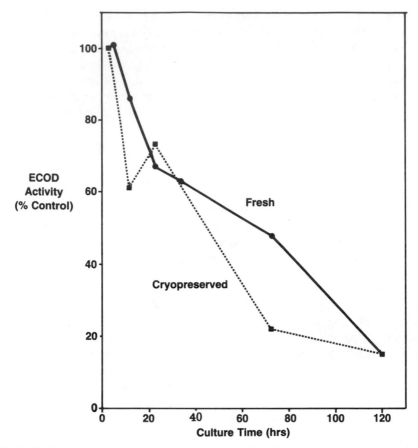

FIG. 3. Decline of 7-ethoxycoumarin-O-deethylase (ECOD) activity for freshly isolated and cryopreserved adult rat hepatocytes after culturing. The cells were cultured on collagen-coated plastic. ECOD activity is commonly measured to represent P450 mixed function oxygenase activity. While a steady drop in activity was observed, at 24 hr post-plating, the cells still retained over 50% of the original activity.

Virtually all studies on xenobiotic metabolism are on the liver parenchymal cells (hepatocytes). The potential activity of nonparenchymal cells are mostly ignored. In our laboratory, we recently compared the potential xenobiotic metabolic activity of rat liver parenchymal and nonparenchymal cells and found that nearly all detectable activities were found in the parenchymal cells (64). Our data therefore suggest that metabolite-induced damage to nonparenchymal cells, often found *in vivo*, are probably a result of the metabolites generated by the neighboring parenchymal cells.

Phase II Conjugation

While the phase I metabolism has been studied in detail in cultured hepatocytes, relatively less information is available for phase II metabolism. In phase II, the highly reactive metabolites generated from phase I metabolism of xenobiotics are "inactivated" via glucuronidation and sulfation. Important phase II enzymes are (a) UDP-glucuronyltransferase, which catalyzes glucuronidation, (b) sulfotransferase, which catalyzes sulfation, and (c) the glutathione-*S*-transferase (GST), which catalyzes glutathione conjugation. All three major conjugation pathways (glucuronidation, sulfation, and glutathione conjugation) have been observed in cultured hepatocytes.

Our study on acetaminophen conjugation illustrates the existence of glucuronidation and sulfation in cultured rat hepatocytes (32). Rat hepatocytes from male and female animals were cultured either on collagen or Matrigel, and both the sulfate and the glucuronide conjugation of acetaminophen were studied. The *in vivo* sex differences in acetaminophen metabolism, with the male rat excreting more acetaminophen sulfate and less acetaminophen glucuronide than the female (22), was apparent in the 1- and 2-day cultures and became less apparent on day 4. We found the hepatocytes cultured on Matrigel to maintain sulfation better than those cultured on collagen, a finding consistent with the general observation that Matrigel is a better substrate for the maintenance of hepatocyte differentiation.

The effect of culturing on GST has been studied. Both GST activity and mRNA levels are found to be affected by medium composition and culture time. But unlike cytochrome P450 isozymes, which tend to diminish with time in culture, GST tends to increase with prolonged culturing. Fetal calf serum appears to maintain GST level, whereas exclusion of fetal calf serum, addition of nicotinamide, or inclusion of DMSO increases GST. A similar trend was observed for hepatocytes co-cultured with liver epithelial cells (49). A later more detailed study showed a more complex picture (67): In conventional culture, after 6 days in culture, there was a decrease in GST subunits 1 and 2, maintenance of subunits 3 and 4, and increase in subunit 7 when fetal calf serum was present. Omission of fetal calf serum led to an increase in subunits 3, 4, and 7. Co-culturing with liver epithelial cells led to increases in all subunits. Exclusion of fetal calf serum in the co-cultures led to a significant reduction in subunit 2.

These findings with phase II metabolism again confirm that freshly isolated hepatocytes are representative of the liver *in vivo*.

Species Comparison Studies

Species difference in xenobiotic metabolism is a well-documented phenomenon and is believed to be one of the major factors accountable for the observed species difference in sensitivity towards chemical toxicants. Because the liver is the major organ for xenobiotic metabolism, hepatocytes cultured from multiple animal species are an attractive experimental system to evaluate this phenomenon, especially as a system to extrapolate data from laboratory animals to humans.

In our laboratory, the parallelogram approach is used to extrapolate data obtained from laboratory animals and cultured animal and human cells to humans *in vivo* (Fig. 4). By understanding the relationship between hepatocytes and *in vivo* results obtained from laboratory animals, one can logically predict human *in vivo* results.

OBJECTIVE: *Prediction Of Human Toxicity*

- Demonstrate *in vitro–in vivo* correlation with experimental animals

- Predict human toxicity from *in vitro* human cell data

In Vivo Toxicity	X	X	X	Predict
In Vitro Toxicity	X	X	X	X

Mouse   Rat   Monkey Human

FIG. 4. The "parallelogram approach" to the extrapolation of human toxicity. Human *in vivo* response (e.g., toxicity, metabolism) is to be derived from *in vitro* human hepatocyte data based on the *in vitro–in vivo* relationship observed in laboratory animals. The key to this approach is to have a thorough understanding of the data derived from laboratory animals, preferably using multiple animal species. A corollary to this approach is that one may use cultured hepatocytes to select an animal species that is the closest to human in xenobiotic metabolism.

Successful application of this approach is dependent on the ability of the cultured hepatocytes to retain the species differences found *in vivo*.

Results with several model chemicals seem to indicate that isolated hepatocytes do retain the species differences in xenobiotic metabolism. One of such compound is amphetamine (AMP). AMP is metabolized via two major pathways: aromatic hydroxylation to parahydroxyamphetamine (pHA) and oxidative deamination (benzoic acid, hippuric acid). Species differences in AMP metabolism is known, with differences existing both in rate of metabolism and in the ratio of metabolites (13). Rabbits metabolize AMP rapidly, with the majority of the metabolites being deamination products. Rats have a moderate rate of metabolism, and unlike most other species they prefer the formation of aromatic hydroxylation products such as pHA. Humans and squirrel monkeys metabolize AMP slowly into mainly deamination metabolites (acids). Green et al. (21) studied AMP metabolism in hepatocytes isolated from rats, rabbits, dogs, squirrel monkeys, and humans and found that isolated hepatocytes retained the species differences found *in vivo*. Similar results were also obtained in our laboratory with freshly prepared and cryopreserved rat and rhesus monkey hepatocytes. After a 4-hr incubation with 10 μM AMP, freshly isolated hepatocytes (5×10^6, in a total volume of 10 ml) from rabbits, rats, and rhesus monkeys were found to metabolize 100%, 32%, and 13%, respectively, of the total AMP. The one human hepatocyte isolate studied showed only 12% metabolism after a 24-hr incubation period. High-performance liquid chromatography (HPLC) analysis of the metabolites showed that rat hepatocytes produced more pHA than acids, whereas rabbits, rhesus monkeys, and humans produced more acids than pHA (Table 2). Our data therefore are consistent with the *in vivo* findings of Dring et al. (13). Other examples of the similarity between freshly isolated hepatocytes and whole animals in xenobiotic metabolism include studies on tolbutamide with rats, rabbits, dogs, and squirrel monkeys (17) and studies on diazepam with rats, rabbits, dogs, guinea pigs, and humans (7). Monteith et al. (48) showed that

TABLE 2. *Metabolism of amphetamine (AMP) by hepatocytes isolated from multiple animal species into p-hydroxyamphetamine (pHA) and deamination-derived benzoic and hippuric acids*

Animal	4 hr			24 hr		
	Acids (%)	pHA (%)	AMP (%)	Acids (%)	pHA (%)	AMP (%)
Rat	10.4	35.2	48.8	23.5	52.9	15.7
Rabbit	54.2	10.0	0.0	Not analyzed		
Monkey	5.7	1.4	86.9	22.1	2.1	68.7
Human	Not analyzed			5.1	3.4	88.1

acetylaminofluorene was metabolized by cultured human hepatocytes in a manner similar to that by humans *in vivo* (68). These studies therefore support the usefulness of isolated hepatocytes in the evaluation of species differences in xenobiotic metabolism. This is especially important in human metabolism studies because experimentation with human *in vivo* is rarely possible.

Discrepancy between hepatocytes and *in vivo* observation also exists. An example is that reported by Humpel et al. (29) with four radiolabeled drugs: lonazolac, bromerguride, lisuride, and terguride. While the metabolite profile generated from hepatocytes for lonazolac and bromerguride were similar to *in vivo* findings, a significantly lower number of metabolites were found for lisuride and terguride in hepatocytes than *in vivo*. Exhepatic metabolism, for instance, by other organs or by gut flora may be a reason for the differences. Hepatocytes isolated from rats, guinea pigs, beagle dogs, and cynomolgus monkeys were used in study. While good correlation was found between hepatocytes and *in vivo* findings in metabolic stability, no quantitative correlation was observed. This illustrates the complexity of data extrapolation. In addition to the lack of nonhepatic tissues and other host factors for the hepatocytes in culture, there are several important differences between the *in vitro* system and the whole animal that most investigators do not consider: While hepatocyte experiments are performed using a static pool of medium containing the drugs, *in vivo* experiments are performed with a bolus injection. The hepatocytes *in vitro* are therefore exposed to a relatively constant concentration of the substrate, whereas the liver *in vivo* is exposed to a continuum of concentrations depending on the route of administration and the rate of clearance. Furthermore, one needs to account for the difference in cell mass between *in vitro* experiments (which usually employ millions of hepatocytes) and *in vivo* experiments with the intact liver (which has a substantially higher number of hepatocytes).

TOXICOLOGY

Hepatocytes are used extensively in hepatotoxicity and carcinogenicity studies. Toxicity assays can be divided into the following main categories: cytotoxicity, genotoxicity, and enzyme induction. As illustrated by the various examples cited below, the advantage of cultured hepatocytes is that one can combine cytotoxicity measurement with various other biochemical measurements and co-treatment of metabolic inhibitors, to allow mechanistic evaluation of toxicity which cannot be easily performed *in vivo* or using cell-free systems such as microsomal preparations.

Cytotoxicity

Measurement of cytotoxicity is probably the most widely used aspect of cultured hepatocytes. A variety of end points have been developed to quantify cytotoxicity.

Morphology

As mentioned earlier, conventional (i.e., on collagen-coated surface) monolayer cultures of hepatocytes exhibit an epithelial cell morphology with a polygonal shape and prominent nuclei (Fig. 2A). With the use of light microscopy, cytotoxicity can sometimes be visualized using a light microscopy by the rounding of the cells, blebbing, and detachment. With the use of electron microscopy, cytotoxicity can be observed by alterations in ultrastructure—for instance, swelling of mitochondrial membranes, appearance of lysosomal inclusion bodies, and so on. The study of Gross et al. (23) illustrates the induction of mitochondrial swelling and lamella inclusion bodies by amiodarone, a hepatotoxic drug (see below). Morphological observation is usually performed as a qualitative, but not quantitative, measurement of cytotoxicity. Sorensen (62) developed a quantitative morphometric analysis procedure with hepatocytes damaged by indomethacin and showed good correlation with cytotoxicity measured by enzyme release (see below). The procedures, however, have not yet been widely applied.

Trypan Blue Uptake

Trypan blue is a high-molecular-weight chemical which is relatively impermeable to viable cells. Cells with damaged plasma membrane, however, will allow rapid permeation of the dye into the cytoplasm, thereby staining the cell nuclei blue. Trypan blue exclusion is commonly used to evaluate cell viability during hepatocyte isolation, and has been applied to short-term suspension cultures to evaluate chemical cytotoxicity. Thompson et al. (65), for instance, evaluated the toxicity of eugenol (4-allyl-2-methoxyphenol), a chemical known to be present in various food and medicinal preparations, in isolated rat hepatocytes. A good correlation between the loss of intracellular glutathione and cell death as measured by trypan blue uptake was obtained. The correlation between glutathione depletion and cytotoxicity induced by eugenol was further confirmed by (a) the prevention of cytotoxicity by *N*-acetylcysteine and (b) the augmentation of cytotoxicity by the glutathione depletion agent, diethylmaleate. This study illustrates the application of cultured hepatocytes, combining metabolism and cytotoxicity studies, toward elucidating the mode of action of a hepatotoxic agent. Trypan blue exclusion can be performed quantitatively but is tedious, requiring manual counting. This is usually performed for experiments with limited numbers of samples. Trypan blue uptake is commonly expressed as the number of cells exhibiting trypan blue, divided by the total cell population counted. A significant increase in this ratio over untreated or solvent-treated controls would indicate cytotoxicity.

Release of Cytoplasmic Enzyme

Assaying for plasma levels of liver specific enzymes, alanine aminotransferase (ALT; also known as serum glutamate pyruvate transaminase, SGPT), and aspartate aminotransferase (AST; also known as serum glutamate oxaloacetate transaminase, SGOT), is an approach well-accepted for the evaluation of liver damage *in vivo*, both in laboratory animals (6) and in humans (70). Although both ALT and AST are present in the cytosol, the mitochondria of hepatocytes contain only AST (31). Analysis of both ALT and AST therefore can allow one to distinguish plasma membrane damage from mitochondria damage.

This analysis of enzyme release has been applied towards cultured hepatocytes. Freshly isolated hepatocytes are allowed to attach, usually overnight. Medium is then changed to that containing the substances to be tested. After another culturing period, usually 24–96 hr, the amount of cytoplasmic enzyme released into the culture medium is determined. In addition to ALT and AST, the release of another cytoplasmic enzyme, lactate dehydrogenase (LDH), is also commonly used. Because of the universal presence of LDH in cells, elevation of plasma LDH for *in vivo* experiments does not necessarily indicate liver damage. Under *in vitro* conditions, however, as only hepatocytes are used, LDH release into culture medium usually reflects plasma membrane damage as well as ALT and AST. Data on enzyme leakage usually is presented as percent of total cytoplasmic enzyme content, using detergent treatment (e.g., triton X-100) to induce 100% lysis.

An example of the application of enzyme release is the evaluation of amiodarone, an iodinated benzofuran widely used for life-threatening cardiac dysrhythmias (61b). Amiodarone is known to induce an elevated level of LDH, ALT, of AST in patients receiving chronic therapy. Cultured rat hepatocytes, when treated with amiodarone and the metabolite desethylamiodarone, were found to release LDH, AST, and ALT into the medium in a dose-dependent and time-dependent manner, thereby reproducing the clinical findings. This study therefore illustrates the application of *in vitro* cytotoxicity in the evaluation of *in vivo* hepatotoxicity.

Because of the availability of automatic clinical analyzers that can accurately measure LDH, ALT, and AST, a large number of samples can be assayed with ease. Enzyme release is therefore widely used to quantify cytotoxic responses of cultured hepatocytes to toxic agents. A point of caution in using enzyme release as an end point is that one needs to ensure that the chemicals tested do not inactivate the enzyme measured. α-Mercapto acids, for instance, are known to inactivate LDH (5).

Other End Points

While the above-mentioned end points are the most commonly used, a variety of other end points can be used to monitor cytotoxicity. Such end points include (a) macromolecular incorporation (mainly measured by radiolabeled amino acid and ribonucleotide incorporation, since hepatocytes in culture have limited DNA synthesis activity) and (b) functional end points, including albumin synthesis, glycogen synthesis, and urea synthesis. Gomez-Lechon et al. (18a) evaluated a variety of hepatotoxins with multiple cytotoxicity end points in cultured rat hepatocytes and found that the sensitivity of each end point varies with each hepatotoxin. While RNA and albumin synthesis were the most sensitive end points for α-amanitin, LDH release was the most sensitive for d-galactosamine and acetaminophen, and ureogenesis was the most sensitive for thioacetamide.

Genotoxicity

Genotoxic chemicals are agents that would interact with DNA, leading to heritable changes (see ref. 37). The role of liver metabolism in the "activation" of nongenotoxic parent compounds (promutagens) to highly reactive electrophiles is well established. Enzymes involved include cytochrome P450 isozymes (see above), peroxidases, monoamine oxidase, and flavin-containing oxygenase (27). Postmitochondrial supernatant (S9) and microsomes prepared from livers of Aroclor-1254-treated rats are commonly used in mutagenesis assays as an exogenous activating system for promutagens (refs. 1 and 35). Hepatocytes themselves are also used as a promutagen activating system, as well as a target cell to measure genotoxicity.

Promutagen Activation

This is accomplished by co-culturing primary hepatocytes with a reporter cell which has little or no P450 metabolism but with which mutation can be quantified. An example is the co-culturing of Chinese hamster ovary (CHO) cells with hepatocytes, followed by mutagen treatment and quantification of mutants at the hypoxanthine-guanine phosphoribosyl transferase (HGPRT) gene locus (38). Using this procedure, we found that rat hepatocytes could be cryopreserved to retain promutagen activating activity (44), and that the parenchymal cells in rat liver had substantial activity while the nonparenchymal cells had virtually no activity in the activation of two promutagens, 3-methylcholanthrene and dimethyl nitrosamine (64). While liver homogenate is routinely used in mutagenicity assays, there is evidence that activation of promutagens by intact hepatocytes provide data more relevant to *in vivo* carcinogenicity. For instance, after comparison of mutagenicity of benzo(*a*)pyrene and four major metabolites in the Ames test, Glat et al. (18) found that the relative mutagenicity of the compounds obtained using intact hepatocytes was closer to the *in vivo* ranking of carcinogenicity than were data obtained with liver homogenate.

Induction of Unscheduled DNA Synthesis (UDS)

After exposure to mutagen, a certain level of DNA repair activity is induced. Some of the DNA lesions are excised and replaced with new DNA, a process known as "unscheduled" DNA synthesis (as opposed to the "scheduled" DNA synthesis during normal DNA replication). This activity can be measured in virtually all mammalian cells, including hepatocytes. The measurement of UDS in hepatocytes as an assay for mutagens was pioneered by Williams (69). After allowing freshly isolated hepatocytes to attach on collagen-coated coverslips, the test substance is added simultaneously with radiolabeled thymidine. Autoradiography is used to quantify radiolabeled thymidine incorporation, with the results expressed as number of grains in the emulsion over the nuclei.

Others

Several other approaches have been used to evaluate the interaction of toxicants with hepatocyte DNA. Using the induction of single-strand breaks as an end point, Liu and Castonguay (43) showed that (+)-catechin, a plant flavonoid, could inhibit the metabolism and genotoxicity of a tobacco-specific carcinogen. Cole et al. (8) measured the binding of aflatoxin B_1 and 2-acetyl-aminofluorene to the DNA of hepatocytes cultured from male and female rats and humans. The known sex and species differences in carcinogenicity were found to correlate well with the DNA binding levels.

Enzyme Induction

The liver contains a host of enzymes that can be up-regulated. From a toxicologist's point of view, the important inducible enzymes are the peroxisomal enzymes and P450 MFO isozymes. As described below, there is often a correlation between the induction of these enzymes and hepatocarcinogenicity. Whether enzyme induction and carcinogenicity are merely coexisting events or mechanistically linked is yet to be elucidated. We have recently hypothesized that some enzyme inducers may also induce the expression of other cellular genes, including cellular oncogenes. Such enzyme inducers therefore have the potential to promote the expression of preexisting mutations in these genes, leading to cancer development (35). Our hypothesis led us to the development of a multiple-end-point hepatocyte assay in which cytotoxicity and enzyme induction (peroxisome induction and P450 induction) were used as toxicity end points (36).

Because of the interanimal variability, the difficulty of quantitation of organ dose, and the activities of extrahepatic factors, it is often difficult to study enzyme induction *in vivo*, especially when mechanistic or quantitative (e.g., dose–response relationship) information is to be obtained. A cell culture system such as cultured hepatocytes maintained in a chemically defined medium is therefore ideal for enzyme induction studies. It is important to emphasize here that cultured hepatocytes remain the only *in vitro* liver system with which enzyme induction can be studied. The relatively long time period (days) required for induction precludes the use of systems such as liver slices or isolated perfused livers, the viability of which can only be maintained for a relatively short time period (hours).

Peroxisomal Induction

Peroxisomes are organelles found ubiquitously in animal and plant cells. The organelle has a diameter of approximately $0.1–1.5$ μm, with a single limiting membrane and a fine granular matrix. In normal hepatocytes, the peroxisome-to-mitochondria ratio is 1:5 or 1:6. The organelles are believed to be involved in fatty acid oxidation, thermogenesis, and respiration. Peroxisome proliferation (increase in peroxisome number) has been known to be induced by high-fat diets, hormonal alterations such as hyperthyroidism, and, as described below, certain chemicals such as some hypolipidemic agents and plasticizers. The biological effects of peroxisome proliferators *in vivo* in rodents include increases in smooth endoplasmic reticulum and P450 MFO activity, hepatomegaly, hypolipidemia, and hepatocarcinogenesis. Peroxisome proliferators have been suggested to be a novel class of hepatocarcinogens (53). These agents include the hypolipidemic agent clofibrate and the plasticizer di-(2-ethylhexyl)phthalate. They are unique in that they do not have genotoxicity as measured by the conventional mutagenicity assays. Peroxisome induction can be measured morphologically by counting numbers of peroxisomes per cell or biochemically by monitoring cyanide-insensitive palmitoyl CoA oxidation. Induction of peroxisomal β-oxidation in cultured hepatocytes by agents known to induce peroxisomes in rodents *in vivo* has been shown (34a).

Whether peroxisome proliferators are human carcinogens is still debatable. Liver biopsies from patients clinically exposed to peroxisomal inducers clofibrate (26a), gemfibrozil (30), and fenofibrate (4) did not show evidence of increased peroxisome proliferation relative to untreated controls. This species difference in response was also observed in cultured hepatocytes. Elcombe and Mitchell (14a) showed that mono(2-ethylhexyl)phthalate and two of its active metabolites significantly induced palmitoyl Co-A oxidation in rat hepatocytes but not in marmoset or human hepatocytes. Foxworthy et al. (16a) showed that monkey hepatocytes were significantly less responsive than rat hepatocytes to the peroxisome induction effects of ciprofibrate, bezafibrate, and LY 171883, thereby supporting the rodent–primate difference observed *in vivo*. In our laboratory, we have evaluated four potent rodent peroxisome proliferators (clofibrate, DEHP, lactofen, and Wy-14,653) and found consistent activation of palmitoyl CoA oxidase activity in rat hepatocytes but not in

TABLE 3. *Effect of peroxisome proliferators on palmitoyl Co-A oxidase activity in cultured human hepatocytes*

| | Palmitoyl CoA oxidase activity (nmol/min/mg·protein)[a] | | |
Treatment	I	II	III
DMSO control	0.07	0.00;0.23	0.20;0.23
Clofibrate (1 mM)	0.06	0.00;0.01	0.26;0.24
DEHP (1 mM)	0.03	0.08;0.13	0.26;0.27
Lactofen (0.1 mM)	—	0.00;0.02	0.20;0.27
Wy-14,643 (0.1 mM)	0.05	—	—

[a]Activity of individual plates shown. Because of the limitation in the number of human hepatocytes available, treatments were performed as duplicates for II and III and as single plates for I. I: 17-year-old female; II: 41-year-old male; III: 35-year-old female. All donors were Caucasian.

three separate isolations of human hepatocytes (Table 3). However, because the carcinogenic mechanism of the peroxisome proliferators is not yet defined, it is difficult to project from these observations to human carcinogenicity.

P450 Induction

As the major organ for xenobiotic metabolism, the cytochrome P450 MFO system in the liver is well characterized. As indicated earlier, cultured hepatocytes are used extensively to study xenobiotic metabolism. The recent findings on the induction of the P450 MFOs are reviewed here.

P450 MFOs exist as isozymes coded for by the P450 gene superfamily. It is often confusing to compare results of different publications because of the multiple names assigned to the isozymes. Recently, a standardized nomenclature for the existing isozymes was proposed based on sequence homology (51). In this review, the previous "nonstandard" nomenclature is converted to this "standardized" nomenclature to allow an easier comparison of results.

Findings from the laboratory of Guzelian and co-workers are probably the most influential for our understanding of P450 induction in cultured hepatocytes. Earlier results from this laboratory showed that P450 IA1 in cultured hepatocytes was induced by 3-methylcholanthrene, β-naphthoflavone, 3,4,3′,4′-tetrachlorobiphenyl, and Aroclor 1254 (14). Incubation of cultured rat hepatocytes with the inducers led to a 5- to 15-fold increase in P450 IA1 protein (measured by immunoprecipitation) accompanied by increases in the synthesis of mRNA and protein for this isozyme. In the same study, the authors showed that safrole, Aroclor 1254, and 3,4,5, 2′,4′,5′-hexachlorobiphenyl prevented the loss of P450 IA2 from the cultured hepatocytes, whereas 3-methylcholanthrene, β-naphthoflavone, and 3,4,3′,4′-tetrachlorobiphenyl had no effect. The authors concluded that modifications of both synthesis and degradation are the major mechanisms for the regulation of P450 isozyme levels, and that different isozymes might be regulated by different mechanisms. The same laboratory also showed that P450 IIIA1 was inducible by glucocorticoids in cultured hepatocytes (55). Dexamethasone was found to be more effective than the other glucocorticoids tested, which include betamethasone, α-methylprednisolone, 16α-carbonitrile, triamcinolone, corticosterone, and hydrocortisone. The induction was shown to be due to an increase in the rate of synthesis of the isozyme, and was reversible upon the withdrawal of the inducers from the cultured medium.

While phenobarbital (PB) is a powerful P450 inducer *in vivo*, its ability to induce cultured hepatocytes is often referred to as "difficult" to demonstrate. An earlier report by Michalopoulous et al. (46) showed that PB induced both P450 content and smooth endoplasmic reticulum in rat hepatocytes cultured on floating collagen gel. Whereas induction by 3-methylcholanthrene required only 2 days, a 5-day induction period was needed for PB. This report was followed by that of Stenberg and Gustaffsson (63), showing that PB induced androstenedione hydroxylation similar to that found *in vivo*. The authors concluded that the inclusion of rat serum in the culture medium was important to study P450 induction. The recent study of Wortelboer et al. (69a) showed that PB only induced a marginal induction of P450 activities in cultured rat hepatocytes measured using a variety of end points such as total P450 content, dealkylation of 7-ethoxyresorufin and 7-pentoxyresorufin, and testosterone hydroxylation. The induction found in the cultured hepatocytes was significantly lower than that found *in vivo*. This finding is consistent with the earlier finding of Schuetz et al. (56) which showed that hepatocytes cultured on collagen were only minimally induced by PB, while cells cultured on Matrigel had significant induction. Via the measurement of mRNA (57) and the measurement of cytochrome P450 activities (61), PB was found to induce mainly the isozymes P450 IIB1/IIB2.

By studying hepatocytes cultured on Matrigel, Schuetz et al. (57) further showed that growth hormone may directly affect the expression of some inducible P450 isozymes. Co-incubation of hepatocytes with phenobarbital and human growth hormone (somatotropin) was shown to completely block the induction of P450 IIB1/IIB2 gene expression. The study was the first to show inhibitory control by growth hormone on P450 induction. This observation demonstrates further the complex mechanisms involved in the regulation of P450 isozymes and the usefulness of the cultured hepatocyte system in the elucidation of the mechanisms.

HUMAN HEPATOCYTES

As stated earlier, one of the powerful applications of hepatocyte culture systems is the extrapolation to humans *in vivo* using data obtained from hepatocytes cultured from laboratory animals and humans and from laboratory animals *in vivo*, an approach we termed the *parallelogram approach* (Fig. 4). The key findings on human hepatocytes with toxicological implications are summarized here.

The establishment of reproducible procedures to isolate and culture human hepatocytes, combined with the characterization of the properties of cultured human hepatocytes, is critical to this application. Many laboratories, including ours, have reported the successful isolation and culturing of human hepatocytes. Guguen-Guillouzo et al. (24) showed the isolation of highly viable hepatocytes from three human livers obtained from kidney donors. By cannulating a portal branch of the left lobe and ligating the arteries, successful perfusion of a small (10% of total) area was achieved, leading to hepatocytes with high viability. In our laboratory, we have experience with the isolation of hepatocytes from whole human livers and surgical fragments. We found that perfusion of small liver portions, preferably 50 g or less, was the most efficient. We have an extremely high success rate (over 90%), yielding hepatocytes with high viability as judged by dye exclusion and attachment (40). The isolated human hepatocytes are responsive to the induction of DNA synthesis by epidermal growth factor (39) and can be transiently transfected with exogenous DNA (41).

Grant et al. (20) studied the stability of P450 isozymes in human hepatocytes cultured as monolayer cells on tissue culture plastic. The results showed that the decline in isozyme activity was apparently slower than that reported for rat hepatocytes. *O*-Dealkylation activities of ethoxyresorufin, pentoxyresorufin, and benzyloxyresorufin at 72 hr after culturing were found to be approximately 64%, 162%, and 100%, respectively, of that found in freshly isolated cells. However, NADPH-cytochrome c reductase and NADH-cytochrome b_5 reductase decreased to 32% and 22% of the level found in fresh cells, respectively. During this time period, glutathione levels remained unaltered. This study represents one of the first to study the phase I oxidative and phase II conjugative metabolism of human hepatocytes in culture.

Several studies illustrated the use of human hepatocytes in the evaluation of species differences in toxicity. Begue et al. (2) compared human and rat hepatocytes, showing that the naturally occurring flavonoid (+)-cyanidanol-3 could protect cultured rat hepatocytes against the cytotoxicity of aflatoxin-Bs, but had no protective effects towards human hepatocytes. The results suggest species differences in metabolism of aflatoxin B_1 and/or (+)-cyanidanol-3. As mentioned earlier, Le Bot et al. (34b) showed differences between rat and human hepatocytes towards the cytotoxicity of anthracycline antibiotics. Using hepatocytes as the exogenous activating system for promutagens, and by the direct measurement of DNA adduct formation, Hsu et al. (28) showed that aflatoxin B_1 was more potent as a mutagen in rat hepatocytes than in mouse hepatocytes, with the potency of human hepatocytes falling somewhere in between. The difference in potency appears to agree with the known rat–mouse difference in carcinogenicity. This finding was later confirmed by ultrastructural studies of human, rat, and mouse hepatocytes, showing a similar order of potency ranking for the induction of nucleolar segregation (9). These studies suggest that human hepatocytes in culture may be a relevant model for the evaluation of the sensitivity of human liver cells to carcinogens.

Donato et al. (11) showed that 3-methylcholanthrene, PB, and ethanol could induce cytochrome P450 MFO in cultured human hepatocytes. The level of induction (1.5- to 2.0-fold) was lower than that reported for cultured rat hepatocytes. Dexamethasone had no induction effect on human hepatocytes. This study is consistent with findings in our laboratory that cultured human hepatocytes are generally less responsive to enzyme inducers than rat hepatocytes.

The most difficult problem with the use of human hepatocytes is the low availability of human liver tissue for research. Access to surgical wastes via collaboration with surgeons and having a laboratory in the vicinity of the operation room are important factors for a fruitful program. One approach to increase the utility of human hepatocytes is to develop a reproducible procedure for cryopreservation so the cells can be stored and transported. We have developed a procedure with which human and rodent hepatocytes could be cryopreserved, with the recovered cells retaining both viability and xenobiotic metabolism (44,45). The cryopreserved cells were later used to study radiopharmaceutical metabolism and found to yield metabolites similar to fresh cells, but at a lower rate (47). Because of the potential complications of cryopreservation-related cellular damages, freshly isolated cells are still preferred over cryopreserved cells in toxicity studies in our laboratory.

INDUSTRIAL APPLICATIONS

Toxicological properties play an important role in industrial product development. Not only do the products need to have the desired efficacy, they must also have the acceptable level of toxicity. It is not an uncommon event to have a potential product with extremely desirable efficacy rejected after the end of the battery of toxicological studies. Product candidates that have an acceptable preclinical toxicological profile may also be rejected because of human toxicity discovered during clinical trials. In fact, hepatotoxicity is one of the toxicity end points easily measured in human subjects, and this has been the demise of a number of potential products.

The challenge is, therefore, how does one predict animal toxicity before expensive and time-consuming toxicology studies, and how does one ensure nontoxicity in human? One approach is to perform short-term toxicology screening assays on related chemical structures that have the desired efficacy. For compounds with a structure which may have hepatotoxic effects, toxicity assays with cultured hepatocytes may be performed. In our laboratory, we have developed a concept called "preference index (P.I.)," which is simply a ranking of preference based on both efficacy and hepatocyte cytotoxicity for these compounds. When a series of structurally related compounds are to be compared, we first develop an efficacy ranking using a quantitative measure called "relative efficacy (R.E.)," where

R.E. = efficacy (chemical X)/efficacy (reference chemical)

This is followed by the calculation of "relative cytotoxicity (R.C.)," where

R.C. = cytotoxicity (chemical X)/cytotoxicity (reference chemical)

The P. I. is then calculated:

$$P.I. = R.E./R.C.$$

The P.I. is therefore simply a ratio of the desired properties to the undesired properties. One can envision adding other factors to the equation, applying weights to each factor, and leading to the development of an equation for P.I. that encompasses all known properties of the potential product. Compounds with high P.I. values should have the highest potential to be developed into a commercializable product.

For pharmaceutical development, metabolic stability and fate are also critical for product development. A chemical with an extremely short half-life may not be a practical drug, because continuous infusion may be required to sustain the therapeutic level. Using cultured hepatocytes, one can compare simultaneously the disappearance rate of a series of structural analogues, allowing the selection of, for instance, a structure with the highest stability. While this approach ignores metabolism by other organs, one has to ensure that the liver is the major organ for metabolism of the chemicals studied. This may be studied via a comparison of *in vivo* and *in vitro* (cultured hepatocytes) metabolite profiles.

Extrapolation of human toxicity is an extremely valuable application. When one encounters a product candidate with obvious species differences in toxicity after testing in multiple species of laboratory animals, one has the question of which animal species is more similar to the human species. Using the parallelogram approach described earlier, data can be developed with cultured hepatocytes from the laboratory animals tested as well as from human hepatocytes. Understanding the correlation between the *in vivo* and *in vitro* studies with laboratory animals and the respective hepatocytes may allow one to evaluate which animal species is the closest to human (Fig. 4).

CONCLUDING COMMENTS

It can be seen from the information presented in this chapter that cultured hepatocytes represent an exciting *in vivo* toxicological system. Hepatocytes can now be isolated and cultured from virtually any mammalian species, including human. Short-term hepatocyte cultures are known to retain most of the liver functions, including species differences in xenobiotic metabolism. Culturing conditions are constantly being refined to allow prolonged maintenance of the differentiated properties, with the most significant finding being the use of reconstituted basement membrane fraction as attachment substratum. Various toxicity end points have been developed to allow research on hepatotoxicity, mutagenicity, and carcinogenicity. Enzyme induction in cultured hepatocytes, including the induction of peroxisomal enzymes and various isozymes, have been demonstrated.

To be able to study metabolism, enzyme induction, and toxicity in one single system is definitely the strength of cultured hepatocytes as compared to other *in vitro* systems. With cultured hepatocytes one can study (a) toxicity mechanisms, (b) correlation of toxicity and metabolism, and (c) the mechanism of enzyme induction under defined experimental conditions. If one were to use liver homogenates, besides the pitfalls in membrane disruption, leading to potential artifacts, one could not study toxicity nor enzyme induction. Problems with liver slices include (a) cell damage during preparation, (b) nonphysiological distribution of oxygen, nutrients, and test chemical to cells at different regions of the slices, and (c) the inability to study enzyme induction because of the short lifespan of the system. However, it is necessary to point out that the nonhepatocyte approaches are also important. With cell homogenate or microsome fractions, one can easily modify cofactor components and substrate concentrations, allowing one to evaluate specific biochemical parameters (e.g., K_m and V_{max}) for individual metabolic pathways. With liver slices, one can evaluate hepatotoxic effects on the nonparenchymal cell populations that are essentially absent in hepatocyte cultures. A successful investigator will be the one who will choose complementary experimental systems that can produce the most comprehensive information.

Besides improving the culturing conditions, there are aspects of the application of hepatocyte culturing system in toxicology that require further development. Based on our increasing knowledge in liver biology, mechanistic-based toxicity end points should be developed and validated with relevant *in vivo* systems. This should include the studying of toxicity towards nonparenchymal cells which is known to occur *in vivo* but which is virtually ignored by *in vitro* toxicologists. Data need to be obtained with more model chemicals, especially with human hepatocytes, to validate the parallelogram approach for the prediction of human health risk. The approach of using cultured hepatocytes in the selection of an animal species that has the highest resemblance to humans in xenobiotic metabolism for *in vivo* toxicology testing should be seriously evaluated. A combination of cultured hepatocytes and other differentiated cells (e.g., intestinal cells) should be evaluated for the development of *in vitro* systems in response to multiorgan metabolism and/or toxicity. Hepatocyte culture as an experimental system already has a significant impact in toxicology. A thorough understanding of the system, knowing both the strengths and limitations, will allow its utilization to the fullest in our continual quest towards the prediction and understanding of chemical toxicity in man.

ACKNOWLEDGMENTS

The author would like to express his gratitude to the following colleagues for their contributions to this chapter: Dale Beck, Don Kaminski, Linda Loretz, Jill Merrill, Asenath Rasmussen, and Annette Teepe.

REFERENCES

1. Ames BN, McCann J, Yamasaki E. Methods for detecting carcinogens and mutagens with the salmonella/mammalian microsome mutagenicity test. *Mut Res* 1975;31:347–364.

1a. Begue JM, Le Bigot JF, Guguen-Guillouzo C, Kiechel JR, Guillouzo A. Cultured human adult hepatocytes: a new model for drug metabolism studies. *Biochem Pharmacol* 1983;32:1643–1646.

2. Begue JM, Baffet G, Campion JP, Guillouzo A. Differential response of primary cultures of human and rat hepatocytes to aflatoxin B_1-induced cytotoxicity and protection by the hepatoprotective agent (+)-cyanidanol-3. *Biol Cell* 1988;63:327–333.

2a. Berry MN, Friend DS. High yield preparation of isolated rat liver parenchymal cells. *J Cell Biol* 1969;43:506–520.

3. Blouin A, Bolender RP, Weibel ER. Distribution of organelles and membranes between hepatocytes and nonhepatocytes in the rat liver parenchyma. *J Cell Biol* 1977;72:441–445.

4. Blumcke S, Schwartzkopff W, Lobeck H, Edmondson NA, Prentice DE, and Blane GF. Influence of fenofibrate on cellular and subcellular liver structure in hyperlipidemic patients. *Atherosclerosis* 1983;46:105–116.

5. Chaffee RRJ, Bartlett WL. Inhibition of lactate dehydrogenase by α-mercaptoacids. *Biochim Biophys Acta* 1960;39:370–372.

6. Charbonneau M, Brodeur J, duSouich P, Plaa GL. Correlation between acetone potentiated CCl_4-induced liver injury and blood concentrations after inhalation or oral administration. *Toxicol Appl Pharmacol* 1986;84:286–294.

7. Chenery RJ, Ayrton A, Oldham HG, Standring P, Norman SJ, Seddon T, Kirbt R. Diazepam metabolism in cultured hepatocytes from rat, rabbit, dog, guinea pig and man. *Drug Metab Dispos* 1987;15:312–317.

7a. Clement B, Guguen-Guillouzo C, Campion J-P, Glaise D, Bourel M, Guillouzo A. Long term cocultures of human hepatocytes with rat liver epithelial cells: Modulation of albumin secretion and accumulation of extracellular material. *Hepatology* 1984;4:373–380.

8. Cole KE, Jones TW, Lipsky MM, Trump BF, Hsu IC. *In vitro* binding of aflatoxin B1 and 2-acetylaminofluorene to rat, mouse and human hepatocyte DNA: the relationship of DNA binding to carcinogenicity. *Carcinogenesis* 1988;9:711–716.

9. Cole KE, Jones TW, Lipsiy MM, Trump B, and Hsu IC. Comparative effects of three carcinogens on human, rat and mouse hepatocytes. *Carcinogenesis* 1989;10:139–143.

10. Decad GM, Hsieh DPH, Byard JL. Maintenance of cytochrome P 450 and metabolism of aflatoxin B1 in primary hepatocyte cultures. *Biochem Biophys Res Commun* 1977;78:279–287.

11. Donato MT, Gomez-Lechon MJ, Castell JV. Effect of xenobiotics on monooxygenase activities in cultured human hepatocytes. *Biochem Pharmacol* 1990;39:1321–1326.

12. Donata MT, Castell JV, Gomez-Lechon MJ. Co-cultures of hepatocytes with epithelial-like cell lines: expression of drug biotransformation activities by hepatocytes. *Cell Biol Toxicol* 1991;7:1–14.

13. Dring LG, Smith RL, Williams RT. The metabolic fate of amphetamine in man and other species. *Biochem J* 1970;116:425–435.

14. Edward AR, Wrighton SA, Pasco DS, Fagan JB, Li D, Guzelian PS. Synthesis and degradation of 3-methylcholanthrene-inducible cytochromes P-450 and their mRNAs in primary monolayer cultures of adult rat hepatocytes. *Arch Biochem Biophys* 1985;241:495–508.

14a. Elcomb CR, Mitchell AM. Peroxisome proliferation due to di(2-ethylhexyl)philhalate (DEHP): Species differences and possible mechanisms. *Environ Health Perspect* 1986;70:211–219.

15. Emi Y, Chijiiwa C, Omura T. A different cytochrome P450 form is induced in primary cultures of rat hepatocytes. *Proc Natl Acad Sci USA* 1990;87:9746–9750.

16. Evarts RP, Marsden E, Thorgeirsson SS. Regulation of heme metabolism and cytochrome P-450 levels in primary culture of rat hepatocytes in a defined medium. *Biochem Pharmacol* 1984;33: 565–569.

16a. Foxworthy PS, White SL, Hoover DM, Eacho PI. Effect of ciprofibrate, bezafibrate and LY171883 on peroxisome beta-oxidation in cultured rat, dog, and rhesus monkey hepatocytes. *Toxicol Appl Pharmacol* 1990;104:386–394.

17. Gee SJ, Green CE, Tyson CA. Comparative metabolism of tolbutamide by isolated hepatocytes from rat, rabbit, dog, and squirrel monkey. *Drug Metab Dispos* 1984;12:174–178.

18. Glat HR, Billings R, Platt KL, Oesch F. Improvement of the correlation of bacterial mutagenicity with carcinogenicity of benzo(*a*)pyrene and four of its major metabolites by activation with intact liver cells instead of cell homogenate. *Cancer Res* 1981;41:270–277.

18a. Gomez-Lechon MJ, Monloya A, Lopez P, Donato T, Larrauri A, Castell JV. The potential use of cultured hepatocytes in predicting the hepatotoxicity of xenobiotics. *Xenobiotica* 1988;18:725–735.

19. Grant MH, Melvin MA, Shaw P, Melvin WT, Burke MD. Studies on the maintenance of cytochromes P-450 and b5, monooxygenases and cytochrome reductases in primary cultures of rat hepatocytes. *FEBS LETT* 1985;190:99–103.

20. Grant MH, Burke MD, Hawksworth GM, Duthie SJ, Engeset J, Petrie JC. Human adult hepatocytes in primary monolayer culture. Maintenance of mixed function oxidase and conjugation pathways of drug metabolism. *Biochem Pharmacol* 1987;36:2311–2316.

21. Green CE, LeValley SE, Tyson CA. Comparison of amphetamine metabolism using isolated hepatocytes from five species including human. *J Pharmacol Exp Ther* 1986;237:931–936.

22. Green MD, Fisher LJ. Age- and sex-related differences in acetaminophen metabolism in the rat. *Life Sci* 1981;29:2421–2428.

23. Gross SA, Bandyopadhyay S, Klaunig JE, Somani P. Amiodarone and desethylamiodarone toxicity in isolated hepatocytes in culture. *Proc Soc Exp Biol Med* 1990;190:163–169.

24. Guguen-Guillouzo C, Clement B, Baffet G, Beaumont C, Morel-Chany E, Glaise D, Guillouzo A. Maintenance and reversibility of active albumin secretion by adult rat hepatocytes co-cultured with another liver epithelial cell type. *Exp Cell Res* 1983;143:47–54.

25. Guzelian PS, Bissel DM, Meyer VA. Drug metabolism in adult rat hepatocytes in primary monolayer culture. *Gastroenterology* 1977;72:1232–1239.

26. Hammond AH, Fry JR. The *in vivo* induction of rat hepatic cytochrome P450-dependent enzyme activities and their maintenance in culture. *Biochem Pharmacol* 1990;40:637–642.

26a. Hanefeld M, Kemmer C, Leonhardt W, Kunze KD, Jaross W, Haller H. Effects of p-dichlorophenoxy-isobutyric acid (CPIB) on the human liver. *Atherosclerosis* 1980;36:159–172.

27. Heflich RH. Chemical mutagens. In: Li AP, Heflich RH, eds. *Genetic toxicology*. Boca Raton, FL: CRC Press, 1990;143–202.

28. Hsu IC, Harris CC, Lipsky MM, Snyder S, Trump BF. Cell and species differences in metabolic activation of chemical carcinogens. *Mutat Res* 1987;177:1–7.

29. Humpel M, Sostarek D, Gieschen H, Labitzky C. Studies on the biotransformation of lonazolac, bromerguride, lisuride and terguride in laboratory animals and their hepatocytes. *Xenobiotica* 1989; 19:361–377.

30. de la Iglesia FA, Penn SM, Lucas J, McGuire EJ. Quantitative stereology of peroxisomes in hepatocytes from hyperlipoproteinemic patients receiving gemfibrozil. *Micron* 1981;12:97–98.

31. Kachman JF, Moss DW. Enzymes. In: Tietz N, ed. *Fundamentals of clinical chemistry*. Philadelphia: WB Saunders, 1976;565–698.

32. Kane RE, Tector J, Brems J, Li A, Kaminski D. Sulfation and glucuronidation of acetaminophen by cultured hepatocytes reproducing *in vivo* sex-differences in conjugation on Matrigel and type 1 collagen. *In Vitro Cell Dev Biol* 1991;27A:953–960.

33. Kleinman HK, McGarvey ML, Hassell JR, Star VL, Cannon FB, Laurie GW, Martin GR. Basement membrane complexes with biological activity. *Biochemistry* 1985;25:312–318.

34. Kocarek T, Schuetz EG, Guzelian PS. Differentiated induction of cytochrome P450b/e and P450p mRNAs by dose of penobarbital in primary cultures of adult rat hepatocytes. *Mol Pharmacol* 1990; 38:440–444.

34a. Lake BG, Evans JG, Gray TJ, Korosi SA, North CJ. Comparative studies on nafenopin-induced peroxisome proliferation in the rat, Syrian hamster, guinea pig, and marmoset. *Toxicol Appl Pharmacol* 1989;99:148–160.

34b. LeBot MA, Begue JM, Kernaleguen D, Robert J, Ratanasarah D, Airau J, Riche C, Guillouzo A. Different cytotoxicity and metabolism of doxorubicin, daunorubicin, epirubicin, esorubicin, and idarubicin in cultured human and rat hepatocytes. *Biochem Pharmacol* 1988;37:3877–3887.

35. Li AP. Hypothesis: modification of oncogene expression as a major mechanism of action of "nongenotoxic" carcinogens. *Environ Mol Mutagen* 1989;14:113–114.

36. Li AP, Merrill JC. Development of a cultured hepatocyte system to study nongenotoxic mechanism of hepatocarcinogenesis. *Toxicologist* 1989;9:63.

37. Li AP, Heflich RH. *Genetic toxicology*. Boca Raton, FL: CRC Press, 1991.

38. Li AP, Gupta RS, Heflich RH, Wassom JS. A review and analysis of the Chinese hamster ovary/hyposanthine guanine transferase assay to determine the mutagenicity of chemical agents. A report of Phase III of the U. S. Environmental Protection Agency Gene-Tox program. *Mutat Res* 1988; 196:17–36.

39. Li AP, Myers CA, Roque MA, Kaminski DL. Epidermal growth factor, DNA synthesis and human hepatocytes. *In Vitro Cell Dev Biol* 1991;27A:831–833.

40. Li AP, Colburn SM, Beck DJ. A simplified method for the culturing of primary adult rat and human hepatocytes as multicellular spheroids. *In Vitro Dev Biol* 1992;28A:673–677.
41. Li AP, Myers CA, Kaminski DL. Gene transfer in primary cultures of human hepatocytes. *In Vitro Cell Dev Biol* 1992.
42. Li AP, Roque MA, Beck DJ, Kaminski DL. Isolation and culturing of hepatocytes from human livers. *J Tissue Culture Methods* 1992.
42a. Li AP, Barker G, Beck DJ, Colburn S, Monsell R, Pellegrin C. Culturing of primary hepatocytes as entrapped aggregates in a packed bed bioreactor: A potential bioartificial liver. *In Vitro Cell Dev Biol* 1993;29A:249–254.
43. Liu L, Castonguay A. Inhibition of the metabolism and genotoxicity of 4-(methylnitrosamino)-1-(3-pyridyl)-1-butanone (NNK) in rat hepatocytes by (+)-catechin. *Carcinogenesis* 1991;12:1203–1208.
44. Loretz LJ, Wilson AGE, Li AP. Promutagen activation by freshly isolated and cryopreserved rat hepatocytes. *Environ Mol Mutagen* 1988;12:335–341.
45. Loretz LJ, Li AP, Flye MW, Wilson AGE. Optimization of cryopreservation procedures for rat and human hepatocytes. *Xenobiotica* 1989;19:489–498.
46. Michalopoulos G, Sattler CA, Sattler G, Pitot H. Cytochrome P-450 induction by phenobarbital and 3-methylcholanthrene in primary cultures of hepatocytes. *Science* 1976;193:907–909.
47. Moerlein SM, Weisman RA, Beck D, Li AP, Welch MJ. Metabolism *in vitro* of radioiodinated *N*-isopropyl-para-iodoamphetamine by isolated hepatocytes. *Nucl Med Biol* 1992.
48. Monteith DK, Michalopoulos G, Strom SC. Metabolism of acetylaminofluorene in primary cultures of human hepatocytes: dose–response over a four-log range. *Carcinogenesis* 1988;9:1835–1841.
49. Morel F, Vanderberghc Y, Pemble S, Taylor JB, Ratanasavanh D, Rogiers V, Ketterer B, Guillouzo A. Regulation of glutathione *S*-transferase subunits 3 and 4 in cultured rat hepatocytes. *FEBS Lett* 1989;258:99–102.
50. Muakkassah-Kelly SF, Bieri F, Waechter F, Bentley P, Staubli W. Long-term maintenance of hepatocytes in primary culture in the presence of DMSO: further characterization and effect of nafenopin, a peroxisome proliferator. *Exp Cell Res* 1987;171:37–51.
51. Nebert DW, Adesnik M, Coon MJ, Estabrook RW, Gonzalez FJ, Guengerich FP, Gunsalus IC, Johnson EF, Kemper B, Levin W, Phillips IR, Sato R, Waterman MR. The P450 gene superfamily: recommended nomenclature. *DNA* 1987;6:1–11.
51a. Niemann C, Gauthier J, Richert L, Ivanov M, Melcion C, Cordier A. Rat adult hepatocytes in primary pure and mixed monolayer culture. Comparison of the maintenance of mixed function oxidase and conjugation pathways of drug metabolism. *Biochem Pharmacol* 1991;42:373–379.
52. Pain AJ. The maintenance of cytochrome P-450 in rat hepatocyte culture: some applications of liver cell cultures to the study of drug metabolism, toxicity and the induction of the P-450 system. *Chem Biol Interact* 1990;74:1–31.
53. Reddy JK, Azarnoff DL, Hignite CE. Hypolipidaemic hepatic peroxisome proliferators form a novel class of chemical carcinogens. *Nature* 1980;283:397–398.
54. Reese JA, Byard JL. Isolation and culture of adult hepatocytes from liver biopsies. *In Vitro* 1981;17:935–940.
55. Schuetz EG, Wrighton SA, Barwick JL, Guzelian PS. Induction of cytochrome P-450 by glucocorticoids in rat liver. 1. Evidence that glucocorticoids and pregnenolone 16α-carbonitrile regulate de novo synthesis of a common form of cytochrome P-450 in cultures of adult rat hepatocytes and in the liver *in vivo*. *J Biol Chem* 1984;259:1999–2006.
56. Schuetz EG, Li D, Omiecinski CJ, Muller-Eberhard U, Kleinman HK, Elswick B, Guzelian PS. Regulation of gene expression in adult rat hepatocytes cultured on a basement membrane matrix. *J Cell Physiol* 1988;134:309–323.
57. Schuetz EG, Schuetz JD, May B, Guzelian P. Regulation of cytochrome P-450b/e and P-450p gene expression by growth hormone in adult rat hepatocytes cultured on a reconstituted basement membrane. *J Biol Chem* 1990;265:1188–1192.
58. Seglen PO. Preparation of liver cells. *Exp Cell Res* 1973;82:391–398.
59. Seglen PO. Preparation of isolated liver cells. In: Prescott DM, ed. *Methods in cell biology*. New York: Academic Press, 1976;30–78.
60. Sinclair PR, Schuetz EG, Bement W, Haugen SA, Sinclair JF, May BK, Li D, Guzelian PS. Role of heme in phenobarbital induction of cytochromes P450 and 5-aminolevulinate synthase in cultured rat hepatocytes maintained on an extracellular matrix. *Arch Biochem Biophys* 1990;282:386–392.
61. Sinclair JF, McCaffrey J, Sinclair PR, Bement WJ, Lambrecht LK, Wood SG, Smith EL, Schenk-

man JB, Guzelian PS, Park SS, Gelboin HV. Ethanol increases cytochromes P450 IIE, IIB1/2, and IIIA in cultured rat hepatocytes. *Arch Biochem Biophys* 1991;284:360–365.

61a. Smedsrod B, Pertoft H. Preparation of pure hepatocytes and reticuloendothelial cells in high yield from a rat liver by means of Percall centrifugation and selective adherence. *J Leokocyte Biol* 1985; 38:213–230.

61b. Somani P, Baudyopadhyay S, Klaunig JE, Gross SA. Amiodarone- and desethylamiodarone-induced myelinoid bodies and toxicity in cultured rat hepatocytes. *Hepatology* 1990;11:81–92.

62. Sorensen EMB. Validation of a morphometric analysis procedure using indomethacin-induced alterations in cultured hepatocytes. *Toxicol Lett* 1989;45:101–110.

63. Stenberg A, Gustaffsson J. Induction of cytochrome P-450-dependent hydroxylases in primary monolayer cultures of rat hepatocytes. *Biochem Biophys Acta* 1978;540:402–407.

64. Teepe AG, Beck DJ, Li AP. A comparison of rat liver parenchymal and nonparenchymal in the activation of promutagens. *Environ Mol Mutagen* 1992.

65. Thompson DC, Constantin-Teodosiu D, Moldeus P. Metabolism and cytotoxicity of eugenol in isolated rat hepatocytes. *Chem Biol Interact* 1991;77:137–147.

66. Tong JZ, De Lagausie P, Furlan V, Cresteil T, Bernard O, Alvarez F. Long-term culture of adult rat hepatocyte spheroids. *Exp Cell Res* 1992;200:326–332.

67. Vandenberghe Y, Foriers A, Rogiers V, Vercruysse A. Changes in expression and "*de novo*" synthesis of glutathione *S*-transferase subunits in cultured adult rat hepatocytes. *Biochem Pharmacol* 1990;39:685–690.

68. Weisburger JH, Grantham PH, Vanhorn E, Steigbigel NH, Rall DP, Weisburger EK. Activation and detoxification of *N*-2-fluorenylacetamide in man. *Cancer Res* 1964;24:475–479.

69. Williams GM. Detection of chemical carcinogens by unscheduled DNA synthesis in rat liver primary cultures. *Cancer Res* 1981;37:1845–1851.

69a. Wortelboer HM, de Kruiff CA, van Iessel AA, Falke HE, Noordhoek J, Blaauboer BJ. Comparison of cytochrome P450 isozyme profiles in rat liver and hepatocyte cultures. The effects of model inducers on apoproteins and biotransformation activities. *Biochem Pharmacol* 1991;42:381–390.

70. Zimmerman HJ. Function and integrity of the liver. In: Henry JH, ed. *Clinical diagnosis and management by laboratory methods*. Philadelphia: WB Saunders, 1984;217–250.

In Vitro Toxicology,
edited by Shayne Cox Gad.
Raven Press, Ltd., New York, © 1994.

11

Application of *In Vitro* Model Systems to the Study of Cardiovascular Toxicity

Kenneth Ramos* and Daniel Acosta†

**Department of Physiology and Pharmacology, College of Veterinary Medicine,
Texas A & M University, College Station, Texas 77843; and
†Division of Pharmacology and Toxicology, College of Pharmacy,
The University of Texas at Austin, Austin, Texas 78712*

The cardiovascular system consists of the heart and blood vessels which form a circuit for (a) the transport of oxygen and nutrients to all tissues throughout the body and (b) the removal of waste products of metabolism. A highly regulated sequence of excitation/contraction coupling cycles from the atria to the ventricles allows the heart to pump blood through the vascular network. Cardiac output is initially received by the aorta, which in turn delivers blood to arterioles, capillaries, and post-capillary venules. Oxygen and nutrient exchange at the tissue level is regulated by discrete changes of microvascular resistance in response to intrinsic metabolic demands. Blood returns to the heart through the capacitance vessels of the venous compartment. In serving these circulatory functions, cardiovascular cells are repeatedly exposed to blood-borne toxins and their metabolic byproducts.

Although cardiovascular function is carried out in a coordinated fashion, the cardiovascular system is characterized by a large degree of structural and functional heterogeneity. From a morphologic standpoint, cardiac muscle consists of nodal tissue, Purkinje tissue, and ordinary muscle. Nodal tissue exhibits a high degree of automaticity, that is, the capacity to depolarize spontaneously, while Purkinje tissue is specialized for the conduction of electrical impulses. Ordinary muscle cells exhibit variable degrees of electromechanical and pharmacomechanical coupling in response to contractile stimuli. The walls of the heart consist of three distinct layers. The *epicardium* is the external layer which originates from visceral connective tissue. The middle layer is referred to as the *myocardium* and consists exclusively of muscle cells. The innermost layer of the heart is the *endocardium*, which is formed by a thin sheet of endothelial cells that extend from the coronary vessels to line the chambers and valves of the heart.

The blood vessel wall of large and medium-sized arteries consists of three distinct layers. The innermost layer, referred to as the *tunica intima*, represents a single layer of endothelial cells which rest on a thin basal lamina. In large vessels such as the human aorta, a distinct subendothelial layer can also be identified. The medial layer consists of several sheets of smooth muscle cells dispersed in a matrix of collagen and elastin. The outermost layer consists of fibroblastic cells which serve to provide structural support to the vessel wall and contribute to the regulation of smooth muscle function. With the exception of capillaries, vessels of small diameter share many of the features described above. However, in these vessels the media is less elastic and often limited to a few layers of smooth muscle cells. Capillaries are endothelial tubes that rest on a thin basal lamina to which pericytes readily attach.

Cardiovascular toxicity can result from excessive accumulation of toxic chemicals within the tissue, cardiovascular-specific bioactivation of protoxicants, and/or chemical interference with specialized physiologic functions. Because cardiotoxic insult interferes with the ability of the heart to pump blood through the vasculature, blood flow to major organs is often compromised. In contrast to the immediacy of cardiotoxic responses, vascular toxicities are often characterized by slow onsets and long latency periods. Angiotoxicity may cause alterations of arterial pressure, blood flow control, and vascular cell growth. The assessment of cardiovascular toxicity *in vivo* is often complicated by the presence of humoral, neuronal, and endocrine influences. The application of *in vitro* model systems to study the toxic responses of cardiovascular cells can overcome some of these limitations. This chapter presents an overview of *in vitro* models commonly used in cardiovascular toxicity testing.

IN VITRO MODEL SYSTEMS IN TOXICITY TESTING

Perfused Organ Preparations

Perfused heart preparations, including the modified Langerdorff technique and the working heart preparation, have been used to evaluate various aspects of myocardial function *in vitro* upon exposure to xenobiotics (1–3). The Langerdorff heart preparation constitutes a beating heart which does not perform work, whereas the working heart preparation is perfused through the left atrium to generate a left-sided working preparation. In the working heart preparation, perfusion fluid passes from the left atrium to the ventricle, where it is ejected via the aorta into a chamber against hydrostatic pressure to mimic physiologic resistance to flow (4). Potassium-arrested hearts can also be used to examine flow-dependent effects in the absence of myocardial function (5). Blood vessel segments from several vascular beds can be isolated and processed for perfusion *in vitro*. Aortic preparations are most often preferred over other macrovascular preparations. Aortic segments can be readily excised and perfused and superfused with appropriate buffered solutions (6). Smaller vessels can also be isolated and processed for perfusion *in vitro* (7). However, the popularity of microvascular preparations in toxicological studies is not yet widespread due to the complexities associated with handling and processing vessels with diameters <100 μm.

Perfused organ systems are probably more representative of the *in vivo* situation than are other *in vitro* preparations. Perfused preparations are particularly advantageous because they retain the level of structural organization found *in vivo* without the influence of extraneous variables. Using these preparations, toxin-induced changes in physiologic/pharmacologic sensitivity and changes in excitability and/or contractility can be readily evaluated. In the case of vascular preparations, studies can be conducted in the presence or absence of endothelial cells to assess the interactions of luminal and medial cells. The most significant limitation of perfused preparations in toxicity testing is that only a small number of replicate preparations can be processed at one time. The time required for isolation and placement of the tissue under physiologic conditions is critical to the preservation of tissue viability. Caution must also be exercised to ensure that initial fiber length (preload) and the force which must be overcome for muscle shortening (afterload) approximate those encountered *in vivo*. Perfused organ systems can only be used for short periods of time due to rapid loss of viability.

Parameters commonly used to evaluate xenobiotic-induced cardiotoxicity include time to peak tension, maximal rate of tension development, and tension development. The oxygen concentration of the perfusate entering the aorta and leaving the pulmonary artery can also be monitored as an index of myocardial oxygen consumption. Coronary flow can be measured by collecting effluent fractions as a function of time, and a latex balloon connected to a pressure transducer can be inserted in the left atria to monitor ventricular pressure. Pin electrodes connected to the right atrium, apex, and pulmonary vessels can be used to obtain electrocardiographic recordings. In the case of vascular preparations, the cannula employed for vessel perfusion can be equipped with side arms for pressure recording. As with cardiac preparations, measurements of contractility and stress development can also be used to evaluate the vascular effects of drugs and chemicals.

Isolated Muscle Preparations

Strips of atrial, ventricular, or papillary muscles (8), as well as segments from various vascular beds (9), can be placed in a bath and superfused with oxygenated physiologic solutions for measurements of tension development. Isolated preparations operate under constant conditions of carbon dioxide exchange, ionic gradients, and diffusion of byproducts of cellular metabolism. In the case of vascular preparations, spiral strips are preferred over longitudinal strips to avoid alterations in the geometry of muscle fibers. Alternatively, simple ring preparations can be prepared from most vessels. After equilibration in a physiologic solution, isolated muscle preparations are subjected to multiple stress/relaxation cycles to define optimal length—that is, the length at which maximal contractility occurs in response to a contractile agonist. The length of the equilibration period is dictated by intrinsic mechanical properties of the tissue. Preparations devoid of plasma membrane restrictions in permeability can be obtained by stripping off the plasmalemma using detergent or mechanical disruption (10–12). Contractions can be elicited using standard solutions of free ionized calcium within the physiologic range as described by Fabiato and Fabiato (13).

As with other *in vitro* models, exogenous influences of neuronal and humoral origin are excluded. The preload and afterload placed upon the tissue *in vitro* can be controlled accurately. Experiments can be conducted to evaluate (a) isometric force development, which precludes muscle shortening, (b) isotonic force development, where the afterload is predetermined and the muscle is able to shorten, and (c) quick-release contractions in which the afterload is varied during contraction (8). Oxygenation of the tissue is due to diffusion, and thus the thickness of the strips and the concentration of oxygen in the bath must be carefully monitored. Concentration–response relationships can be constructed for selected contractile agonists in the absence or presence of toxin (14,15). These relationships are obtained by cumulative increases in the concentration of each agonist without intervening washout until attainment of maximal developed force. However, before subsequent agonist addition, preparations should be allowed to reach steady state. In the case of vascular preparations, the effects of relaxing agents can also be evaluated. The vessel segment is precontracted to about 70–80% of the maximal contraction, and then challenged with the relaxing agent. Isolated preparations can be controlled with precision, but their stability is limited to brief periods of time.

Organ Culture

Ingwall et al. (16) have described the use of whole fetal hearts in culture to study processes associated with myocardial cell injury. A variation of the method using the right atria has been reported by Speralakis and Shigenoubu (17) and by Tanaka et al. (18). A similar approach has recently been reported by Gotlieb and Boden (19), who described the preparation of organ cultures of aortic tissue. Organ culture preparations offer long-term stability relative to other *in vitro* preparations. In the case of aortic preparations, evidence of persistent tissue edema, primarily in the first layers of the aorta, has been documented (19). The application of organ culture techniques facilitates the study of cellular interactions. However, more work is required to fully exploit the application of these preparations in toxicology.

Single-Cell Suspensions

Various combinations of physical, enzymatic, and chelating agents have been successfully employed to isolate cardiovascular cells. Suspensions of embryonic or neonatal cells derived from ventricular, atrial, or whole heart tissue can be easily prepared by enzymatic and/or mechanical dissociation. Isolation of cardiac myocytes typically requires the use of calcium-free solutions to weaken the connective tissue matrix. The isolation of adult myocytes which exhibit tolerance to physiologic calcium concentrations requires the use of more sophisticated techniques. Jacobson (20) has described the use of a dissociation apparatus consisting of finger-like projections (bristles) which provide abrasive action for the isolation of adult heart cells. Bkailey et al. (21) have suggested replacement of calcium with stronium or barium to prevent loss of physiologic regulation. Adult hearts can also be dissociated by a modified recirculating Langerdorff perfusion (22) that yields a high proportion of cells which remain rod shaped and are quiescent in medium containing physiologic calcium levels. Welder et al. (23) have reported a method for the isolation of adult rat cardiac myocytes using a custom-made glass apparatus for even perfusion of multiple hearts.

The anatomic distribution of cells within the mammalian vessel wall of large and medium-sized vessels facilitates the isolation of relatively pure suspensions of fibroblastic, endothelial, or smooth muscle cells. In contrast to cardiac preparations, vascular cells from embryonic, neonatal, and adult vessels can be efficiently isolated in calcium- and magnesium-containing solutions. This discrepancy may be based on differences in metabolic demand which allow vascular cells to remain viable under hypoxic conditions for longer periods. Endothelial cells are typically isolated by collagenase perfusion of intact cylinders, whereas collagenase/elastase mixtures or trypsin are employed to isolate medial smooth muscle cells or fibroblasts. Enzymes, temperature, osmolarity/pH, and time of incubation are important determinants of cell viability immediately after isolation. Most investigators agree that purified collagenase alone is not adequate for the isolation of cardiovascular cells. This suggests that other constituents present in the crude enzyme preparation are essential to the isolation process. Caution must be exercised when purchasing commercially available enzyme preparations because different lots and suppliers may exhibit different activities. Other proteolytic enzymes such as trypsin or papain have been successfully used to isolate neonatal cardiac myocytes and adult vascular myocytes. Although trypsin is useful for the isolation of myocytes, caution must be exercised to avoid deleterious effects such as increased cellular aggregation, removal of surface enzymes, reduction in receptor binding sites, and chromosomal damage. Cell damage during the isolation procedure can be minimized by carrying out the enzymatic digestion at an optimal low temperature. In most experimental systems the use of trypsin in the isolation of endothelial cells is avoided to minimize cellular injury.

Myocardial cell suspensions represent a heterogeneous population of muscle and nonmuscle cells. Neonatal myocytes are remarkably resistant to injury and exhibit variable degrees of beating shortly after isolation. In contrast, spontaneous beating of adult cardiac myocytes is thought to be due to the uncontrolled leakage of calcium through a permeable plasma membrane. This phenomenon is thought to represent a calcium-paradox phenomenon similar to that originally described by Zimmerman and Hulsmann (24). Under these conditions, cellular injury is characterized by release of intracellular protein, accumulation of calcium and sodium within the cell, and loss of intracellular potassium. These cells are said to be calcium-intolerant and often can be identified by their rounded appearance. However, assessment of cell shape alone may be misleading because rod-shaped myocytes may display abnormal resting membrane potentials (21). Viable adult myocytes should exhibit normal sarcomere length and remain quiescent at low external calcium concentrations and contract in response to increasing calcium concentrations. The fact that adult cardiac myocytes are mechanically at rest when isolated properly suggests that a fundamental difference exists between adult and neonatal cells.

Isolated cells can be microinjected with fluorescent dyes for the assessment of multiple cellular functions upon exposure to toxic chemicals. Muscle cells in suspension can also be voltage-clamped to evaluate spontaneous and chemically induced electrophysiologic changes. In general, toxic responses may be of slower onset or differing magnitude relative to those observed *in vivo*. The viability of cells in suspension decreases rapidly as a function of time. The density of saturable beta-adrenergic binding sites and coupling efficiency are significantly reduced in cardiac cell suspensions (25).

Cell Culture Systems

Because cells in suspension exhibit short-term stability, cell culture systems are preferred to evaluate chemical toxicity after prolonged exposures or following multiple challenges *in vitro*. Primary cultures can be established with relative ease from cell suspensions of cardiac and vascular tissue. Vascular endothelial and smooth muscle cultures can also be established by the explant method in which pieces of tissue are placed in a culture vessel to allow for cellular migration and proliferation *in vitro*. The usefulness of this approach may be questionable because the explant technique affords cells of enhanced migratory potential a selective growth advantage *in vitro* (26). Neonatal and embryonic cells of cardiac origin proliferate readily under appropriate conditions *in vitro* (27). Although cardiac myocytes from adult animals do not divide in culture, recent studies have suggested that the ability of cardiac myocytes for cell division is repressed but not completely lost (28). This is consistent with studies showing that some atrial myocytes synthesize large amounts of DNA and undergo complete cell division after an infarct to the ventricle (29). Myocardial cell division can also be stimulated by insertion of the large tumor antigen from the SV40 virus into the myocyte genome (30). Wang et al. (31) have recently described the establishment of a human fetal cardiac myocyte cell line by co-transfection of human cardiac myocytes with the SV40 large T antigen. These cells preserve many of the morphologic and functional features of human fetal cardiac myocytes in primary culture.

Vascular endothelial and smooth muscle cells derived from large and medium-sized vessels of embryonic, neonatal, or adult animals proliferate readily under appropriate conditions *in vitro* (32). Thus, cultures can be propagated *in vitro* to prepare cell lines which retain variable degrees of differentiation as a function of growth conditions *in vitro*. Although an early report on the isolation of endothelial cells from the heart microvasculature was presented by Simionescu and Simionescu (33), little information is available on the influence of toxic chemicals on the microvasculature. In this regard, Obeso et al. (34) have recently described the development of a stable murine cell line derived from a mouse hemangioendothelioma as a model to study the responses of microvascular endothelial cells. These endothelioma cells synthesize angiotensin converting enzyme, express surface receptors for acetylated low-density lipoprotein, produce thrombospodin, and show intracellular staining with an antibody to von Willebrand antigen. However, the application of such a model in toxicity testing may be limited because these cells express properties of a neoplastic phenotype. Of particular interest from a toxicologic perspective is that cytochrome P4501A1 activity is present in vertebrate cardiac endothelial cells of the marine scup (35). This P450 activity appears to be induced in animals from contaminated environments, suggesting that endothelial P450 may be important in the toxicologic effects of xenobiotics affecting the vasculature of the heart and other organ systems.

In the preparation of primary cultures, cardiac myocytes can be separated from nonmuscle cells by a differential pour-off technique based on the rate of attachment of cells in suspension to the substratum (36). Most of the nonmuscle cells attach to the dishes within 3 hr, whereas muscle cells remain in suspension for 16–19 hr. Because the percentage of fibroblasts in culture increases logarithmically, if no attempt is made to separate individual cell types, fibroblasts will eventually dominate the culture. This is a particular problem for cultures of pre- or postnatal myoblasts because the cells resemble fibroblasts in their physical appearance. A monoclonal antibody to cell surface adhesion factors has been used to enrich preparations of cultured myocardial cells (37). The addition of mitotic inhibitors and the maintenance of cultures in glutamine-free or serum-free media can also be used to enhance culture purity (38). By taking advantage of the anatomic distribution of cells within the vascular wall of large and medium-sized arteries, relatively pure suspensions of vascular endothelial cells and smooth muscle cells can be prepared. Under most experimental conditions, vascular smooth muscle cells do not exhibit spontaneous contractility, but contract in response to pharmacologic stimulation (39). Endothelial cells subjected to fluid mechanical forces associated with blood flow become elongated and orient themselves in the direction of shear stress (40). Growth of endothelial cells on extracellular matrix components, on layers of smooth muscle cells, and under flow may mimic some aspects of the vascular wall not found when grown on plastic.

The maintenance of most cells *in vitro* requires either serum or plasma for attachment, proliferation, and survival. Sato (41) has demonstrated that the serum or plasma requirement for cell growth of several cell lines can be satisfied by addition of specific hormones and growth factors to synthetic media. The growth environment of cells in culture is an important determinant of cellular behavior *in vitro*. Until recently, the extracellular matrix consisting of a mixture of collagens, noncollagen proteins, and carbohydrate-rich molecules was considered a static support for the cells *in vivo*. However, the matrix consists of molecules which can modulate cellular behavior and, thus, toxicologic responsiveness. Recent studies in this laboratory have shown that the matrix regulates the phenotypic expression of aortic smooth muscle cells in culture (42). Another important consideration is that the presence of serum modulates the antioxidant capabilities of cells *in vitro* (43). The identity of cells in culture must be carefully evaluated before toxicity studies are initiated. Cultures may be characterized at the morphologic, ultrastructural, biochemical, or functional level. Cardiovascular cells in culture undergo variable degrees of dedifferentiation, including loss of defined contractile features and cell-specific functions (44–46).

The occurrence of gross morphologic changes is routinely used to screen chemicals of unknown toxic potential and to assess potentially significant toxic interactions. Flow cytometry and computerized evaluation of cell images has greatly expanded the usefulness of microscopic analysis in toxicity testing (47). In the case of cardiac myocytes, toxicity can also be evaluated based on the arrhythmogenic potential of chemicals (48,49). Arbitrary or computer-assisted grading systems can be implemented to evaluate these responses (50). Because toxicity is often due to interactions with or disruption of antioxidant defense systems, measurements of the glutathione status of cells may be particularly useful in the elucidation of mechanisms of toxicity (51). Ionic homeostasis can also be used as an index of disturbances in the structural and functional integrity of the plasma membrane (52,53). Of particular interest is the application of co-culture systems of muscle and nonmuscle cells to the assessment of cardiovascular toxicity. Co-cultures of vascular endothelial and smooth muscle cells have been successfully used to study cell–cell interactions *in vitro* (54,55). Cardiac myocytes have also been co-cultured in the presence of neurons to attempt to replicate some of the relationships observed *in vivo*. These systems reconstruct the complexities of the cellular environment *in vivo*, but retain the advantages inherent to cell culture. The complexity of co-culture systems is exemplified by studies which show that endothelial cells modulate the extent of binding, internalization, and degradation of low-density lipoproteins by arterial smooth muscle cells (56) and produce growth factors for both smooth muscle cells and fibroblasts.

CONCLUDING REMARKS

The successful application of *in vitro* model systems to evaluate the cardiovascular toxicity of drugs and chemicals has evolved from many years of coordinated research effort. Experiments using any one of the *in vitro* model systems described here can be conducted using tissues from naive animals which have been challenged with test chemicals *in vitro* or from animals which have been dosed *in vivo* and then processed for *in vitro* measurements. Finally, it must be recognized that if systems are used as *in vitro* predictors of the human response, the preparations should be derived from species which respond with fidelity to the toxic challenge.

REFERENCES

1. Pilcher GD, Langley AE. The effects of perfluoro-*n*-decanoic acid in the rat heart. *Toxicol Appl Pharmacol* 1986;85:389–397.

2. Hale PW, Poklis A. Cardiotoxicity of thioridazine and two steroisomeric forms of thioridazine 5-sulfoxide in the isolated perfused rat heart. *Toxicol Appl Pharmacol* 1986;86:44–55.
3. Khatter JC, Agbanyo M, Navaratnam S, Nero B, Hoeschen RJ. Digitalis cardiotoxicity: cellular calcium overload a possible mechanism. *Basic Res Cardiol* 1989;84:553–563.
4. Neely JE, Liebermeister H, Battersby EJ, Morgan HE. Effect of pressure development on oxygen consumption in isolated rat hearts. *Am J Physiol* 1967;212:804–814.
5. McFaul SJ, McGrath JJ. Studies on the mechanism of carbon monoxide-induced vasodilation in the isolated perfused rat heart. *Toxicol Appl Pharmacol* 1987;87:464–473.
6. Crass MF, Hulsey SM, Bulkley TJ. Use of a new pulsatile perfused rat aorta preparation to study the characteristics of the vasodilator effect of parathyroid hormone. *J Pharmacol Exp Ther* 1988; 245:723–734.
7. Granger HJ, Schelling ME, Lewis RE, Zaweija DC, Meininger CJ. Physiology and pathobiology of the microcirculation. *Am J Otolaryngol* 1988;9:264–277.
8. Foex P. Experimental models of myocardial ischemia. *Br J Anaesth* 1988;61:44–55.
9. Hester RK, Ramos K. Vessel cylinders. In: Tyson C, Frazier J, eds. *Methods in toxicology*. San Diego, CA: Academic Press, 1991.
10. Ramos K. Sarcolemmal dependence of isosorbide dinitrate-induced relaxation of vascular smooth muscle. *Res Commun Chem Pathol Pharmacol* 1986;52:195–205.
11. Chatterjee M, Murphy RA. Calcium-dependent stress maintenance without myosin phosphorylation in "skinned" smooth muscle cells. *Science* 1983;221:464–466.
12. Fabiato A, Fabiato F. Activation of skinned cardiac cells. Subcellular effects of cardioactive drugs. *Eur J Cardiol* 1973;1:143–155.
13. Fabiato A, Fabiato F. Calculator programs for computing the composition of the solutions containing multiple metals and ligands used for experiments with skinned muscle cells. *J Physiol* 1979; 75:363–505.
14. Gibbs CL, Woolley G, Kotsanas G, Gibson WR. Cardiac energetics in daunorubicin-induced cardiomyopathy. *J Mol Cell Cardiol* 1984;16:953–962.
15. Togna G, Dolci N, Caprino L. Inhibition of aortic vessel adenosine diphosphate degradation by cadmium and mercury. *Arch Toxicol* 1984;7:378–381.
16. Ingwall JS, DeLuca M, Sybers HD, Wildenthal K. Fetal mouse hearts: a model for studying ischemia. *Proc Natl Acad Sci USA* 1975;72:2809–2813.
17. Speralakis N, Shigenoubu R. Organ cultured chick embryonic heart cells of various ages. Part I. Electrophysiology. *J Mol Cell Cardiol* 1974;6:449–471.
18. Tanaka H, Kasuya Y, Saito H, Shigenobu K. Organ culture of rat heart: maintained high sensitivity of fetal atria before innervation to norepinephrine. *Can J Physiol Pharmacol* 1987;66:901–906.
19. Gotlieb AI, Boden P. Porcine aortic organ culture: a model to study the cellular response to vascular injury. *In Vitro* 1984;20:535–542.
20. Jacobson SL. Culture of spontaneously contracting myocardial cells from adult rats. *Cell Struct Funct* 1977;2:1–9.
21. Bkailey G, Speralakis N, Doane J. A new method for preparation of isolated single adult myocytes. *Am J Physiol* 1984;247:H1018–H1026.
22. Piper HM, Probst I, Schwartz P, Hutter FJ, Spieckermann PG. Culturing of calcium stable adult cardiac myocytes. *J Mol Cell Cardiol* 1982;14:397–412.
23. Welder A, Grant R, Bradlaw J, Acosta D. A primary culture system of adult rat heart cells for the study of toxicological agents. *In Vitro Cell Dev Biol* 1991;27:921–926.
24. Zimmerman ANE, Hulsmann WG. Paradoxical influences of calcium ions on the permeability of the cell membranes of the isolated heart. *Nature* 1966;211:646–647.
25. Welder AW, Machu T, Leslie SW, Wilcox RE, Bradlaw JD, Acosta D. Beta adrenergic receptor characteristics of postnatal rat myocardial cell preparations. *In Vitro Cell Dev Biol* 1988;24:771–777.
26. Alipui C, Ramos K. Tenner T. Alteration of aortic smooth muscle cell proliferation in diabetes mellitus. *Cardio Res* (in press).
27. Kasten FR. Rat myocardial cells *in vitro*: mitosis and differentiated properties. *In Vitro* 1972;8:128–149.
28. Barnes DM. Joint Soviet–U.S. attack on heart muscle dogma. *Science* 1988;242:193–195.
29. Rumyantsev PP. Interrelations of the proliferation and differentiation processes during cardiac myogenesis and regeneration. *Int Rev Cytol* 1977;51:187.
30. Claycomb WC, Lanson NA Jr. Proto-oncogene expression in proliferating and differentiating cardiac and skeletal muscle. *Biochem J* 1987;247:701–706.

31. Wang Y-C, Neckelmann N, Mayne A, Herskoqit A, Srinivasan A, Sell KW, Ahmed-Ansair A. Establishment of a human fetal cardiac myocyte cell line. *In Vitro Cell Dev Biol* 1991;27:63–74.
32. Ramos K, Cox LR. Primary cultures of rat aortic endothelial and smooth muscle cells: an *in vitro* model to study xenobiotic-induced vascular cytotoxicity. *In Vitro Cell Dev Biol* 1987;23:288–296.
33. Simionescu M, Simionescu N. Isolation and characterization of endothelial cells from the heart microvasculature. *Microvasc Res* 1978;16:426–452.
34. Obeso J, Weber J, Auerbach R. A hemangioendothelionia-derived cell line: its use as a model for the study of endothelial cell biology. *Lab Invest* 1990;63:259–269.
35. Stegeman JE, Miller MR, Hinton, DE. Cytochrome P4501A1 induction and localization in endothelium of vertebrate (teleost) heart. *Mol Pharmacol* 1989;36:723–729.
36. Ramos K, Acosta D. The heart. Primary cultures of newborn myocardial cells as a model system to evaluate the cardiotoxicity of drugs and chemicals. In: McQueen C, ed. *In vitro models in toxicology*. Caldwell, NJ: Telford Press, 1989.
37. McDonagh JC, Cebrat EK, Nathan RD. Highly enriched preparations of cultured myocardial cells for biochemical and physiological analyses. *J Mol Cell Cardiol* 1987;19:785–793.
38. Wenzel DG, Cosma GN. A model system for measuring comparative toxicities of cardiotoxic drugs with cultured rat heart myocytes, endothelial cells and fibroblasts. I. Emetine, chloroquine and metronidazole. *Toxicology* 1984;33:103–115.
39. Cox LR, Ramos K. Allylamine-induced phenotypic modulation of aortic smooth muscle cells. *Br J Exp Pathol* 1989.
40. Ives CL, Eskin SG, McIntire LV. Mechanical effects on endothelial cell morphology: *in vitro* assessment. *In Vitro Cell Dev Biol* 1986;22:500–507.
41. Sato GH. The growth of cells in serum-free hormone supplemented media. *Methods Enzymol* 1979;58:94–109.
42. Ramos K, Weber TJ, Liau G. Vascular smooth muscle cell proliferation: influence of substratum and growth conditions *in vitro*. *Biochem J* 1993;289:57–63.
43. Bishop CT, Mirza Z, Crapo JD, Freeman BA. Free radical damage to cultured porcine aortic endothelial cells and lung fibroblasts: modulation by culture conditions. *In Vitro Cell Dev Biol* 1985; 21:21–25.
44. Owens GK, Thompson MM. Developmental changes in isoactin expression in rat aortic smooth muscle cells *in vivo*. *J Biol Chem* 1986;261:13373–13380.
45. Simpson P, Savion S. Differentiation of rat myocytes in single cell cultures with and without proliferating non-myocardial cells. *Circ Res* 1982;50:101–116.
46. Ramos K. Cellular and molecular basis of xenobiotic-induced cardiovascular toxicity: application of cell culture systems. In: Acosta D., ed. *Focus on cellular molecular toxicology and in vitro toxicology*. Boca Raton, FL: CRC Press, 1990;139–155.
47. Luckhoff A. Measuring cytosolic free calcium concentration in endothelial cells with indo-1: the pitfalls of using the ratio of two fluorescence intensities recorded at different wavelengths. *Cell Calcium* 1986;7:233–248.
48. Wenzel DG, Innis JD. Arrhythmogenic and antiarrhythmic effects of lipolytic factors on cultured heart cells. *Res Commun Chem Pathol Pharmacol* 1983;41:383–396.
49. Aszalos A, Bradlaw JA, Reynaldo EF, Yang GC, El-Hage AN. Studies on the action of nystatin on cultured rat myocardial cells and cell membranes. *Biochem Pharmacol* 1984;33:3779–3786.
50. Yarom R, Hasin S, Raz S, Shimoni Y, Fixler R, Yagen B. T-2 toxin effect on cultured myocardial cells. *Toxicol Lett* 1986;31:1–8.
51. Ramos K. Combs AB, Acosta D. Cytotoxicity of isoproterenol to cultured heart cells: effects of antioxidants on modifying membrane damage. *Toxicol Appl Pharmacol* 1983;70:317–323.
52. Ramos K, Combs AB, Acosta D. Role of calcium in isoproterenol cytotoxicity to cultured myocardial cells. *Biochem Pharmacol* 1984;33:1989–1992.
53. McCall D, Ryan K. The effect of ethanol and acetaldehyde on Na pump function in cultured rat heart cells. *J Mol Cell Cardiol* 1987;19:453–463.
54. Horrigan S, Campbell JH, Campbell GR. Effect of endothelium on VLDL metabolism by cultured smooth muscle cells of differing phenotype. *Atherosclerosis* 1988;71:57–69.
55. Weinberg CB, Bell E. A blood vessel model constructed from collagen and cultured vascular cells. *Science* 1986;231:397–399.
56. Davies PF, Truskey GA, Warren HB, O'Connor SE, Eisenhaure BA. Metabolic cooperation between vascular endothelial cells and smooth muscle cells in coculture: changes in low density lipoprotein metabolism. *J Cell Biol* 1985;101:871–879.

In Vitro Toxicology,
edited by Shayne Cox Gad.
Raven Press, Ltd., New York, © 1994.

12

Gastrointestinal Toxicology:
In Vitro Test Systems

Shayne Cox Gad

Toxicology, SYNERGEN, Boulder, Colorado 80301

The gastrointestinal (GI) tract is a frequently overlooked potential target organ system for toxic effects. Specific GI toxicity is widely thought to be relatively rare and limited in forms. Yet for many potentially toxic agents, the length of the GI tract is not only the region of first contact, but also the route of entry into the body. The structure and function of the tract are also much more complex than generally thought.

Two reasons why the GI tract has been thought of as a relatively insensitive target organ are as follows: (a) it cannot be easily observed directly *in vivo*, and (b) alterations in its functions are rarely expressed in a manner that implicates the tract solely and directly. However, methodology does exist for studying GI function *in vivo*, and the tract is the primary target organ for some toxicants. Indeed, the tract expresses toxicity in a rich variety of manners.

Interest in various forms of GI toxicology has increased significantly since the mid-1980s. The reader is referred to reviews on the subject by Walsh (18,19) and Schiller (12) to gain a better understanding of the background, history, and methodology of the field.

At the same time, interest in having effective *in vitro* models for identifying and studying GI toxicity has arisen from both the organ-system-specific problems with the *in vivo* model cited above and with a set of perceived general advantages for *in vitro* models. (These are discussed in detail elsewhere in this volume.)

TYPES OF GI CELLS AND TOXICITY

The GI tract is not a monocytic structure of one or a few cell types, but rather a connected series of organs each composed of a complex of multifunctional cell types. This organ system is made even more complex in its function by its resident symbiotic population of bacteria. The three large organs which make up the tract—

the stomach and large and small intestines—serve not just as a highway for the passage of nutrients and water into (and waste out of) the body, but also have significant metabolic homeostatic and immunologic functions. The GI tract has a range of expressions of toxicity. These include irritation, cytotoxicity, malabsorption (of electrolytes, fluids, and nutrients), altered motility, altered secretion, and neoplasia. Each of these can actually be subdivided further, and such can be expressed in a range of the cell types present in the tract.

Each of the expressions or types of toxicity in the GI tract deserves some specific consideration. As will be clear, some of the divisions between them are not cut and dried, with a range of interactions existing between each of the major toxicity types. However, the major types of toxicity can be considered as follows:

Irritation   A range of agents irritate the GI tract, causing erythemia, disrupting membrane integrity, and serving to alter both absorption and GI motility. Some necrosis (cell death) may be present, in more advanced stages leading to ulceration.

Cytotoxicity   GI cell populations may be killed selectively (one or two cell types affected) or generally (either a broad range or all types of cells dying). What will be observed is a range of cells displaying stages of disfunction and structural breakdown, becoming increasingly more severe with some dying or dead. As some of the cell types "turn over" regularly, timing of "sampling" (observation) will influence the ability to detect and characterize responses to acute insults.

Malabsorption   Materials are absorbed by the GI tract by a range of mechanisms of both passive and active nature. Electrolytes (sodium, potassium and chloride ions, largely), fluids (mostly water), nutrients, and pharmaceutical agents have the tract as their chief route of entry into the body.

Altered secretory activity   A primary function of the GI tract is secretion of various entities into its contents (the major example being secretion of hydrogen ions by the parietal cells into the stomach). Agents which irritate the mucosa can produce gastritis, leading to reduced secretion. Other agents can stimulate gastric secretion, which can lead to acid-induced erosions and ulcers in the stomach and duodenum.

Altered motility   GI motility *in vivo* is influenced by the smooth muscle cells, entrinsic nervous system inputs, extrinsic nervous system input, hormone, and the constituents and volume of luminal content. Proper motility is essential for both absorptive functions and in influencing the potential of toxicants to do harm.

Neoplasia   The transformation of constituent cell types to proliferative, nonfunctional forms. Some animal model GI neoplasias (such as rodent forestomach cancer) do not appear to have true human analogues. Some of the high-turnover-rate cell populations in the GI tract are particularly prone to neoplasia.

Symbiotic population alteration   Proper functioning of the GI tract, particularly in terms of absorption and metabolism, is dependent on there being a stable population (in terms of both organism types and numbers) of micro-organisms in portions of the tract. Well-recognized are the adverse effects of some antibiotics on tract function due to their altering the balance of the resident microbial population. These same populations play significant roles in the toxicity and carcinogenicity of a number of agents (10).

IN VITRO MODELS

The models available for use in toxicity testing can be classified in various ways. Table 1 presents one classification of models in general based on complexity, with intact organisms being the most complex and computer simulation the least. As the table broadly points out, each of these levels has advantages and disadvantages.

More specifically, we should consider models (both *in vivo* and *in vitro*) designed to address the classes of end points that were presented in the preceding section.

Irritation

Irritation is usually evaluated by gross or microscopic evaluation of the surface of the tract after the selected test species has received or been exposed to the material of interest for a predetermined period of time. Such examinations are usually performed after terminal sacrifice of the test animals. One can also monitor the rate of

TABLE 1. *Levels of models for toxicity testing and research*

Level/Model	Advantages	Disadvantages
In vivo (intact higher organism)	Full range of organismic responses similar to target species.	Costs. Ethical/animal welfare concerns. Species-to-species variability.
Lower organisms (earthworms, fish)	Range of integrated organismic responses.	Frequently lack responses of higher organism. Animal welfare concerns.
Isolated organs	Intact yet isolated tissue and vascular system. Controlled environmental and exposure conditions.	Donor organism still required. Time-consuming and expensive. No intact organismic responses. Limited length of viability.
Cultured cells	No intact animals directly involved. Ability to carefully manipulate system. Low costs. Wide range of variables can be studied.	Instability of system. Limited enzymatic capabilities and viability of system. No or limited integrated multicell and/or organismic responses.
Chemical/ biochemical systems	No donor organism problems. Low cost. Long-term stability of prep. Wide range of variables can be studied. Specificity of response.	No *de facto* correlation to *in vivo* system. Limited to investigation of single defined mechanism.
Computer simulations	No animal welfare concerns. Speed and low per evaluation cost.	Problematic predictive value beyond narrow range of structures. Expensive to establish.

loss of cells from the GI surface into the luminal fluid. As irritation is more a tissue response than cell response, it is harder to model *in vitro*

Cytoxicity

In vivo, the same methods used to evaluate irritation can be and are used to evaluate cytotoxicity. These can also be considered under the alternate label of "assessment of structural integrity" of the tract or portion of interest of the tract. Another gross measure of such integrity *in vivo* is fecal blood loss, which tells if significant damage has been done.

In vitro, assessment of cytoxicity to either single-cell-type populations or mixed cultures is one of the most basic methodologies for all target tissues.

Malabsorption

What is actually assessed is the absorptive function. The simplest approach is to measure how much of a labeled material which is administered shows up in the systemic fluids. Accurate measurement requires consideration of appropriate pharmacokinetic considerations.

In vitro methods available include the inverted intestinal sac (20) and the use of rings cut from the whole wall of the intestine (23), which provides a better oxygenated tissue model but is generally limited to measurement of accumulation of materials of interest in the ring tissue. There is also the Ussing chamber (11,14), which allows measurement of electrolyte flux across the intestinal membranes.

Altered Secretory Activity

There are both invasive and noninvasive *in vivo* techniques. The invasive requires surgical implantation of a sampling tube (16). The noninvasive method requires quantitation of how much azure A is released from an azure A–resin complex in the stomach (13). Available *in vitro* methods have been very useful in understanding mechanisms. The Ussing chamber and isolated parietal cells from gastric glands (11,14,15) are useful for both mechanistic and some limited test material screening-specific questions.

Altered Motility

The continued motility of the GI tract serves to move contents steadily through its length and out of the body. *In vivo*, one can simply measure the transit of one of a number of nonabsorbable intraluminal markers. Isolated superfused ileum can be used to evaluate specific test material responses (5), while isolated rabbit jejunum preparations (4) or cultured myocytes (1) can be used to study transit times and mechanistic questions, respectively.

Neoplasia

What is actually measured specific to the GI tract is the proliferation of mucosal cells. *In vivo* this can be measured by rates of incorporation of ^{3}H-thymidine. It can also now be measured using flow cytometry.

Symbiotic Population Alternation

There are methodologies for evaluating bacterial metabolism of gut flora *in vitro* (with gut contents having been collected and incubated) and *in vivo*, and the *in situ* bacterial flora of the intestine. The actual study of effects on the flora itself is best done *in vitro* using variations on traditional microbiology techniques, but it is difficult to model the complex interactions between these organisms and a host organism using an *in vitro* methodology.

Table 2 presents an overview of eight different *in vitro* test systems available (and used for) evaluating GI toxicity. Each focuses on one or two specific functional end points of toxicity, with either perfused/superfused tissues or organs or cultured cells

TABLE 2. In vitro *test systems for gastrointestinal toxicity*

System	End point	Evaluation	References
Isolated perfused intestines (M)	Functional: biochemical and metabolic	Correlation with *in vivo* finding for methylprednisolone	Mehendale (9)
Isolated perfused intestines (M)	Functional: biochemical and metabolic	Limited	Mehendale (9)
Isolated superfused ileum (S)	Functional: pharmacologic responses and biochemical	Correlation with *in vivo* findings for antitoxidants and receptor-mediated agents	Gad et al. (5)
Stomach wall in a Ussing chamber (M)	Functional: gastric secretion (acid secretion), electrolyte flux	Correlation for pharmacological agents	Soll (14) Sachs and Berglingh (11)
Parietal cells from gastric glands (M, S)	Functional: hydrogen ion secretion measurement	Good correlation for ulcerogens	Soll (14) Sachs and Berglingh (11) Soll and Berglingh (15)
Inverted intestinal sac (M)	Functional: energy-mediated carrier transport process	Well studied	Wilson and Wiseman (20)
Isolated rabbit jejenum (M)	Functional: motility measurement	Well studied and correlated	Edinburgh (4)
Cultured myocytes (M)	Functional: motility	Limited	Bitar and Makhlouf (1)

NOTE: Letters in parentheses indicate primary employment of system: (S), screening system; (M), mechanistic tool.

as models. These are categorized, somewhat arbitrarily, as either screening or mechanistic systems, depending on the emphasis of their use to date.

SPECIFIC PROBLEMS/LIMITATIONS OF *IN VITRO* GI MODELS

Though components of many of the functions of the GI tract are expressions of the function of a specific cell or tissue type, the overall functions of interest are largely expressions of an integrated physiological and biochemical function. The chief limitation of *in vitro* assessment of GI toxicity is that it is either not possible or only possible on a very limited basis to model the organ-system-wide nature of such functions as motility (mass transport) and absorption. Similarly, effects on the microbial populations/ecologies of the GI tract regions are very complex. Aspects of these can be studied *in vitro*, as Table 2 establishes, but not the entire functionality.

Similarly, modeling the *in vivo* modes (and characteristics) of exposure to environmental agents in *in vitro* models is particularly difficult. In part this is because there are so many sources of potential toxicants—ingestion (which can include inhaled, particularly water, contaminants, dietary components and contaminants, drugs, etc.), tract secretions (both plasma and biliary toxicants), microbial products, and the products of GI biotransformation of environmental agents.

REFERENCES

1. Bitar KN, Makhlouf GM. Receptors on smooth muscle cells: characterization by contraction and specific antagonists. *Am J Physiol* 1982;242(4):G400–G407.
2. Crane RK, Mandelstam P. The active transport of sugars by various preparations of hamster intestine. *Biochim Biophys Acta* 1960;45:460–476.
3. Crane RK, Wilson TH. *In vitro* method for the study of the rate of intestinal absorption of sugars. *J Appl Physiol* 1958;12:145–146.
4. Department of Pharmacology, University of Edinburgh. *Pharmacological experiments on isolated preparations* Edinburgh: E&S Livingstone, 1970.
5. Gad SC, Leslie SW, Acosta D. Inhibiting actions of butylated hydroxytoluene (BHT) on isolated rat ileal, atrial and perfused heart preparations. *Toxicol Appl Pharmacol* 1979;48:45–52.
6. Hohenleitner FJ, Senior JR. Metabolism of canine small intestine vascularly perfused *in vitro*. *J Appl Physiol* 1969;26:119–128.
7. Howdle PD. Organ culture of gastrointestinal mucosa. *Postgrad Med J* 1984;60:645–652.
8. Kimmich GA. Intestinal absorption of sugar. In: Johnson LR, ed. *Physiology of the gastrointestinal tract*, vol 2. New York: Raven, 1981:1035–1062.
9. Mehendale HM. Application of isolated organ techniques in toxicology. In: Hayes AW, ed. *Principles and methods of toxicology*. New York: Raven, 1989:699–740.
10. Rowland IR. *Role of the gut flora in toxicity and cancer*. New York: Academic Press, 1988.
11. Sachs G, Berglingh T. Physiology of the parietal cell. In: Johnson LR, ed. *Physiology of the gastrointestinal tract*. New York: Raven, 1981:570–574.
12. Schiller CM. *Intestinal toxicology:* New York; Raven, 1984.
13. Segal HL, Miller LL, Plumb EJ. Tubeless gastric analysis with an azure A ion-exchange compound. *Gastroenterology* 1955;28:402–408.
14. Soll AH. Secretagogue stimulation of ^{14}C-aminopyrine accumulation by isolated canine parietal cells. *Am J Physiol* 1980;238:G366–G375.
15. Soll AH, Berglingh T. Physiology of isolated gastric land and parietal cells: receptors and effectors

regulating function. In: Johnson LR, ed. *Physiology of the gastrointestinal tract.* New York: Raven, 1987:883–909.

16. Szabo S, Reynolds ES, Lichtenberger LM, Haith LR, Dzau VJ. Pathologenesis of duodenal ulcer: gastric hyperacidity caused by propionitrile and cysteamine in rats. *Res Commun Chem Pathol Pharmacol* 1977;16:311–323.

17. Ussing HH, Zerahn K. Active transport of sodium as the source of electric current in the short-circuited isolated frog skin. *Acta Physiol Scand* 1951;23:110–127.

18. Walsh CT. *Mechanisms of gastrointestinal toxicology.* Society of Toxicology, 1988.

19. Walsh T. Methods in gastrointestinal toxicology. In: Hayes AW, ed. *Principles and methods of toxicology.* New York: Raven, 1989:659–675.

20. Wilson TH, Wiseman G. The use of sacs of everted small intestine for the study of the transference of substances from the mucosal to the serosal surface. *J Physiol (Lond)* 1954;123:116–125.

In Vitro Toxicology,
edited by Shayne Cox Gad.
Raven Press, Ltd., New York, © 1994.

13

Strategy and Tactics for Employment

Shayne Cox Gad

Toxicology, SYNERGEN, Boulder, Colorado 80301

The test methods designed and used to evaluate the potential of man-made materials to cause harm to the people who make, transport, use, or otherwise come in contact with them hold a unique and ambivalent place in our society. On one hand, our society not only is critically dependent on technological advances to improve and/or maintain standards of living, but is also intolerant of risks (real or potential) to life and health—for example, diseases like acquired immunodeficiency syndrome (AIDS) and multiple sclerosis and illness or disability caused by household products, pesticides, or waste products. At the same time, the traditional tests (with both their misuse and misunderstanding of their use) have served as the rallying point for those concerned about the humane and proper use of animals. This has caused the field of testing for potential to cause irritation or damage to the eyes to become both the most active area for the development of alternatives and innovations and the most sensitive area of animal testing and use in research. But all testing using animals has come under question.

In recent years tremendous progress has been made in our understanding of biology down to the molecular level. This has translated to multiple modifications and improvements in *in vitro* testing procedures which now give us tests which (a) are more reliable, reproducible, and predictive of potential hazards in humans, (b) use fewer animals, and (c) are considerably more humane than earlier test forms. At the same time, a number of *in vitro* test systems have been proposed, developed, and validated to at least some extent. Yet the perception persists that little has changed in how safety assessment is performed by or for industry. Why?

It is the intent of this volume to make more scientists aware of the full range of new techniques which are available. But more importantly it is hoped that the whole process involved in testing can be modified so that only what needs to be done will be and that such tests will answer the desired questions in a manner which maximizes efficiency, effectiveness, and animal welfare.

The entire product safety assessment process, in the broadest sense, is a multistage process in which none of the individual steps is overwhelmingly complex, but the integration of the whole process involves fitting together a large complex pattern of pieces. This volume as a whole seeks to address the questions of the use of *in vitro* test methods. How the data generated by the various test systems and models described elsewhere in this volume can be integrated into programs for government and private enterprise to provide for a safe product life cycle is the subject of this chapter. As will be seen, this calls for a significant conceptual modification of the approach to the general product safety assessment problem, and it will be addressed by starting with the current general case and progressing to plans and a means for changing the process in an interative fashion. Along the way, limitations of current models and approach and places where testing and research data could be made more practically useful will be pointed out. Particularly with an understanding of mechanisms becoming increasingly important in both product design and evaluating the relevance of findings, the integration of *in vitro* methodologies into the product safety assessment process has become essential.

The entire safety assessment process which supports new product research and development is a multistage process in which none of the individual steps is overwhelmingly complex, but for which the integration of the whole process involves fitting together a large complex pattern of pieces. In this chapter an approach is proposed in which integration of *in vitro* test systems calls for a modification of the approach to the general product safety assessment problem. This modification can be addressed by starting with the current general case and progressing to a means for changing the process in an iterative fashion. Particularly with an understanding of mechanisms becoming increasingly important in both candidate drug selection and the design and evaluation of the relevance of findings, the integration of *in vitro* methodologies, particularly into the pharmaceutical safety assessment process, has become essential.

The single most important part of any product safety evaluation program is, in fact, the initial overall process of defining and developing an adequate data package on the potential hazards associated with the product life cycle (the manufacture, sale, use and disposal of a product and associated process materials) (2). To do this, one must ask a series of questions in a very interactive process, with many of the questions designed to identify and/or modify their successors. The first is, What information is needed?

Determining what information is needed calls for understanding the way in which the chemical is to be made and used, as well as understanding the potential health and safety risks associated with exposure of humans who will be either using the drug or associated with the processes involved in making it. This is on the basis of a hazard and toxicity profile. Once such a profile is established (as illustrated in Fig. 1), the available literature is searched to determine what is already known. Much of the necessary information for support of safety claims in registration of a new drug is regulatorily mandated. This is not the case at all, however, for those safety studies done (a) to select candidate products for development, or (b) to design pivotal safety studies to support registration, or (c) to pursue mechanistic questions.

Taking into consideration this literature information and the previously defined exposure profile, a tier approach (Fig. 2) has traditionally been used to generate a

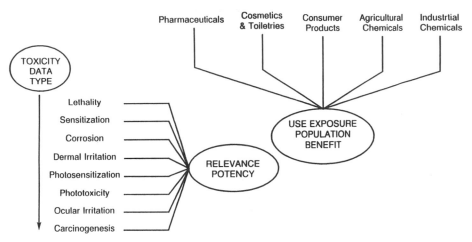

FIG. 1. Multidimensional matrix for hazard assessment. What are the hazards associated with a new product is a multidimensional problem depending on (a) the product's intended use, its innate toxicity, and its physiochemical properties and (b) the potential human and environmental exposure. This matrix diagrammatically illustrates the key questions involved in developing the final hazard assessment profile.

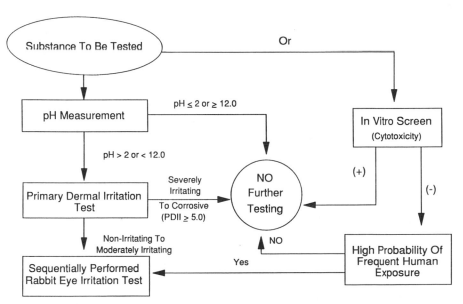

FIG. 2. Alternative tier approaches for eye irritation testing. The usual plan for characterizing the toxicity of a compound or product is to develop information in a tier approach. More information is required (a higher tier level is attained) as the volume of production and the potential for exposure increase. A common scheme is shown.

list of tests or studies to be performed.[1] What goes into a tier system is determined by (a) regulatory requirements imposed by government agencies, (b) the philosophy of the parent organization, (c) economics, and (d) available technology. How such tests are actually performed is determined on one of two bases. The first (and most common) is the menu approach: selecting a series of standard design tests as "modules" of data. The second is an interactive/iterative approach, where strategies are developed and studies are designed based both on needs and on what has been learned to date about the product.

DEFINING TESTING OBJECTIVES

The initial and most important aspect of a product safety evaluation program is the series of steps that leads to an actual statement of the problem or of the objectives of any testing and research program. This definition of objectives is essential and, as proposed here, consists of five steps: (i) defining product or material use, (ii) estimating or quantitating exposure potential, (iii) identifying potential hazards, (iv) gathering baseline data, and (v) designing and defining the actual research program to answer outstanding questions. Later, we will look at the specific application of this to dermal and ocular toxicity cases, where the concept of *communities of interest* (that is an understanding of the needs of the organization producing the material and the users) will become essential. This concept will be discussed in detail later.

Objectives Behind Data Generation and Utilization

To understand how product safety and toxicity data are used, and how the data generation process might be changed to better meet the product safety assessment needs of society, it is essential to understand that different regulatory organizations have different answers to these questions. The ultimate solution is in the form of a multidimensional matrix, with the three major dimensions of the matrix being (i) the toxicity data type (lethality, sensitization, corrosion, irritation, photosensitization, phototoxicity, etc.), (ii) exposure characteristics (extent, population size, population characteristics, etc.) and (iii) the stage in the research and development process we are dealing with.

What is called for is a careful zero-based consideration of what the optimum product safety assessment strategy for a particular problem should be. A framework for such a strategy which integrates both *in vitro* and *in vivo* tests is as shown in Fig. 1. Before formulating such a strategy and deciding what mix of tests should be used, it is first necessary to decide criteria for what would constitute an ideal (or acceptable) test system.

---

[1]There is also the special case of pharmaceutical and pesticide products, where there are regulatory mandated minimum test batteries.

Any useful test system must be sufficiently sensitive that the incidence of false-negatives is low. Clearly a high incidence of false-negatives is intolerable. In such a situation, large numbers of dangerous chemical agents would be carried through extensive additional testing only to find that they possess undesirable toxicological properties after the expenditures of significant time and money. On the other hand, a test system which is overly sensitive will give rise to a high incidence of false-positives which could have the deleterious consequence of rejecting potentially valuable drugs. The "ideal" test will fall somewhere between these two extremes and thus provide adequate protection without unnecessarily stifling development.

The "ideal" test should have an end-point measurement which provides data such that dose–response relationships can be obtained. Furthermore, any criterion of effect must be sufficiently accurate in the sense that it can be used to reliably resolve the relative toxicity of two compounds which produce distinct (in terms of hazard to humans) yet similar responses. In general, it may not be sufficient to classify compounds into generic toxicity categories, such as "intermediate" toxicity, since a candidate chemical which falls in a given category, yet is borderline to the next more severe toxicity category, should be treated with more concern than a second candidate which falls at the less toxic extreme of the same category. Therefore it is useful for a test system to be able to rank compounds with potentially similar uses accurately within any general toxicity category.

The end-point measurement of the "ideal" test system must be objective. This is important so that a given compound will give similar results when tested using the standard test protocol in different laboratories. If it is not possible to obtain reproducible results in a given laboratory over time or between various laboratories, then the historical database against which new compounds are evaluated will be time/laboratory-dependent. Along these lines, it is important for the test protocol to incorporate internal standards to serve as quality controls. Thus, test data could be represented utilizing a reference scale based on the test system response to the internal controls. Such normalization, if properly documented, could reduce intertest variability.

The test results for any given compound should be reproducible both intrinsically (within the same laboratory over time) and extrinsically (between laboratories). If this condition is not satisfied, then there will be significant limitations on the application of the test system because it would potentially produce conflicting results. From a regulatory point of view, this possibility would be highly undesirable (and perhaps indefensible).

Alternatives to current *in vivo* test systems basically should be designed to evaluate the subject toxic response in a manner as closely predictive of that in man as possible while also reducing animal use and avoiding inhumane treatments.

From a practical point of view, there are several additional features of the "ideal" test which should be satisfied. The test should be rapid so that the turnaround time for a given compound is reasonable. Obviously the speed of the test and the ability to conduct tests on several chemicals simultaneously will determine the overall productivity. The test should be inexpensive so that it is economically competitive with current testing practices. And finally, the technology should be easily transferred from one laboratory to another without excessive capital investment for test implementation. It should be kept in mind that although some of these practical considerations may appear to present formidable limitations for a given test system at the present time, the possibility of future developments in testing technology could overcome these obstacles.

This brief discussion of the characteristics of the "ideal" test system provides a general framework for evaluation of alternative test systems in general. No test system is likely to be "ideal."

Therefore, it will be necessary to weigh the strengths and weaknesses of each proposed test system in order to reach a conclusion on how "good" a particular test is. The next section will present the basis for the specific test evaluation.

In both theory and practice, both *in vivo* and *in vitro* tests have potential advantages. Tables 1 and 2 summarize these advantages.

DESIGNING THE RESEARCH PROGRAM

The next step, given that no data are found from any literature sources (and that it has been determined that data are needed), is to perform appropriate predictive tests. The bulk of this volume addresses specifics of performing such tests using *in vitro* models. Before considering how to design and conduct a testing program, we must first consider how the practice of safety assessment came to its current state in the employment of such tests.

To understand how product safety and toxicity data are used, and how the data generation process might be changed to better meet the product safety assessment needs of society, it is essential to understand that different commercial and regula-

---

TABLE 1. *Rationale for using* in vivo *test systems*

1. Provides evaluation of actions/effects on intact animal and organ/tissue interactions.
2. Either pure chemical entities or complete formulated products (complex mixtures) can be evaluated.
3. Either concentration or diluted products can be tested.
4. Yields data on the recovery and healing processes.
5. Required statutory tests for agencies such as the Food and Drug Administration (for "pivotal" safety studies) and the European Economic Community (EEC).
6. Quantitative and qualitative tests with scoring system, generally capable of ranking materials as to relative hazards.
7. Amenable to modifications to meet the requirements of special situations (such as multiple dosing or exposure schedules).
8. Extensive available database and cross-reference capability for evaluation of relevance to human situation.
9. The ease of performance and relative low capital costs in many cases.
10. Tests are generally both conservative and broad in scope, providing for maximum protection by erring on the side of overprediction of hazard to man.
11. Tests can be either single end point (such as lethality, pyrogenicity, etc.) or shot-gun [also called multiple end point (including such test systems as a 13-week oral toxicity study)].

TABLE 2. *Rationale for seeking* in vitro *alternatives for toxicity tests*

1. Avoid complications (and potential confounding or masking findings) or animal and tissue/organ *in vivo* evaluation.
2. *In vivo* systems may only assess short-term site of application or immediate structural alterations produced by agents. Note, however, that tests may only be intended to evaluate acute local effects.
3. Technician training and monitoring are critical (particularly if the evaluation called for is subjective in nature).
4. If our objective is either the total exclusion of a particular type of agent or the identification of truly severe acting agents on an absolute basis (that is, without false-positives or false-negatives), *in vivo* tests in animals do not perfectly predict results in humans.
5. Clearly, there are structural and biochemical differences between test animals and humans which make extrapolation from one to the other difficult.
6. Lack of standardization of *in vivo* systems.
7. Variable correlation with human results.
8. Large biological variability between more complex experimental units (i.e., individual animals).
9. Large, diverse and fragmented databases which are not readily comparable.

tory organizations have different answers to these questions. The ultimate answer is a multidimensional matrix, with the three major dimensions of the matrix being (i) the toxicity data type (lethality, sensitization, corrosion, irritation, photosensitization, phototoxicity, etc.), (ii) exposure characteristics (extent, population size, population characteristics, etc.) and (iii) type of commercial organization (or organizations) regulated (which we will call the "community of interest"). This matrix was shown in Fig. 1.

Communities of interest are defined by how the products are to be used, who regulates their use, and what benefits are expected for the consumer. There are a number of ways of classifying such communities, but for our purposes we will divide and define them as follows.

Pharmaceuticals: Materials of concern are agents intended as therapeutics (or medical devices) where the production worker or health care provider (doctor, nurse or pharmacist) may have a significant chance of exposure, but the major concern is for those patients who receive or use the drug or device. The Food and Drug Administration (FDA) is the primary United States (US) regulator.

Cosmetics and Toiletries: The materials are cosmetics, fragrances, shampoos, hand and body soaps, hair dyes, and other materials intended to improve appearance and personal presentation. These are intended to be applied to the skin (or other body surface) or to be applied or used in a manner that makes dermal or ocular exposure (at least) unavoidable. The major US regulators are the FDA and the Consumer Product Safety Commission (CPSC).

Consumer Products: Products intended to be used by the average person in and around their home can be divided into those that have a high potential for exposure (dish and laundry detergents, for example), those that have low potential for such exposure (drain cleaners, oven cleaners, etc.), or those that are somewhere in a wide range in between (such as window and carpet cleaners). The primary regulators are the CPSC and the Department of Transportation (DOT), but the Environmental Protection Agency (EPA) also is important in terms of new chemical entities and disposal and waste management.

Agricultural Products: These products are pesticides, herbicides, fertilizers, and other international food additives (such as preservatives, sterilants, etc.). The extent of dermal, inhalation, oral, and other routes of exposure will vary widely in use. Note that these could be subdivided into those agents used in the field (that is, actually used in agriculture), those for home or inside use, and those agents used in the storage and processing of foods. Regulatory oversight is vested primarily in the EPA [under the Federal Insecticide, Fungicide and Rodenticide Act (FIFRA)], with secondary considerations by DOT and FDA. The third group (those used on foods) has the FDA as the primary driving force, with EPA and DOT concerns secondary.

Industrial Chemicals: These are materials to which the major exposure is to workers involved in the manufacture and transportation of products. In a sense, all the materials (e.g., the above categories) fall into this group at some time, plus a number of other chemicals that never appear (as such) in those categories (such as hydrofluoric acid and plasticizers). These are handled by a smaller population relative to most other products. Direct contact is never intended; in fact, active measures are taken to prevent it. The use of safety assessment data in these cases is to fulfill labeling requirements for shipping (DOT) and protecting workers (OSHA) and to provide hazard assessment information for accidental exposures and its treatment (DOT and OSHA). The results of such tests do not directly affect the economic future of a material.

Each of these communities have different needs and uses for each of the kinds of data produced, and these must be considered independently.

What is called for is a careful consideration of what the optimum product safety assessment strategy would be. A framework for such a strategy is as shown in Fig. 3. The components that constitute each of the data generation tool boxes shown (screens, confirmatory tests, higher-tier tests, and mechanistic evaluations) are common to all safety assessment programs in some form. But what is actually used for each of these tasks is not common to all of these programs, nor is how the judgement ovals (here labeled acceptance criterion and risk/benefit judgement) operate. The selection of these details are what constitutes the actual formulation of a strategy. Before formulating such a strategy and deciding what mix of tests should be used, it is first necessary to decide criteria for what would constitute an ideal (or acceptable) test program.

Considerations in Adopting New Test Systems

Conducted toxicological investigations in two or more species of laboratory animals is generally accepted as being a prudent and responsible practice in developing a new chemical entity, especially one that is expected to receive widespread use and

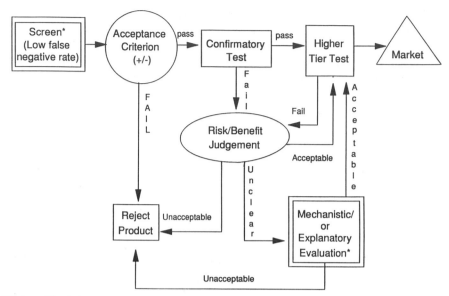

*Points For Initial Employment of In Vitro Tests

FIG. 3. Iterative approach to a tiered product safety assessment. Within a tiered product safety assessment approach, it is possible to ask each question to a different degree of detail. If an early evaluation provides sufficient information, testing may be complete with relatively low expense. Conversely, it may also be determined that a more detailed (or specific) assay must be performed. Shown here is such an iteractive approach which identifies points where *in vitro* systems could readily be utilized in place of *in vivo* systems.

to have exposure potential over human lifetimes. Adding a second or third species to the testing regimen offers an extra measure of confidence to the toxicologist and the other professionals who will be responsible for evaluating the associated risks, benefits, and exposure limitations or protective measures. Although it undoubtedly broadens and deepens a compound's profile of toxicity, the practice of enlarging on the number of test species is, as has been demonstrated in multiple points in the literature (ref. 5 for example), an indiscriminate scientific generalization. Moreover, such a tactic is certain to generate the problem of species specific toxicoses; that is, a toxic response or an inordinately low biological threshold for toxicity is evident in one species or strain, whereas all other species examined are either unresponsive or strikingly less sensitive. The investigator confronting such findings must be prepared to address the all-important question "Are humans likely to react positively or negatively to the test agent under similar circumstances"?

Assuming that numerical odds prevail and that humans automatically fit into the predominant category, whether on the side of being safe or at risk, would be scientifically irresponsible. Far from being an irreconcilable nuisance, however, such a confounded situation can be an opportunity to advance more quickly into the heart of the search for predictive information. Species-specific toxicosis can frequently contribute toward better understanding of the general case if the underlying biological mechanism either causing or enhancing toxicity is defined, especially if it is discovered to uniquely reside in the sensitive species.

A mention of species-specific toxicoses usually implies that either different metabolic pathways for converting and excreting xenobiotics or anatomical differences are involved. The design of our current safety evaluation tests appear to serve society reasonably well (i.e., significantly more times than not) in identifying hazards that would be unacceptable in a confirmatory manner. However, the process can just as clearly be improved from the standpoints of both improving our protection of society and performing necessary screening and exploratory research in a manner that uses fewer animals and uses these fewer animals in a more humane manner.

In Vitro Models

In vitro models, at least as screening tests, have been with us in toxicology for some 20 years now. The last 5–10 years has brought a great upsurge in interest in such models. This increased interest is due to economic and animal welfare pressures and technological improvements.

It should be noted that, in addition to potential advantage, *in vitro* systems per se

TABLE 3. *Possible interpretations when* in vitro *data do not predict results of* in vivo *studies*

1. Compound is not absorbed at all or is poorly absorbed in *in vivo* studies.
2. Chemical is well absorbed but is subject to first-pass effect in liver.
3. Compound is distributed so that less (or more) reaches the receptors than would be predicted on the basis of its absorption.
4. Chemical is rapidly metabolized to an active or inactive metabolite that has a different profile of activity and/or different duration of action than the parent drug.
5. Compound is rapidly eliminated (e.g., through secretory mechanisms).
6. Species of the two test systems used are different.
7. Experimental conditions of the *in vitro* and *in vivo* experiments differed and may have led to different effects than expected. These conditions include factors such as temperature or age, sex, and strain of animal.
8. Effects elicited *in vitro* and *in vivo* by the particular case in question differ in their characteristics.
9. Tests used to measure responses will probably differ greatly for *in vitro* and *in vivo* studies, and the types of data obtained may not be comparable.
10. The *in vitro* study did not use adequate controls (e.g., pH, vehicle used, volume of test agent given, samples taken from sham-operated animals).
11. *In vitro* data cannot predict the volume of distribution in central or in peripheral compartments.
12. *In vitro* data cannot predict the rate constants for movement of drug agent between compartment.
13. *In vitro* data cannot predict the rate constants of chemical elimination.
14. *In vitro* data cannot predict whether linear or nonlinear kinetics will occur with specific dose of a drug *in vitro*.
15. Pharmacokinetic parameters (e.g., bioavailability, peak plasma concentration, half-life) cannot be predicted based solely on *in vitro* studies.
16. *In vivo* effects of chemical are due to an alteration in the higher order of an intact animal system, which cannot be reflected in a less complex system.

also have a number of limitations which can contribute to their not being acceptable models. Some of these reasons are detailed in Table 3.

At the same time, as demonstrated throughout this volume, there are substantial potential advantages in using *in vitro* system. These advantages of using cell or tissue culture in toxicological testing are (a) isolation of test cells or organ fragments from homeostatic and hormonal control, (b) accurate dosing, and (c) quantitation or results. It is important to devise a suitable model system which is related to the mode of toxicity of the compound. Tissue and cell culture has the immediate potential to be used in two very different ways by industry. Firstly, it has been used to examine a particular aspect of the toxicity of a compound in relation to its toxicity *in vivo* (i.e, mechanistic or explanatory studies). Secondly, it has been used as a form of rapid screening to compare the toxicity of a group of compounds for a particular form of response. Indeed, the pharmaceutical industry has used *in vitro* test systems in these two ways for years in the search for new potential drug entities.

The author has already addressed the theory and use of screens in toxicology (3). Mechanistic and explanatory studies are generally called for when a traditional test system gives a result that is unclear or whose relevance to the real-life human exposure is doubted. *In vitro* systems are particularly attractive for such cases because they can focus on very defined single aspects of a problem or pathogenic response, free of the confounding influence of the multiple responses of an intact higher-level organism. Note, however, that first one must know the nature (indeed the existence of) the questions to be addressed.

Short-Term Advances: A Mixed Battery

1. Product safety assessment should not continue to be performed as it traditionally has been.
2. There are no generally accepted *in vitro* test systems immediately available to completely replace all (or, indeed, any) of the *in vivo* testing requirements.
3. There are some steps which can be taken to move development and acceptance of *in vitro* systems along.
4. There are some modifications to current *in vivo* testing methods which both can and should be adopted.

Before developing these points, however, one must consider the needs of the communities of interest responsible for testing and understand the basic concept of a screen (as opposed to a definitive test).

Concept of Screens

Screens are simple tests which try to answer single questions with great sensitivity (but not necessarily marked specificity). Many of the currently proposed *in vitro* systems show immediate promise as screens. As such, they would be employed to rapidly and efficiently identify those materials which were clearly strong irritants or corrosives—for example, those which would therefore not need further evaluation.

Until *in vitro* tests are further developed and accepted, the appropriate strategy (or mix or tests) for industrial safety assessment should be mixed tier approach (such as Fig. 3) utilizing *in vitro* tests as screens. The tier approach presented in Table 4 is one form which can be (and is being) utilized currently (for ocular irritation), but this can be improved on. For the short term, a better system could be used which employs a mixed series of screening steps. Such a system would have the following stages (using the particular case of evaluation of potential eye irritants as an example).

I. *In Vitro* Screen

a. Extremely active compounds in any assay (such as one of the cytotoxicity test systems) should be considered strong irritants (or worse) and classified/handled as such. Note that this should also serve to identify (among others) the same compounds as the current pH screen, and therefore that step is not required.

b. Less active or inactive compounds would pass on, unless the testing need was only to identify I(a)-type compounds (in which case testing is complete).

TABLE 4. *Tier testing[a,b]*

Tier testing	Mammalian toxicology	Genetic toxicology	Remarks
0	Literature review	Literature review	Upon initial identification of a problem, a database of existing information and of particulars of use of materials is established
1	Cytotoxicity screens Dermal sensitization Acuted systemic toxicity Lethality screens	Ames tests *In vitro* SCE *In vitro* cytogenetics Forward mutation/CHO	R&D materials and low-volume chemicals with severe limited exposure
2	Subacute studies Metabolism Primary dermal irritation Eye irritation	*In vivo* SCE *In vivo* cytogenetics	Medium-volume materials and/or those with a significant chance of human exposure
3	Subchronic studies Reproduction Teratology Chronic studies Mechanic studies		Any material with a high volume or a potential for widespread repeated human exposure or one which gives indications of specific long-term effects

[a]Shown here is a now widely adopted example of an iterative/tier approach to toxicity testing which utilizes a range of test systems (physicochemical, *in vitro*, and *in vivo*) to minimize both cost and animal usage and distress.

[b]Abbreviations: CHO, Chinese hamster ovary; R&D, research and development; SCE, Sister Chromatid Exchange.

II. Primary Dermal Irritation
   a. Severely irritating to corrosive compounds should be treated as I(a) above.

   b. Mild to nonirritant should be treated as I(b).

III. Staggered Eye Irritation Test
   Using a low-volume-type test, materials would be evaluated using a single animal. If no irritation was seen at 24 h, a second (and 24 h later, a third) rabbit would be added to the test. Clear positive findings would stop the test.

Far Horizons: How to Get Them

Clearly great progress has been made both in practices as to the conduct of safety assessment tests in intact animals and in developing an array of promising *in vitro* candidates for replacement of the *in vivo* test.

Where we would like to be is to have in place (that is, accepted and used by industry and regulation agencies) one or a battery of *in vitro* systems which would reduce the need for intact animal testing to necessary cases. And we would also like to have duplicate or unnecessary testing of materials reduced to a minimum. These goals are dictated as much by economic reasons and the need to do better science as they are by ethical and humane concerns. The efficient and effective safety assessment/toxicology laboratory of the very near future will have as its "front door" an *in vitro* screening shop which will "draw" validated specific target organ screens from a library, as needed, to perform the initial go/no go evaluations on new compounds (or at least provide guidance as to where further evaluation is required). This same shop would also provide (again, from its established collection) *in vitro* system models to elucidate mechanistic questions later in the assessment process. Some would say that this is the current state-of-the-art. Clearly much of the necessary library could be assembled (4).

Though substantial progress has been made in improving the design and conduct of *in vivo* tests, it does not appear that we are currently closer to achieving the one optimum case than we were in 1980 (though we clearly understand it better), and minimal progress towards the specific objectives of improved strategy is immediately apparent. How does the science and practice of toxicology go about getting to this point?

There are two critical steps that must be taken for the eventual fulfillment of these objectives. The first of these is the need for acceptance of a scientific approach to the problem of safety assessment. The second is to develop an operative validation and acceptance process for new test procedures.

A scientific approach to safety assessment, such as the one presented in this chapter, does have proponents and adherents. Such an approach requires those involved in both the management and conduct of the safety assessment process to continually question (and test) both the efficiency and the validity of their evaluation systems and processes. More to the point, it requires recognition of the fact that "we have always done it this way" is not a reason for continuing to do so. This approach asks first what is the objective behind the testing, and then it asks how well is our testing meeting this objective. Such questions are exemplified by efforts such as those that are questioning if the information given by using six rabbits in an eye irritation test is more predictive than that given by using two or three (1,7).

The second necessary step which is currently totally absent is that there needs to be a collaborative process involving industrial, academic, and regulatory agencies for the validation and "acceptance" of new test systems. The general model of peer recognition leading to acceptance by the scientific community (6) is not working in this case, as should have been expected from a situation where politics, social policy, and litigation have as much influence as science itself.

CONCLUSION

The first principle in hazard assessment is to have your real data as near as possible to the real-life situation you are concerned about. That is, the nearer the model to man, the better the quality of the prediction of any potential hazards.

The second principle should now also be clear: To be able to translate toxicity to hazard, and to be able to manage such hazards, it is essential to know how the agent is to be used and the marketplace it is to be a part of. It is hoped that this chapter has made these relationships clear.

Finally, alternatives of both *in vitro* and *in vivo* types are in the process of development for almost all the different end points of concern in safety assessment. Many of these have great promise, and could be used as screens for many of the uses presented here or as mechanistic tools. But complete replacement is clearly not near at hand, particularly for the more complicated end points. How these then can (and should) be integrated into strategies for product safety assessment is the key scientific and managerial challenge for the next decade. For not only are there strong reasons making it adverse to continue where we are, but there are also the potentials for tremendous competitive advantage to those who successfully manage to integrate *in vitro* tools as both efficient screens and effective means of isolating and understanding the mechanistic underpinning for toxic and pathogenic processes. At the same time, each practicing toxicologist should feel both a moral and ethical compulsion to reduce the number of animals used in research and testing to the fullest extent possible, and to ensure that those that are used are maintained and used in as humane a manner as possible.

REFERENCES

1. DeSousa DJ, Rouse AA, Smolon WJ. Statistical consequences of reducing the number of rabbits utilized in eye irritation testing: data on 67 petrochemicals. *Toxicol Appl Pharmacol* 1984;76:234–242.
2. Gad SC. *Product safety evaluation handbook*. New York: Marcel Dekker, 1988.

3. Gad SC. An approach to the design and analysis of screening data in toxicology. *J Am Coll Toxicol* 1988;7(2):127–138.
4. Gad SC. A tier testing strategy incorporating *in vitro* testing methods for pharmaceutical safety assessment. *Humane Innovation and Alternatives In Animal Experimentation* 1989;1:75–79.
5. Gad SC, Changelis CP. *Acute Toxicology*. Caldwell, NJ: Telford Press, 1988.
6. Greim H, Andrae U, Forster U, Schwarz L. Application, limitation and research requirements of *in vitro* test systems in toxicology. *Arch Toxicol [Suppl]* 1986;9:225–236.
7. Talsma DM, Leach CL, Hatoum NS, Gibbons RD, Roger JC, Garvin PJ. Reducing the number of rabbits in the Draize eye irritancy test: a statistical analysis of 155 studies conducted over 6 years. *Fundam Appl Toxicol* 1988;10:146–153.

In Vitro Toxicology,
edited by Shayne Cox Gad.
Raven Press, Ltd., New York, © 1994.

14

Scientific and Regulatory Considerations in the Development of *In Vitro* Techniques in Toxicology

Patricia D. Williams

Investigative Toxicology, Medical Research Division, American Cyanamid Company, Pearl River, New York 10965

The application of *in vitro* techniques in toxicology has received much attention over the past 10 years. The impetus for this growing interest has come from multiple sources. The *in vitro* "movement" has been driven by scientific, economic, and societal demands. Scientifically, the state of technological developments in biochemistry and pharmacology (e.g., cellular biology, receptor pharmacology) has had an influence on the model systems available. Economic and societal pressures within academic and industrial institutions have also contributed to the interest in reducing animal use. The rising costs of drug development within industry and increasingly lean sources of funding for academic research have had an impact on limiting the use of animals from an economic perspective. At the same time, public opinion and involvement in animal welfare and use issues have provided additional impact and impetus to the practicing toxicologist/pharmacologist to consider alternatives to animal use.

While considerable activity in *in vitro* toxicology has occurred and is still occurring, significant hurdles remain in the evolution of alternative procedures. The most significant issues are of a scientific and regulatory nature. While scientific and regulatory areas are often considered exclusive, the present discussion will address the need for scientific and regulatory acceptance of *in vitro* alternatives to proceed in parallel. Indeed, the separation of scientific and regulatory issues poses a major obstacle to the continued advancement and integration of *in vitro* techniques in toxicologic assessment.

SHARED GOALS: PREDICTABILITY AND RESPONSIBILITY

Let's first discuss the scientific and regulatory issues relative to the proximate and ultimate goals of the toxicologist both within industry and within the various regulatory agencies. Scientifically, challenges remain in defining what specific *in vitro* systems can do in terms of modeling events occurring *in vivo*. Thus, in the short term, the goal of fully characterizing the *in vitro* models in terms of their morphological, biochemical, and functional capacity is paramount. Ultimately as well, the development of systems that can more accurately predict *in vivo* events is a key scientific goal and challenge. From a regulatory perspective, the issue of what will be acceptable in terms of alternative procedures remains unresolved. However, the regulatory goal of providing data predictive of *in vivo* toxic liabilities is quite similar to the ultimate scientific challenge and objective *in vitro* test development. Thus, the goals of the scientist working in the alternatives area are congruent with the objectives of the regulatory agencies—that is, to develop model systems that can accurately predict events occurring *in vivo*. The congruence between scientific and regulatory issues in alternative test development has also been noted in a publication from the Division of Toxicology of the FDA in which Dr. Sidney Green stresses the need for test systems which correlate with *in vivo* end points and objectives (3).

ISSUES: WHEN AND HOW TO USE *IN VITRO* SYSTEMS

Assuming, as discussed above, that the scientific and regulatory needs to develop accurate and relevant *in vitro* models for safety assessment are congruent, what measure, if any, can be taken at present to utilize existing techniques?

The Drug Discovery Process

Toxicology is an important participant in the early stages of drug discovery and selection. *In vitro* systems designed to monitor adverse or toxic properties are used alone and in concert with *in vivo* testing to evaluate and select against specific target organ effects and liabilities. These test systems are often similar to those used in examining pharmacological properties, employing subcellular and cellular models. The use of *in vitro* systems as prescreens for toxicity assessments is an application which is generally well accepted by the scientific and regulatory communities (4). At these early stages of chemical synthesis and evaluation, *in vitro* toxicologic models can also assist in drug design via structure–activity relationship studies. Secondly, the identification of structures that can potentially improve the toxicity profile of existing drugs (e.g., toxicity inhibitors) is facilitated by the use of *in vitro* systems. In this fashion, toxicology can play an intimate and key role in the discovery process. A broader recognition and acceptance of *in vitro* toxicologic techniques at the early stages of compound discovery and selection is certainly evolving within the drug industry. The need to make early assessments of toxicologic properties prior to commitment of resources to develop new drugs provides continuing impetus to apply *in vitro* toxicologic techniques in parallel with discovery efforts (which also frequently employ *in vitro* pharmacologic techniques).

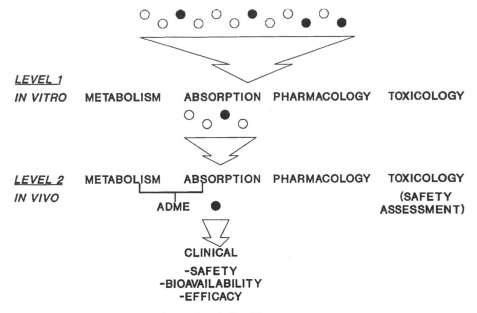

FIG. 1. Preclinical evaluation of new chemical entities.

At the preliminary stages of compound selection, *in vitro* systems can be and are used to make such decisions on the fate of a compound. Typically, compounds selected via *in vitro* screening procedures are subsequently tested in definitive *in vivo* testing prior to project commitment, or within the safety assessment process itself (Fig. 1). Thus, the evidence or decision of product safety prior to the clinical introduction of new drug entities would not be made on the basis of an *in vitro* test alone. An exception would be in the area of genotoxicity, where positive *in vitro* results might well deter the development of a new product.

The Safety Assessment Process

During the conduct of preclinical safety assessment studies, *in vitro* systems are most commonly used to assist in resolving issues that arise. In this capacity, *in vitro* systems offer unique opportunities in exploring mechanisms of toxicity and in performing species comparisons. Such problem-solving can also occur at the clinical phase of drug development, where issues arise in man. To a limited extent, *in vitro* testing also contributes directly in the product safety profile at the preclinical state of development. The use of genotoxicity assays is an example of this application. In the future, it is possible that *in vitro* systems will play an even greater role in the preclinical safety assessment process; however, the extent will depend on the level of scientific advancement and validation of *in vitro* techniques in toxicology.

Selection of Test Procedures

The most reliable tests are those for which there exists a large database of experimental and mechanistic data on a variety of drugs/chemicals. The isolated hepatocyte, for example, has emerged as a powerful tool for evaluating drug-induced hepatotoxicity and for establishing metabolic profiles and has also emerged as an adjunct to other *in vitro* systems (e.g., metabolic supplementation). In addition, there are numerous *in vitro*/biochemical assays that have multiple uses in pharmacology and toxicology. Many of these test systems have not been as extensively applied to toxicology as they could be. Examples of such systems would include (a) central nervous system/cardiovascular receptor assays in isolated membranes, cells, and tissues, (b) enzyme assays (e.g., cholinesterase), and (c) simple *in vitro* assays that measure specific processes (e.g., histamine release in mast cells). It must also be noted that reliability and acceptance of test will be determined to some degree by the specific application. For example, there is a vast difference in the acceptability of tests for screening purposes as compared to tests designed to potentially replace an *in vivo* procedure.

ISSUES: WHERE DO WE GO FROM HERE?

Proactive Versus Reactive Behavior

The saying "If you're not part of the solution, you're part of the problem" never rang truer. Toxicologists cannot expect scientific or regulatory acceptance of *in vitro* systems unless they become involved:

- Involved in the appropriate use of *in vitro* systems in screening and mechanistic investigations.
- Involved in the submission of *in vitro* data in conjunction with definitive *in vivo* data to appropriate regulatory agencies.
- Involved in addressing scientific and regulatory needs for predictive model systems, namely, research and development of advanced technologies.

As discussed above, there are numerous avenues for the *immediate* reduction in animal use in toxicology screening and mechanistic investigations. But it is up to the toxicologist to use these tools more extensively and creatively. Toxicologists cannot simply "default" to government agencies to make these decisions for them.

Government Proactiveness

In parallel, the need for federal agencies such as the Food and Drug Administration (FDA) and the Environmental Protection Agency (EPA) to become more involved in *in vitro* test development is painfully evident. Outside the United States, governmental agencies have been more visibly supportive of alternative research and development. Recently, for example, the Health Protection Branch of Health and Welfare Canada published an information report entitled *Report on the Status and Trends in In Vitro Toxicology and Methodology Modifications for Reducing Animals Use* (2). Similarly, the Organisation for Economic Co-operation and Development (OECD) sponsored a review entitled *Scientific Criteria for Validation of In Vitro Toxicity Tests* (1). Thus, governmental agencies can contribute directly to the continuing dialogue and discussion of alternative procedures.

Scientific/Regulatory Collaboration

Perhaps most critical to the advancement of alternative procedures is the establishment of mechanisms whereby active communication, debate, and guidance can occur between industrial and governmental agencies. Furthermore, the evolution of true collaborative efforts between scientists and regulators, in designing and supporting testing strategies, both in the present and future, offers the potential to accelerate the integration of alternatives into the safety assessment process.

An example of the type of collaborative effort that could be initiated might involve conducting retrospective *in vitro* analyses of key compounds identified in historical databases at FDA, EPA, or industry. Such analyses would provide information on the predictive value of proposed test systems on compounds for which there exists a great deal of data on target organ effects *in vivo*.

VALIDATION

Validation, it is said, has different meanings to different people. One aspect, however, is clear: Validation by any definition is meaningless without sound science. An alternative that is simple, reproducible, and transferable means *nothing* unless it is relevant to the physiological or biochemical end point one is seeking to predict or model. Thus, a key factor in the validation of *in vitro* techniques in toxicology involves the degree of correlation between events occurring *in vitro* and those which the toxicologist evaluates in the intact animals. This correlation determines (a) the ultimate scientific value of the techniques and (b) the level of confidence associated with a particular test in terms of its predictability from a safety perspective. The scientific criteria that determine the degree of correlation or level of confidence in a given test are predictability, identity, mechanisms of injury, and compensatory factors (Fig. 2). Unfortunately, test reproducibility, simplicity, and transferability are frequently viewed as the critical ingredients to test validation, at the expense of any mechanistic or scientific validity. It can be argued that such components, though important in test standardization and acceptance, have little bearing on the true scientific validation and rigor of new test procedures.

The degree to which an *in vitro* test fulfills the scientific and regulatory criteria outlined in Fig. 2 will determine its level of utility in the drug discovery and safety assessment process. The more empirical the test procedure, the greater the risk that

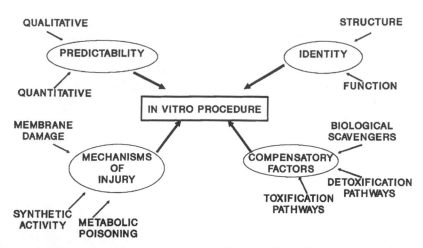

FIG. 2. Scientific and regulatory criteria for establishing validity of *in vitro* test procedures.

such a test will fail to accurately predict *in vivo* events. Thus, the usefulness of certain tests may be limited to early selection and screening of new chemical entities prior to *in vivo* evaluation. More mechanistically sound and scientifically valid models can be utilized as adjuncts to resolve *in vivo* issues that arise preclinically or clinically.

SUMMARY

Considerable interest and activity has evolved over the past decade in the development and application of *in vitro* techniques for risk assessment. At the same time issues of a scientific and regulatory nature persist and must be addressed in parallel for the continued evolution and acceptance of *in vitro* techniques. From a scientific perspective, challenges remain in the development and application of model systems that accurately reflect events occurring *in vivo*. While some of the scientific challenges involve advancing the existing technologies to meet the needs for mechanistically relevant systems, the potential to apply long-established biochemical and pharmacological techniques has not been fully exploited. From a regulatory perspective, confidence that *in vitro* tests can either reduce or replace existing *in vivo* procedures presents both scientific and political challenges. Because of the responsibility to the public, regulatory acceptance of alternatives requires demonstration of scientific validity and predictability in order to bridge the confidence gap. At the same time, avenues for the broad use of *in vitro* techniques for preclinical screening activities as well as in resolving key regulatory issues in drug development are immediately available. The successful evolution of *in vitro* techniques will require open communication and collaboration between industrial and governmental scientists on advances in *in vitro* systems as they develop scientifically.

REFERENCES

1. Frazier JM. *Scientific criteria for validation of in vitro toxicity tests*. OECD environment monograph no. 36, 1990;62pp.
2. Gilman JPW. *Report on status and trends in in vitro toxicology and methodology modifications for reducing animal use*. Health and Welfare Canada, 1991;107pp.
3. Green S. Regulatory issues associated with use of alternative tests. In: Mehlman MA, ed. *Advances in modern environmental toxicology, vol X. Safety Evaluation: toxicology, methods, concepts and risk assessment*. Princeton, NJ: Princeton Scientific Publishing Company, 1987;107–116.
4. Green S. Animal alternatives in toxicology. *J Am Coll Toxicol* 1988;7(4):459–462.

In Vitro Toxicology,
edited by Shayne Cox Gad.
Raven Press, Ltd., New York, © 1994.

15

Safety Issues in the Use of Human Tissue by *In Vitro* Toxicology Laboratories

Katherine L. Allen

Human Liver Research Facility, SRI International, Menlo Park, California 94025

The past few years have seen an increasing use of human tissue in toxicology studies that had previously been conducted exclusively with laboratory animals (1,2). Hospital staff, who have been trained to properly protect themselves, are more aware of the dangers of viral infections and other human pathogens than are most toxicology researchers. With every use of human tissue, researchers incur risk of infection and illness. To minimize the chance of infection, strict policies and procedures should be established by every research laboratory using human tissue. Grizzle and Polt (3) and the National Disease Research Interchange (5) have outlined some excellent guidelines that should be reviewed carefully before introducing human tissue into a laboratory. Another source of information is the Occupational Safety and Health Administration (OSHA) which has recently published guidelines for procedures that protect against exposure to hepatitis B virus (HBV) and human immunovirus (HIV) (6). In general, these guidelines are very similar to those normally followed in a laboratory using carcinogens, with a few minor modifications.

All human tissue should be treated as potentially infectious, because it is impossible to identify all the hazardous agents associated with each specimen. As a general rule, all human primary cell and tissue cultures should be treated as if they were contaminated with viral agents from the donor. Herpes B and SV40 viruses have been known to be a problem in rhesus kidney cell cultures, and human cells are unlikely to be any different. Some of the viruses that can be associated with human cells and tissue are described below. Additionally, products derived from human tissue, such as human serum, are also a potential risk to researchers.

This chapter is designed to suggest to researchers precautions which should be taken when using human tissue. It is not intended to replace standard procedures appropriate for each laboratory, which must be established based on the type of research to be performed. Many of the suggestions are common sense. Those that may appear to be overzealous actually are not, but are designed to be convenient and ensure worker safety without jeopardizing the laboratory efficiency.

Perhaps the most significant aspect of using human tissue is the researcher's lack of perception of the danger involved in this work. Most accidents occur during routine procedures such as diluting and plating cell cultures. The laboratory must be organized in such a way that the rules of worker safety are convenient and can be followed easily at all hours of the day, even by tired investigators. Every supervisor and technician working in laboratories that perform experiments with human tissue must be constantly aware of the importance of proper attitude in the prevention of contamination accidents.

For more than 10 years, SRI International has used human liver in studies ranging from hepatotoxicity and metabolic activation to comparative metabolism of pharmaceuticals in numerous species. During this time, we have established a workable routine that ensures technician safety when processing human tissue.

SEROLOGY

The three common sources of human tissue—biopsy specimens, cadaver donor, and organ donor—must have extensive serology tests performed on them before they are used in research. Tests that are routinely performed include those for HIV, hepatitis B and C (HBV, HCV), syphilis, and cytomegalovirus (CMV). Many human tissue specimens will test positive for CMV but are still acceptable for use. Any tissue testing positive for HIV, HBV, HCV, or syphilis, however, should not be used unless specifically required by the project.

In our laboratory, without exception, all personnel working with human tissue must be inoculated against HBV before they are allowed to work in the laboratory. This is an excellent policy, because viral hepatitis is far more infectious than HIV. Researchers should also be inoculated against HCV when a vaccine becomes available for it.

Regardless of the serology results, all human tissue should be treated as if it were infectious. Serology tests are very limited in scope and do not provide information on other infectious and rare diseases such as kuru, Creutzfeldt–Jakob disease, scrapie, transmissible mink encephalopathy, measles, and papovavirus.

LABORATORY PROCEDURES AND GENERAL PRECAUTIONS

This section, as well as the one that follows, briefly describes some recommended laboratory policies. Most of these can be readily implemented without any inconvenience to the laboratory staff. Others may require changing personal habits and laboratory practices.

The door(s) to the laboratory designated for human tissue studies should always be properly labeled with the universal biohazard sign and kept closed while experiments are in progress. Incubators used to culture human cells, as well as refrigerators and freezers used to store samples from human cultures, should also be labeled with the universal biohazard sign.

The human tissue should be handled whenever possible in a biological safety cabinet (Class II) with a *vertical* laminar air flow hood (horizontal flow hoods provide absolutely no protection). In this way, spills and aerosols can be localized to a single area that can be decontaminated easily and other personnel working in the laboratory area are not at risk. Also, all specimens of human tissue, including cell cultures and tissue homogenates, should be labeled prominently with a special warning that alerts other laboratory personnel to potentially infectious material.

When transferring human tissue from one location to another, use a secondary container to prevent liquid from spilling across the floor and counters; cell cultures, too, which must be carried back and forth between the incubator and the safety flow hood should be placed in a plastic container in case the medium is spilled across the tray and onto the floor.

Most viruses can remain infective in blood, body fluids, and tissues even after they have dried. For this reason, the laboratory area must be cleaned frequently. Laboratory records should always be kept only in clean areas, away from human tissue. Papers contaminated with blood, media, or serum can transfer the infection to an unsuspecting technician who touches them (7). Be very careful where you keep your paperwork!

When working with human tissue that is frozen, it is best to wait until it has thoroughly thawed before cutting it because stray pieces of tissue can shoot off into every direction. If frozen tissue must be used, be sure to work in a biological safety cabinet, use barrier protection, and warn other people in the laboratory. Barrier protection includes disposable caps and hoods, face shields, water-impermeable labcoats, double gloves, and shoe covers.

LABORATORY PROCEDURES THAT MINIMIZE RISK OF INFECTION

There are numerous ways in which the researcher is exposed to infectious agents associated with human tissue and cells, including inhalation, ingestion, needle sticks, and dermal absorption.

Inhalation

Aerosol

Although needle sticks and dermal absorption are the most direct routes of infection in clinical settings, inhalation of aerosols is probably more significant to researchers who will be processing the human tissue into primary cell cultures, tissue homogenates, and microsomal fractions. Any procedure that causes a break in a film of fluid generates aerosols and scatters the tiny droplets. The tiniest of these droplets dry out almost immediately, and the organisms they contain become airborne on the air currents in the laboratory. Many procedures, such as sonication and homogenization, will create droplets and aerosols that can be easily inhaled, not only by the technician performing the manipulation but also by anyone else in the laboratory. Extra care must be taken when performing procedures with human tissue that are known to produce aerosols, and these procedures should also be conducted in a biological safety cabinet.

Pipetting

Ejection of fluids from pipettes or syringes must be performed in a controlled flow to produce a gentle stream. Forceful pressure causes aerosols. All pipetting of human tissue specimen fluids should be done in hood, because there is always some aerosol formation. The discharge from the pipette should be released as close as possible to the plate, or the contents should be allowed to run down the wall of the tube or bottle, not dropped from a height above it (causing splashing or viral transfer to air components). *Never* use a syringe and needle as a substitute for a pipette when diluting biohazardous fluids.

Centrifuging

Centrifuging creates aerosols and droplets, so samples should be contained in either capped centrifuge tubes or safety cups. Also, the tubes should never be filled to the point that liquid is in contact with the lip of the tube, because the high G forces will drive the liquid past the cap seal and over the outside of the tube. Although many clinical laboratories maintain centrifuges in biological safety cabinets, this precaution is not practical in most research laboratories and so researchers must be careful to keep the centrifuge away from active areas of the laboratory. The lid of the centrifuge should always be closed when the unit is in motion. Serofuges, the type used in blood banks, should be oriented so that the air exhausting from the vent located at the base of the centrifuge is directed away from the operator. The centrifuge should be properly labeled with a universal biohazard sign and should be cleaned thoroughly after every use, as described below.

Homogenization

This process will create the largest volume of aerosols. When homogenizing with either a mortar-and-pestle-type apparatus or a Polytron homogenizer, this procedure must *always* be conducted in a biological safety cabinet. Blenders also should be used only in a hood.

Cell Sorters

Droplets will be generated by fluorescent activated cell sorters and represent potentially infectious material. Because these apparatuses are too large to be located in a hood, plastic shielding should be placed between the droplet-collecting area and the technician to reduce contamination.

Other Routes of Aerosol Formation

The vacuum tubes that are used to collect blood specimens frequently retain vacuum, making it difficult to remove the rubber stopper. Aerosols are formed by "popping" the cork, so the preferred method of opening the tube is by first covering it with absorbent paper or cloth and then twisting the cork gently. Stirring and shaking also produce aerosols, particularly if the media contains material that produces bubbles or foam, such as bovine serum albumin or fetal bovine serum. Sonication and lyophilization produce aerosols and should always be performed in a hood.

Ingestion

This is a route of contamination that is easy to avoid. Standard laboratory safety procedures, as well as common sense, should be followed to prevent ingestion of infectious agents. Never pipet by mouth. Don't eat, drink, or apply makeup in the laboratory. Many research facilities have limited office space, and frequently desks are located in the laboratory. It's tempting to have a cup of coffee or to eat a snack while doing calculations at the desk, but don't do it. Also, do not keep food in the laboratory refrigcrator, even if it is used only for storage of culture medium.

Needle Sticks

Syringes

Use needles and syringes only when absolutely necessary, and if they must be used, avoid sudden, jerky movements. Use only needle-locking syringes or, preferably, disposable syringe–needle units. Fill the syringe carefully to minimize air bubbles and frothing of the inoculum, and expel excess air vertically into a cotton pledget moistened with disinfectant. Disposable syringe–needle units should be placed in a puncture-resistant container after use and should be incinerated with all contaminated waste, as described below. Needles should *not* be clipped, recapped, purposely bent, or broken before disposal. The needle should be removed from the syringe carefully in a way that minimizes aerosol production. Needle holders are available from must surgical supply houses and are invaluable for handling needles that do not have their own individual plastic sheaths. Needles should *never* be removed from syringes by hand.

Sharp Items

Scalpel blades used to cut, slice, and apportion the human tissue will probably be more commonly used by researchers than needles. They must be handled with extraordinary care to prevent skin puncture. Broken or chipped glassware should be discarded immediately in puncture-resistant containers (one for contaminated waste disposal and another for routine waste disposal). This source of contamination can be avoided by using only plasticware, rather than glass, when working with human tissue.

Skin Absorption

Hand Washing

Hands and wrists should be washed frequently and always immediately after removing gloves when working with potentially hazardous materials. Tests have shown that it is not unusual for microbial or chemical contamination to be present despite the use of gloves, because of unnoticed small holes, abrasions, tears, or entry at the wrist. This risk is substantially reduced by wearing two pairs of gloves. It is especially important to wash your hands and wrists before eating, smoking, drinking, or using the bathroom after working with human tissue. Hand washing should be done with gentle rubbing, not vigorous scrubbing.

Gloves

The importance of wearing gloves during all procedures that require exposure to human tissue cannot be overemphasized. The selection of a glove appropriate for the work that is to be performed is crucial. Gloves made of polyethylene or polyvinyl chloride are ineffective barriers to virus particles (4). Latex is a far superior barrier to virus permeation.

Gloves should be worn at all times while handling human tissue or equipment or materials that have come into contact with human tissue. The most difficult thing about wearing gloves is to resist touching any unprotected area of the body. It is important not to touch anything else when wearing gloves, such as the telephone or doorknobs (use a paper towel). All gloves should be disposed of properly immediately after use (into plastic biohazard waste) to avoid contaminating other surfaces in the laboratory.

Personnel with open wounds should not work with human tissue until the wound has healed. A bandage is not a sufficient barrier against viruses!

Labcoats should always be worn in the laboratory and should be appropriately stored or discarded before leaving the laboratory. Disposable labfrocks or coveralls are indispensable when working with human tissue, because the contaminated garment can be discarded along with contaminated waste. It's also a good idea to wear disposable shoe covers in case blood or media are spilled on the floor.

PERSONAL HYGIENE

The importance of keeping hands away from mouth, nose, eyes, face, and hair has already been stressed. This habit must be developed. In some circumstances, a beard may be undesirable because it retains particulate contamination more persistently than does clean-shaven skin. Also, if the research requires a face mask or respirator, a clean-shaven face is essential for a proper fit. Those with long hair should wear a head covering that can easily be decontaminated to protect the hair from fluid splashes and reduce facial contamination caused by adjusting the hair.

LABORATORY CLEANUP

Every counter and every surface of every apparatus, chair, and floor area should be wiped after use with 0.525% sodium hypochlorite (10% household bleach). The outside of every tube and every container should also be wiped clean. All reusable surgical instruments and glassware should be soaked and rinsed thoroughly in 10% bleach, 0.1% Duponal, or some other disinfectant detergent (at least 10 min) before washing and sterilization. Reusable pipettes should be laid flat in a container of the disinfectant (rather than being dropped vertically, which produces aerosols as the fluid rapidly rises to the pipette lumen). Every doorknob, switch, and surface that has been touched with a contaminated glove should also be wiped clean; this cleanup can be most conveniently done by maintaining a squirt bottle of 10% bleach or 0.1% Duponal (properly labeled with the concentration and date) at convenient locations in the laboratory. A routine cleaning schedule, in addition to the cleanup immediately after an experiment, is also advised.

Note. Bleach must be used within 6 months after opening, because hypochlorite breaks down and chlorine escapes as a gas, causing the solution to slowly lose its potency after the container has been opened. We generally date and initial each jug at the time of opening it. Also, bleach reacts with proteins in general, so if an area is contaminated by blood, full-strength bleach must be used to decontaminate the area. Because of the toxic potential of these disinfectant agents, use of quaternary ammonium compounds or iodoform or phenolic solutions is regulated by the Environmental Protection Agency (EPA) and requires extensive record-keeping and training.

WASTE DISPOSAL

Waste disposal is a critical issue in our laboratory, and special care should be taken by all researchers to dispose of human tissue correctly so that neither company employees nor residents of the community are endangered by infectious human tissue. Three containers should be prepared: one for needles and sharp objects (this container must be puncture-proof); one for plastics (which produce toxic gases when incinerated); and one for tissue, blood, and heavily contaminated gauze. A fourth category of waste, liquids such as culture medium, must be decontaminated with 10% bleach for 10 min, then poured down the drain.

Sharp waste includes hypodermic needles, scalpel blades, needles with attached tubing, broken glass, Pasteur pipettes, blood vials, and anything else that could puncture the standard biohazard bag. Plastics include gloves, disposable labcoats, unbroken plastic pipettes, culture dishes and flasks, centrifuge tubes, syringes (without the needle), and so on.

The three human waste containers should be kept separate from other waste in the laboratory and should be clearly labeled as biohazardous (we use bright orange bags labeled "Biohazard Bag" with the universal biohazard emblem, which can be purchased from most large laboratory store suppliers and several smaller, specialized vendors). This area should be clearly marked with signs that can be read 25 feet away. Our limited-access area sign reads (in both English and Spanish) "Caution: Biohazardous Waste Storage Area—Unauthorized Persons Keep Away." The orange biohazard bags should be kept in rigid containers for storage, handling, or transport and should be moved only after they have been tied closed. The rigid containers must be leak-resistant and have tight-fitting lids. Like the bags, special containers labeled "Biohazardous Waste" can be purchased from several sources. The containers should be properly washed and disinfected each time they are emptied unless they are disposable.

All human tissue waste is regulated under the Medical Waste Management Act, and they recommend that the "Sharps" and "Plastics" containers should be stored at room temperature for only 7 days before disposal. This is accomplished by first autoclaving the containers in their orange biohazard bags, and the contents, now rendered noninfectious, may be removed from the orange bags and landfilled as industrial waste. In California, the autoclave must be dedicated to treatment of medical waste and registered with the county for this purpose. Infectious materials are completely inactivated by autoclaving for 1 hr at 121°C and 20 psi. "Tissue" waste must be stored at or below $-20°C$ until incineration. All disposal of human waste must be coordinated by the Health and Safety division of each institution using human tissue.

ACKNOWLEDGMENTS

The author would like to gratefully acknowledge Drs. Colette Rudd, Charles Tyson, and Carol Green for their comments and discussion during the preparation of this manuscript. The author would also like to gratefully acknowledge the Health and Safety Department at SRI International.

REFERENCES

1. Frazier JM, Tyson CA. *The third international conference on the use of human cells, tissues and organs in research.* The National Disease Research Interchange, pp. 1–4, September 17–18, 1990.
2. Frazier JM, Tyson CA, McCarthy C, McCormick JJ, Meyer D, Powis G, Ducat L. Contemporary issues in toxicology: potential use of human tissues for toxicity research and testing. *Toxicol App Pharmacol* 1989;97:387–397.
3. Grizzle WE, Polt SS. Guidelines to avoid personnel contamination by infective agents in research laboratories that use human tissues. *J Tissue Cult Methods* 1988;11:191–200.
4. Klein RC, Party E, Gershey EL. Virus penetration of examination gloves. *BioTechniques* 1990;9: 196–199.

5. National Disease Research Interchange. *Guidelines for handling human tissues and body fluids used in research*. Prepared by the NCI Cooperative Human Tissue Network, 1987.
6. Occupational Safety and Health Administration. Compliance Assistance Guideline for the February 27, 1990 OSHA Instruction CPL 2-2.44B. *Enforcement procedures for occupational exposure to hepatitis B virus and human immunodeficiency virus*.
7. Pattison CP, Boyer DM, Maynard JE, Kelly PC. Epidemic hepatitis in a clinical laboratory: possible association with computer card handling. *JAMA* 1974;230:854–857.

Subject Index

NOTE: Page numbers followed by t or f denote tables or figures, respectively.

Validation, 20, 38–41, 71–78
  early studies, 73–74
  scientific and regulatory criteria for,
    259–260, 260f
Vascular cells
  culture of, 226–228
  single-cell suspensions derived from,
    225
  smooth muscle, preparations of,
    223–224
Vasoactive intestinal peptide (VIP),
    127–128
V_d. *See* Volume of distribution
Ventricular tissue
  muscle preparations, 223–224
  single-cell suspensions derived from,
    224–226
Viability, assessment of, 63–65, 77
Viruses, in human tissue, protection
    against, 263–271
Voltage-clamp techniques,

  neurotoxicological studies with,
    129–130
Volume of distribution, 79

W

Waste disposal, and safety concerns,
    269–270
Whole-animal systems, developmental
    toxicity assay in, 106–110
Whole-embryo culture, developmental
    toxicity assays in, 109–110
Working heart preparation, 222

X

Xenobiotic, total concentration of, in
    organ, calculation of, 80
Xenobiotic metabolism, 195–196,
    201–205
  species comparison studies of, 203–205
Xenopus laevis, developmental toxicity
    assay in, 107